LASER DIODE TECHNOLOGY AND APPLICATIONS

Volume 1043

CONTENTS

Conference Committee vi
Symposium Organizers vii
Introduction viii

PLENARY SESSION

1043-02 **Recent advances in high power semiconductor lasers** 2
D. R. Scifres, W. Streifer, D. F. Welch, M. Sakamoto, G. H. Harnagel, Spectra Diode Labs., Inc.

SESSION 1 — NOVEL SEMICONDUCTOR LASER STRUCTURES AND PROCESSING

1043-03 **Extremely low threshold InGaAsP DFB laser diode by the MOCVD/LPE (Invited Paper)** 10
S. Kakimoto, K. Ikeda, H. Namizaki, W. Susaki, K. Shibayama, Mitsubishi Electric Corp. (Japan).

1043-04 **Monolithic four-beam semiconductor laser array with built-in monitoring photodiodes** 17
T. Yamaguchi, K. Yodoshi, K. Minakuchi, Y. Inoue, N. Tabuchi, K. Komeda, H. Hamada, T. Niina, Sanyo Electric Co., Ltd. (Japan).

1043-05 **Focused-ion-beam micromachined diode laser mirrors (Invited Paper)** 25
R. K. DeFreez, J. Puretz, R. A. Elliott, G. A. Crow, H. Ximen, D. J. Bossert, G. A. Wilson, J. H. Orloff, Oregon Graduate Ctr.

1043-06 **Laser-patterned desorption of GaAs in an inverted MOCVD reactor (Invited Paper)** 36
J. E. Epler, D. W. Treat, H. F. Chung, T. L. Paoli, Xerox Palo Alto Research Ctr.

1043-07 **Monolithically integrated two-dimensional arrays of optoelectronic threshold devices for neural network applications** 44
J. H. Kim, Jet Propulsion Lab.; S. H. Lin, California Institute of Technology; J. Katz, Jet Propulsion Lab.; D. Psaltis, California Institute of Technology.

SESSION 2 — HIGH POWER SEMICONDUCTOR LASERS

1043-08 **High power single-mode laser diodes (Invited Paper)** 54
D. F. Welch, W. Streifer, D. R. Scifres, Spectra Diode Labs., Inc.

1043-09 **Quantum well ridge waveguide lasers optimized for high power single spatial mode applications** ... 61
D. R. Daniel, D. Buckley, B. Garrett, STC Defence Systems (UK).

1043-10 **Monolithic two-dimensional arrays of diode lasers (Invited Paper)** 69
W. W. Simmons, E. R. Anderson, L. R. Eaton, L. O. Heflinger, J. Huang, M. Jansen, S. S. Ou, M. Sergant, J. Z. Wilcox, J. J. Yang, TRW Space and Technology Group.

1043-11 **Long-life GaAlAs high power lasers with nonabsorbing mirrors (Invited Paper)** 75
H. Shimizu, Matsushita Electronics Corp. (Japan).

1043-12 **Transverse-mode-controlled wide-single-stripe lasers with loading modal filters** 81
K. Ikeda, K. Shigihara, T. Aoyagi, S. Hinata, Y. Nagai, N. Kaneno, Y. Mihashi, Y. Seiwa, W. Susaki, Mitsubishi Electric Corp. (Japan).

1043-13 **Fundamental lateral-mode operation in broad-area lasers having built-in lens-like refractive index distributions** 87
S. Nakatsuka, K. Tatsuno, Hitachi Ltd. (Japan).

1043-14 **Two-dimensional surface-emitting arrays of GaAs/AlGaAs diode lasers (Invited Paper)** 92
J. P. Donnelly, K. Rauschenbach, C. A. Wang, W. D. Goodhue, R. J. Bailey, Lincoln Lab./MIT.

(continued)

LASER DIODE TECHNOLOGY AND APPLICATIONS

Volume 1043

1043-15	Mode control of an array of AlGaAs lasers using a spatial filter in a Talbot cavity F. X. D'Amato, E. T. Siebert, C. Roychoudhuri, Perkin-Elmer Corp.	100
1043-16	High power AlGaAs broad-area laser diodes for a light-triggered thyristor valve system S. Nakatsuka, R. Iyotani, C. Tanaka, Hitachi Ltd. (Japan).	107
1043-52	Optical cavity design for wavelength-resonant surface-emitting semiconductor lasers (Invited Paper) S. R. J. Brueck, M. Y. A. Raja, M. Osinski, C. F. Schaus, M. Mahbobzadeh, J. G. McInerney, K. J. Dahlhauser, Univ. of New Mexico.	111
1043-17	Scanning single-slit and double-slit phase measurements of grating surface emitter diode laser arrays S. L. Reinhold, J. M. Finlan, J. G. Lehman, Jr., S. M. Hamilton, General Electric Co.	123
1043-18	Phase control of coherent diode laser arrays using liquid crystals W. J. Cassarly, J. M. Finlan, M. DeJule, C. Stein, General Electric Co.	130
1043-19	Coupling of index-guided lateral modes in three-stripe gain-guided laser diode arrays D. G. Heflinger, W. R. Fenner, The Aerospace Corp.	138

SESSION 3 — SEMICONDUCTOR LASER MODELING AND DESIGN

1043-20	Analysis of double-heterostructure and quantum well lasers using effective index techniques (Invited Paper) J. K. Butler, Southern Methodist Univ.; G. A. Evans, David Sarnoff Research Ctr.	148
1043-21	Computer modeling of GRIN-SCH-SQW diode lasers S. R. Chinn, General Electric Co.; P. S. Zory, Univ. of Florida; A. R. Reisinger, General Electric Co.	157
1043-23	Semiconductor laser stabilization by external optical feedback D. R. Hjelme, A. R. Mickelson, Univ. of Colorado/Boulder; R. G. Beausoleil, J. A. McGarvey, R. L. Hagman, Boeing High Technology Ctr.	167
1043-24	Measurement of semiconductor laser linewidth enhancement factor using coherent optical feedback K.-H. Chung, J. G. McInerney, M. Osiński, Univ. of New Mexico.	175
1043-25	Effects of fabricational variations on quantum wire laser gain spectra and performance H. Zarem, K. J. Vahala, A. Yariv, California Institute of Technology.	184
1043-26	Design of multiple quantum well lasers for surface-emitting arrays J. Z. Wilcox, W. W. Simmons, G. P. Peterson, J. J. Yang, M. Jansen, S. S. Ou, TRW Space and Technology Group.	192
1043-27	Leaky-guided channeled substrate planar laser with reduced substrate radiation and heating S. J. Lee, R. V. Ramaswamy, Univ. of Florida; L. Figueroa, Boeing Electronics High Technology Ctr.	197

SESSION 4 — LOW THRESHOLD AND HIGH FREQUENCY LASERS

1043-28	Short-pulse and high frequency signal generation in semiconductor lasers (Invited Paper) K. Y. Lau, Columbia Univ.	206
1043-29	Laser-based optoelectronic integrated circuits for communications (Invited Paper) R. M. Ash, R. C. Goodfellow, A. C. Carter, Plessey Research Caswell Ltd. (UK).	214
1043-31	High performance 1.3-μm buried crescent lasers and LEDs for fiber optic links R. J. Fu, E. Y. Chan, C. S. Hong, Boeing Electronics High Technology Ctr.	221

SESSION 5 — NOVEL SEMICONDUCTOR LASER APPLICATIONS I

1043-32	Diode laser radar system analysis and design for high precision ranging M. de La Chapelle, J. D. McClure, E. J. Vertatschitsch, R. G. Beausoleil, J. G. Bull, J. A. McGarvey, Boeing Electronics High Technology Ctr.	228
1043-33	Compound-cavity lasers for medium-range lidar applications D. A. Cohen, Z. M. Chuang, E. M. Strzelecki, L. A. Coldren, Univ. of California/Santa Barbara; K. Y. Liou, C. A. Burrus, AT&T Bell Labs.	238

PROCEEDINGS
SPIE—The International Society for Optical Engineering

Laser Diode Technology and Applications

Luis Figueroa
Chair/Editor

18–20 January 1989
Los Angeles, California

Sponsored by
SPIE—The International Society for Optical Engineering

Cooperating Organizations
Applied Optics Laboratory/New Mexico State University
Center for Applied Optics Studies/Rose-Hulman Institute of Technology
Center for Applied Optics/University of Alabama in Huntsville
Center for Electro-Optics/University of Dayton
Center for Excellence in Optical Data Processing/Carnegie Mellon University
Center for Microwave-Lightwave Engineering/Drexel University
Center for Research in Electro-Optics and Lasers/University of Central Florida
Jet Propulsion Laboratory/California Institute of Technology
Optical Sciences Center/University of Arizona
Optoelectronic Computing Systems Center/University of Colorado, Colorado State University

Published by
SPIE—The International Society for Optical Engineering
P.O. Box 10, Bellingham, Washington 98227-0010 USA
Telephone 206/676-3290 (Pacific Time) • Telex 46-7053

Volume 1043

SPIE (The Society of Photo-Optical Instrumentation Engineers) is a nonprofit society dedicated to advancing engineering and scientific applications of optical, electro-optical, and optoelectronic instrumentation, systems, and technology.

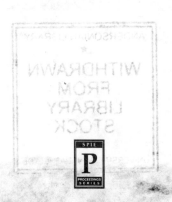
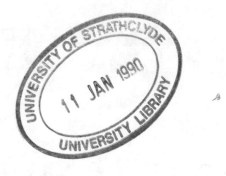

The papers appearing in this book comprise the proceedings of the meeting mentioned on the cover and title page. They reflect the authors' opinions and are published as presented and without change, in the interests of timely dissemination. Their inclusion in this publication does not necessarily constitute endorsement by the editors or by SPIE.

Please use the following format to cite material from this book:
   Author(s), "Title of Paper," *Laser Diode Technology and Applications,* Luis Figueroa, Editor, Proc. SPIE 1043, page numbers (1989).

Library of Congress Catalog Card No. 89-60005
ISBN 0-8194-0078-5

Copyright © 1989, The Society of Photo-Optical Instrumentation Engineers.

Copying of material in this book for sale or for internal or personal use beyond the fair use provisions granted by the U.S. Copyright Law is subject to payment of copying fees. The Transactional Reporting Service base fee for this volume is $2.00 per article and should be paid directly to Copyright Clearance Center, 27 Congress Street, Salem, MA 01970. For those organizations that have been granted a photocopy license by CCC, a separate system of payment has been arranged. The fee code for users of the Transactional Reporting Service is 0-8194-0078-5/89/$2.00.

Individual readers of this book and nonprofit libraries acting for them are permitted to make fair use of the material in it, such as to copy an article for teaching or research, without payment of a fee. Republication or systematic or multiple reproduction of any material in this book (including abstracts) is prohibited except with the permission of SPIE and one of the authors.

Permission is granted to quote excerpts from articles in this book in other scientific or technical works with acknowledgment of the source, including the author's name, the title of the book, SPIE volume number, page number(s), and year. Reproduction of figures and tables is likewise permitted in other articles and books provided that the same acknowledgment of the source is printed with them, permission of one of the original authors is obtained, and notification is given to SPIE.

In the case of authors who are employees of the United States government, its contractors or grantees, SPIE recognizes the right of the United States government to retain a nonexclusive, royalty-free license to use the author's copyrighted article for United States government purposes.

Address inquiries and notices to Director of Publications, SPIE, P.O. Box 10, Bellingham, WA 98227-0010 USA.

LASER DIODE TECHNOLOGY AND APPLICATIONS

Volume 1043

1043-34	Utilizing GaAlAs laser diodes as a source for frequency-modulated cw coherent laser radars A. R. Slotwinski, F. E. Goodwin, D. L. Simonson, Digital Signal Corp.	245
1043-35	Novel device functions and applications of two-electrode distributed feedback lasers (Invited Paper) K.-Y. Liou, AT&T Bell Labs.	252
1043-37	Semiconductor laser-based multichannel analog video transmission using FDM and WDM over single-mode fiber P. S. Natarajan, P. S. Venkatesan, C. W. Lundgren, C. Lin, Bell Communications Research.	260
1043-38	High stability frequency and timing distribution using semiconductor lasers and fiber optic links G. F. Lutes, Jet Propulsion Lab.	263

SESSION 6 NOVEL SEMICONDUCTOR LASER APPLICATIONS II

1043-39	Applications and requirements of laser diodes for free-space laser communications (Invited Paper) D. L. Begley, Ball Aerospace Systems Group.	274
1043-40	All fiber laser low cost "rangefinder" for small vibration measurements Y. N. Ning, City Univ. (UK); B. T. Meggitt, Kings College London (UK); K. T. V. Grattan, A. W. Palmer, City Univ. (UK).	284
1043-42	Radiation pattern of a laser diode collimator as a function of driving current and frequency J. C. Cabrita Freitas, F. Carvalho Rodrigues, LNETI (Portugal); V. M. Silvestre, EID (Portugal); R. D. Prina, INDEP (Portugal); L. Cadete, M. da Silva, Estado Maiordo Exercito (Portugal).	291

SESSION 7 SEMICONDUCTOR LASER OPTOELECTRONICS PACKAGING AND RELIABILITY

1043-43	High frequency characteristics of 1.3-μm lasers (Invited Paper) D. S. Renner, W. H. Cheng, J. Pooladdej, A. Appelbaum, K. L. Hess, S. W. Zehr, Rockwell International Corp.	300
1043-44	Influence of In on the performance of (Al)GaAs single quantum well lasers (Invited Paper) R. G. Waters, C. M. Harding, B. A. Soltz, McDonnell Douglas Astronautics Co.; P. K. York, J. N. Baillargeon, J. J. Coleman, Univ. of Illinois/Urbana-Champaign; S. E. Fischer, D. Fekete, J. M. Ballantyne, Cornell Univ.	310
1043-45	Reliability of single-element diode lasers for high performance optical data storage applications M. K. Benedict, C. B. Morrison, A. J. Tzou, IBM Corp.; A. D. Gleckler, Kaman Aerospace; D. W. Fried, K. J. Giewont, IBM Corp.	318
1043-46	Packaging considerations for semiconductor laser diodes A. J. Perryman, J. D. Regan, R. T. Elliott, STC Defence Systems (UK).	330
1043-47	Optomechanical packaging for extended temperature performance S. Enochs, Tektronix Inc.	338
1043-48	Self-consistent heat load evaluation of laser diode modules for high temperature operation E. Y. Chan, C. C. Chen, Boeing Electronics High Technology Ctr.	344
1043-49	Laser diode cooling for high average power applications D. C. Mundinger, R. J. Beach, W. Benett, R. W. Solarz, V. Sperry, Lawrence Livermore National Lab.	351
1043-50	Wafer thin coolers for cw AlGaAs/GaAs monolithic linear diode laser arrays S. M. Stazak Kastigar, R. E. Hendron, J. R. Lapinski, Jr., G. R. Hertzler, McDonnell Douglas Astronautics Co.	359
1043-51	Screening test procedure for long-life single-mode step index separate confinement heterostructure single quantum well laser diodes W. J. Fritz, McDonnell Douglas Astronautics Co.	368
	Addendum	376
	Author Index	377

LASER DIODE TECHNOLOGY AND APPLICATIONS

Volume 1043

CONFERENCE COMMITTEE

Chair
Luis Figueroa
Boeing Electronics High Technology Center

Program Committee
David L. Begley, Ball Aerospace Systems Group; **Dan Botez,** TRW Space and Technology Group; **Robert D. Burnham,** Amoco Research Center; **James J. Coleman,** University of Illinois/Urbana-Champaign; **Gary A. Evans,** David Sarnoff Research Center; **Gary T. Forrest,** *Laser Focus*; **Robert C. Goodfellow,** Plessey Research Caswell Limited (UK); **Chi-Shain Hong,** Boeing Electronics High Technology Center; **Kenji Ikeda,** Mitsubishi Electric Corporation (Japan); **Dae M. Kim,** Oregon Graduate Center; **Kam Y. Lau,** Columbia University; **Chinlon Lin,** Bell Communications Research; **Randy Randall,** Tektronix, Inc.; **Daniel S. Renner,** Rockwell International Corporation; **Chandrasekhar Roychoudhuri,** Perkin-Elmer Corporation; **Richard W. Solarz,** Lawrence Livermore National Laboratory; **James N. Walpole,** Lincoln Laboratory/Massachusetts Institute of Technology; **Peter S. Zory,** University of Florida

Session Chairs
Plenary Session
Peter S. Zory, University of Florida

Session 1—Novel Semiconductor Laser Structures and Processing
Chi-Shain Hong, Boeing Electronics High Technology Center

Session 2—High Power Semiconductor Lasers
Dan Botez, TRW Space and Technology Group

Session 3—Semiconductor Laser Modeling and Design
Gary A. Evans, David Sarnoff Research Center

Session 4—Low Threshold and High Frequency Lasers
James N. Walpole, Lincoln Laboratory/Massachusetts Institute of Technology

Session 5—Novel Semiconductor Laser Applications I
Luis Figueroa, Boeing Electronics High Technology Center

Session 6—Novel Semiconductor Laser Applications II
David L. Begley, Ball Aerospace Systems Group

Session 7—Semiconductor Laser Optoelectronics Packaging and Reliability
Randy Randall, Tektronix, Inc.

Symposium on Lasers and Optics

This conference was part of a 19-conference symposium on Lasers and Optics held at SPIE's OE/LASE '89 Symposium on Optics, Electro-Optics, & Laser Applications in Science & Engineering, 15–20 January 1989, Los Angeles, California. The conferences were:

Conference 1040, *High Power and Solid State Lasers II*
Conference 1041(I), *Metal Vapor Laser Technology and Applications*
Conference 1041(II), *Deep Blue and Ultraviolet Lasers: Technology and Applications*
Conference 1042, *CO_2 Lasers and Applications*
Conference 1043, *Laser Diode Technology and Applications*
Conference 1044, *Optomechanical Design of Laser Transmitters and Receivers*
Conference 1045, *Modeling and Simulation of Laser Systems*
Conference 1046, *Pulse Power for Lasers II*
Conference 1047, *Mirrors and Windows for High Power/High Energy Laser Systems*
Conference 1048, *Infrared Fiber Optics*
Conference 1049, *Recent Trends in Optical Systems Design and Computer Lens Design Workshop II*
Conference 1050, *Infrared Systems and Components III*
Conference 1051, *Practical Holography III*
Conference 1052, *Holographic Optics: Optically and Computer Generated*
Conference 1053, *Optical Pattern Recognition*
Conference 1054, *Fluorescence Detection III*
Conference 1055, *Raman Scattering, Luminescence, and Spectroscopic Instrumentation in Technology*
Conference 1056, *Photochemistry in Thin Films*
Conference 1057, *Biomolecular Spectroscopy*

Lasers and Optics Symposium Chair
James J. Ewing, Spectra Technology, Inc.

Technical Organizing Committee

Fran Adar, Instruments SA Inc.
Stephen A. Benton, Media Laboratory/MIT
Robert R. Birge, Syracuse University
Donald L. Bullock, TRW Space and Technology Group
Tom R. Burkes, Texas Tech University
Robert L. Caswell, Rockwell International Corporation
Ivan Cindrich, Environmental Research Institute of Michigan
George Dubé, McDonnell Douglas Astronautics Company
James D. Evans, Teledyne Brown Engineering
Luis Figueroa, Boeing Electronics High Technology Center
Robert E. Fischer, Ernst Leitz Canada Limited
Gary Forrest, FYI Reports
Thomas F. George, State University of New York/Buffalo
James E. Griffiths, Instruments SA Inc. and Armstrong State College
James A. Harrington, Heraeus LaserSonics, Inc.
Tung H. Jeong, Lake Forest College
Richard C. Juergens, Optical Research Associates
Abraham Katzir, Tel Aviv University (Israel) and MIT
Jin J. Kim, University of Central Florida
Randy Kimball, Liconix, Inc.
Claude A. Klein, Raytheon Research Division
Sing H. Lee, University of California/San Diego
Jeremy M. Lerner, Instruments SA Inc.
Hua-Kuang Liu, Jet Propulsion Laboratory
Edward V. Locke, Avco Research Laboratory, Textron
Henry H. Mantsch, National Research Council Canada
Glen McDuff, Texas Tech University
E. Roland Menzel, Texas Tech University
Leon J. Radziemski, New Mexico State University
Bernard D. Seery, TRW Space and Defense
Jeff Steinfeld, MIT
Hugo Weichel, Defense Nuclear Agency
P. Jeffrey Wisoff, Rice University

LASER DIODE TECHNOLOGY AND APPLICATIONS

Volume 1043

INTRODUCTION

This is the second SPIE semiconductor laser technology conference to be held in Los Angeles and, like last year's conference, we believe it was a great success.

The conference began with two outstanding plenary talks by distinguished scientists in the field of semiconductor lasers. In the first presentation, Professor A. Yariv of the California Institute of Technology provided an overview of quantum well semiconductor laser technology (paper 1043-01, not available).

Quantum well technology is revolutionizing the design of low threshold, high frequency, and high power laser diodes. Threshold current densities as low as 88 A/cm^2 with differential efficiencies approaching 90% (wall plug efficiencies in excess of 50%) have been achieved with these structures. The most common geometry used is the graded-index separate carrier and optical confinement heterostructures (GRIN-SCH).

In the area of high speed, time delays of < 18 ps have been measured with quantum well structures. Coupled with their inherently low threshold currents, these delays will permit the operation of these lasers with no bias current and thus they function like LEDs but at much higher efficiencies. One of the most important applications involves computer interconnects.

One of the key features of quantum well lasers that permits low threshold current densities, high efficiencies, and narrow spectral linewidth is the low optical absorption losses compared to conventional lasers (2 to 3 cm^{-1} compared to ~30 cm^{-1}).

The second plenary talk by Dr. D. Scifres of Spectra Diode Labs provided an overview of high power laser diode arrays using quantum well technology. At the present time, these laser arrays have achieved more than 50 W cw from a 1-cm bar (20% packing density) and an ~36% total efficiency (the best is >50%). Mean time to failure in excess of 5000 h for powers of 5 W cw at $T = 25°C$ have been measured. Two-dimensional laser arrays used as solid-state replacements for flashlamps have achieved powers in excess of 800 W and total efficiencies of 35% (150-μs pulses, 40-Hz repetition rates). The projected lifetime is in excess of 10^{13} pulses. More recently, the quantum well technology has been used to fabricate high power ($P > 100$ mW) single-mode lasers with relatively narrow spectral linewidths (<5 MHz).

The first session was on Novel Semiconductor Laser Structures and Processing. In an invited paper (1043-03) K. Ikeda, from Mitsubishi Electric, described a low threshold p-substrate PPI BH distributed feedback laser ($\lambda \cong 1.3$ μm). The lowest threshold current obtained was ~3 mA cw, which is a record according to the speaker. Side-mode suppression was greater than 40 dB. With such a low threshold, "0" bias, rz modulation is possible up to 1 Gb/s.

In another invited paper (1043-05) presented by R. DeFreez, Oregon Graduate Center, focused ion beam technology was reviewed. Micromachined semiconductor structures have been used to fabricate C^3-type lasers, surface emitting lasers, curved mirrors, etc. Recent results indicate lifetimes in excess of 5000 h ($T = 50°C$) for micromachined TJS-type lasers. A novel approach for fabricating lasers with variable wavelength emission using laser-assisted MOCVD was presented by J. Epler from the Xerox Palo Alto Research Center (1043-06). Quantum well lasers with J_{th} ~330 A/cm^2 has been produced with this process. In addition, the aluminum composition can vary from $x = 0.04$ to $x = 0.08$ in ~4 mm of horizontal distance.

The afternoon session on High Power Semiconductor Lasers offered several exciting results in the area of high power single-mode lasers. Researchers from both Spectra Diode Labs. and STC Technology have been able to design quantum well lasers with single-mode output power in excess of 150 mW. STC researchers (1043-09) use a ridge waveguide geometry with a two-active-layer GRIN-SCH structure. The use of the two active layers apparently improves the T_0 of the structure. The Spectra Diode Labs laser (1043-08) offers a maximum power of 500 mW (n_D ~90%, n_{total} ~60%), while the STC device can produce powers in excess of 300 mW. It has a burnoff power in excess of 9 MW/cm^2. The spectral linewidth is <5 MHz. One of the more interesting features of the Spectra Diode Labs device is the ability to tune continuously over an ~8°C temperature range, which is considerably larger than most conventional laser structures.

In an invited paper (1043-11), H. Shimuzu, Matsushita Electronics, described recent progress on pushing the power limits for conventional semiconductor laser technology using LPE. He described a nonabsorbing mirror (NAM) version of the p-substrate TRS laser that uses LPE for the laser and MOCVD for the NAM. A maximum output power of 300 mW (nondestructive) was obtained under cw and greater than 1.25 W under short-pulse conditions. Maximum power in a single longitidunal mode is ~120 mW cw. Reliability measurements indicate an MTTF in excess of 6000 h for $P = 100$ mW and $T = 50°C$. Another exciting high power laser structure (1043-12) was described by K. Ikeda, Mitsubishi Electric. He described the wide-stripe SBA (W ~150 μm) laser, which uses a mode-selective mirror at the laser facets. Preliminary results indicate output powers in excess of 300 mW into a narrow FF (2 to 3°). Two invited papers described recent work on surface-emitting GaAlAs/GaAs laser diodes. (1043-10) W. Simmons (1043-10) from TRW described phase locking of a two-dimensional laser array. J. Donnelly (1043-14) of Lincoln Labs described a hybrid surface-emitting laser array that uses chemically etched mirrors in silicon to redirect the beams to the surface. The researchers have obtained pulse powers in excess of 65 W with differential efficiencies in excess of 75%.

Session 3, Semiconductor Laser Modeling and Design, opened with J. K. Butler (1043-20) from Southern Methodist University described detailed modeling results on the CSP-type laser. S. Lee (1043-27), University of Florida, described his results on a modified version of the CSP laser that has a GaAlAs buffer layer and thus provides for "leaky" mode operation. Such "leaky" mode structures have recently become of interest in the fabrication of stable and diffraction-limited arrays. P. Zory (1043-21), University of Florida, described a detailed model for predicting the performance of quantum well lasers. In particular, the T_0 of the quantum well laser is a strong function of the active layer thickness. N. W. Carlson (1043-22), David Sarnoff Research Center, provided an overview of the coherence properties of diode laser arrays including both edge-and surface-emitting devices.

H. Zarem and K. Vahala (1043-25), California Institute of Technology, described their modeling work on two-dimensional quantum well structures. Their modeling calculations

(continued)

predict threshold currents in the tens of microamps and a factor of 2 increase in the maximum modulation frequency for quantum wire lasers.

Session 4 on Low Threshold and High Frequency Lasers included an invited paper (1043-28) by K. Lau, Columbia University, who provided an overview of short-pulse and high frequency signal generation. One conclusion predicts that semiconductor lasers may be mode-locked at frequencies as high as 80 GHz. A. C. Carter (1043-29) of Plessey Research provided an overview of optoelectronics research at Plessey. Laser drivers operating at frequencies in excess of 2 Gb/s have been fabricated. P. D. Dapkus (1043-30), University of Southern California, described the use of the atomic layer and selective epitaxy for the fabrication low-threshold QW laser structures.

Two sessions on Novel Semiconductor Laser Applications included detailed modeling results on the use of semiconductor lasers in laser radar systems [M. de la Chapelle (1043-32), Boeing High Technology Center]. A complete semiconductor laser radar system using FMCW was described by A. R. Slotwinski (1043-34) from Digital Signal Corporation. The use of multielectrode lasers for laser radar and logic operations was described in two papers. Semiconductor laser technology (1043-37) in combination with wavelength division multiplexing is being used for transmission of high definition TV signals. High speed analog modulated semiconductor lasers in combination with fiber optics appears to be the medium of choice for transmitting precise frequency standards (1043-38). However, lasers with lower noise (RIN) will be required. Last, applications and requirements of laser diodes in free-space laser communications was provided by D. Begley (1043-39) of Ball Aerospace.

The last session covered Semiconductor Laser Optoelectronics Packaging and Reliability. In an invited paper, D. Renner (1043-43), Rockwell International, provided an overview of the development of high frequency DC-PBH laser structures. Lasers with modulation bandwidths in excess of 10 GHz have been developed. R. Walters, McDonnell Douglas, described work (1043-44) on strained layer $In_xGa_{1-x}As/GaAs$ pseudomorphic quantum well structures. For lasers having $x = 0.37$ ($\lambda \sim 1.01$ μm), relatively low degradation rates (~2%/KHR increase in drive current) have been observed in life tests conducted with $P = 70$ mW, $T = 30°$C. In addition, no sudden failures were observed.

Two papers (1043-45 and 1043-46) were presented on laser packaging. Laser welding for fiber optics attachment is used and one of the primary goals is to increase the usable operating temperature range of the package to beyond 100°C.

Last, two papers (1043-49 and 1043-50) were given on external coolers for high power lasers. D. Mundinger described the Lawrence Livermore approach, which used either etched or sawed silicon grooves. For a 3-mm package, the package can be used to provide 5 W of average optical power (10 to 11 W peak). McDonnell Douglas researchers have used grooves cut in either copper or BeO to achieve a maximum temperature rise of ~1°C between the cooler and the array.

An evening panel discussion on Emerging Applications for Laser Diodes in the 1990s was held. Topics of discussion included laser space communications, semiconductor laser-based LIDAR, diode laser-pumped solid-state lasers, microwave fiber optic transmission, optical computer interconnects, and advanced video transmission. Some of the highlights included: (1) The strong need for a 1- to 2-W single-mode laser for laser space communications. (2) The potential for merging laser space communications and laser radar technology. (3) The potential use of diode-pumped solid-state lasers for low noise optical-microwave and coherent fiber optic links. However, one of the biggest potential applications is in the graphics market for full-color printers. (4) In the area of optical computer interconnects, the need for a tunable surface-emitting laser for a reconfigurable geometry was described. Again, the trend is toward the use of quantum well laser technology.

In conclusion, the program committee would like to extend its sincere appreciation to all the speakers for their presentations and published materials. In addition, the participants of the evening panel discussion are to be thanked for their valuable inputs and for taking the time to participate.

Luis Figueroa
Boeing Electronics High Technology Center
for the Program Committee

LASER DIODE TECHNOLOGY AND APPLICATIONS

Volume 1043

PLENARY SESSION

Chair
Peter S. Zory
University of Florida

RECENT ADVANCES IN HIGH POWER SEMICONDUCTOR LASERS

Don Scifres, William Streifer, David Welch,
Masamichi Sakamoto and Gary Harnagel

1. INTRODUCTION

Recent advances in high power semiconductor lasers can be divided into two categories. These are partially coherent semiconductor lasers and coherent laser diodes. This paper will review advances in the operation of both such laser devices.

2. PARTIALLY COHERENT LASER DIODES

Partially coherent devices can emit a diffraction limited output beam perpendicular to the plane of the p-n junction of the laser but exhibit multimode behavior parallel to the junction plane. This multimode behavior of the lateral laser direction limits these lasers to applications which do not require fully diffraction limited output beams. Examples of applications for such lasers include a) optical pumping of solid state lasers such as Nd:YAG b) infrared illumination 3) laser soldering 4) eye surgery and other applications requiring high power launched into a multimode fiber. Examples of partially coherent devices include broad area gain guided lasers (stripe widths greater than ~6 um), multistripe arrays, laser bars and 2-D stacked arrays.

The earliest demonstrated CW laser diode device operating reliably at cw power levels in excess of 100 mw was the multistripe array shown in Fig.1.[1] This laser consists of 10 gain guided emitters fabricated on 10 um center to center spacings. The active region in this case consists of a single quantum well approximately 80 Å thick. Owing to the enhanced gain of quantum well active region devices, low threshold, high power conversion efficiency and high reliability can be obtained in a single device. The device is grown by MOCVD.

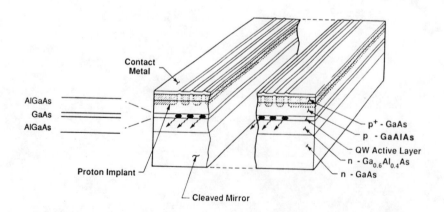

Fig.1 Single Quantum Well-Separate Confinement
Heterostructure Laser Diode Array

Shown in Fig.2 is the output power versus DC drive current for both a 10 stripe (100 um aperture) and 20 stripe (200 um aperture) SQW laser array.[2] As shown, output powers reach 6 W cw and 8 W cw for these lasers respectively. At high power, a thermally induced rollover is observed to limit the output power.

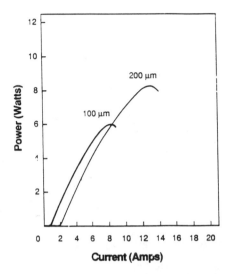

Fig 2 Output power limits from a 10 stripe (6 W cw) and 20 stripe (8.2 W cw) linear laser array

Such SQW lasers can also be optimized to achieve high electrical to optical power conversion efficiency. Shown in Fig.3 is an L versus I plot demonstrating a 54% front facet power conversion efficiency for a single quantum well separate confinement heterostructure 10 stripe laser array. Although the back facet of the array is HR coated (~95% reflectivity), some of the light is also radiated from the rear facet yielding an overall power conversion efficiency in excess of 56%. Note that there is an optimal operating point which maximizes power conversion efficiency. At low operating current the efficiency is low due to the laser threshold current. Above threshold, the efficiency rises rapidly based on the high differential efficiency of the device. However, at high current the power conversion efficiency rolls over owing to series resistance and junction heating. Because of the high power conversion efficiency, reliable operation (>10,000 hours) of such lasers has been obtained at 0.5 W cw and 1 W cw for 100 um and 200 um aperture devices respectively.[3]

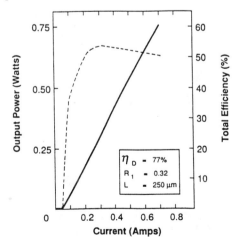

Fig. 3 High Efficiency SQW 10 stripe Laser Array

If such 10 stripe lasers are fabricated on 500 um centers to form a 1 cm long laser bar with a 20% packing density (see Fig.4) output powers as great as 55 W cw have been obtained.[4] This bar was fabricated on a copper heat sink and was thermally limited. When cooled to 0°C a similar laser bar has reached 75 W cw with a power conversion efficiency of 40%.

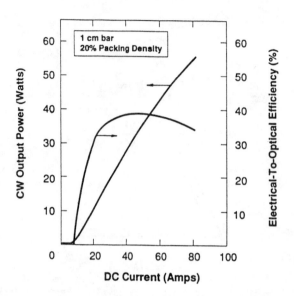

Fig 4. CW output power and efficiency versus DC current from a monolithic 1 cm long laser bar

Owing to thermal limitations 100% packing density bars have not yet been operated CW. However, under long pulse quasi cw operation (150 usec pulse width, 100Hz) up to 134 watts of output power were obtained several years ago.[5] Such data is shown in Fig.5. Even in this monolithic bar form power conversion efficiencies as high as 50% were obtained.

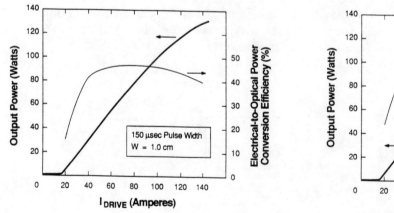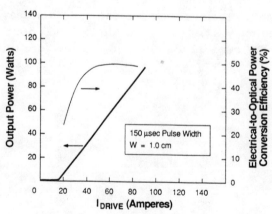

Fig. 5 Quasi CW (150 usec) pulsed operation of a 1 cm long linear monolithic laser bar

Using such laser bars mounted on thin plates as many as 33 bars can be stacked together to form a 2-D array of laser bars. A three bar stack of such devices emitted 300 W and radiated an optical power density of 3.6 KW/cm^2 under quasi-cw conditions.[6] Further increases in incoherent optical pump power density could be obtained by coupling such arrays to ribbon optical fibers. Depending on fiber core diameter and diode bar operating conditions, optical power densities up to 20 KW/cm^2 are potentially available with fiber ribbon coupled geometries.

3. COHERENT LASER DIODES

Coherent laser diodes are those which exhibit single mode behavior both parallel and perpendicular to the plane of the p-n junction. These lasers can be utilized in applications requiring diffraction limited operation. Examples of such uses are a) optical recording b) satellite communications c) telecommunications via single mode fibers, and d) printing, as well as others. Clearly it is the aim of much diode laser research to fabricate high power coherent laser diodes if possible since they can generally be used for applications requiring partially coherent lasers as well.

The most common form of coherent laser diode is the single stripe index guided laser. This device is found in millions of CD audio players around the world. The CD laser diode emits only 3 mw of cw output power enabling it to be fabricated with high yield and high reliability thus allowing low cost mass production. As the output power of such lasers is increased, reliability and yield are decreased.

Coherent index guided laser diodes have been fabricated at wavelengths between 0.67 um and 1.55 um. To date, the highest CW output power obtained from an index guided device was 500 mw at which time the laser mirror failed due to catastrophic facet damage.[7] This laser however maintained single transverse mode operation to only 170 mw. Characteristics of such a coherent index guided laser are shown in Figs.6 and 7. A remarkable feature of the laser is its operation in a single longitudinal mode (no longitudinal mode hops) over a power range of 0-70 mw cw.

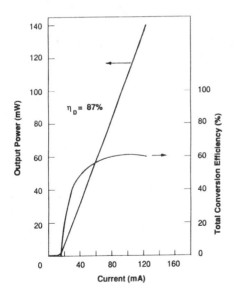
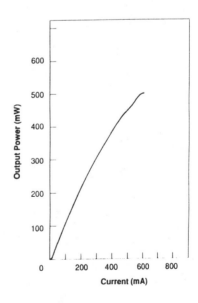

Fig. 6 Illustrating L vs I curves for index guided lasers having a 60 % total power conversion efficiency and >500 mw cw catastrophic damage limit.

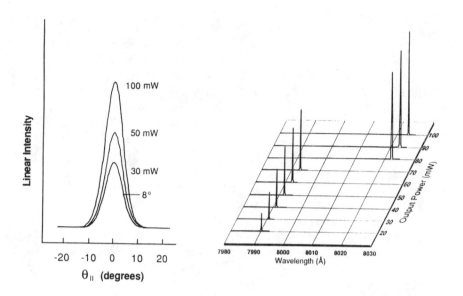

Fig. 7 Far field pattern and spectral output from an index guided high power laser

Because of the power limits associated with catastrophic facet damage, it is desirable to spread the light on the laser output facet while maintaining beam coherence. One method for achieving this performance is shown in Fig.8. As shown, a Y-coupled array of real refractive index waveguides are utilized to force the laser array to operate in the lowest order mode of the array. This yields a narrow diffraction limited output beam in the lateral direction to approximately 150 mw cw.[8] Above this level multimode operation and phase distortions owing to spatial hole burning cause a broadening of the output beam.

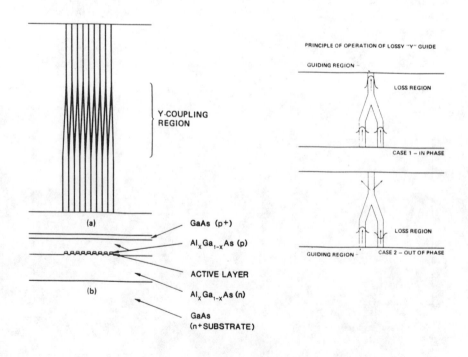

Fig. 8 Y-coupled coherent BH laser array

Monolithic 2-D coherent arrays are also being explored. Two types of such arrays include 1) those with angled facet etched reflectors to direct the light upward out of the junction plane,[9,10,11] and 2) grating beam deflectors radiating in the 2nd order diffraction mode.[12-14] To date, coherent operation of a grating coupled 2-D array has been demonstrated to greater than 1.4 W of peak pulsed (~100usec pulse width) power.[13]

Still another form of coherent laser diode array is an external cavity laser. Such devices (shown in Fig.9) were operated to ~700 mw (200ns pulse width) in a very compact and stable GRIN lens cavity.[15] However, apparently owing to thermal gradients along the p-n junction, the maximum CW power obtained with diffraction limited output is approximately 300 mw. Recently, Lincoln Labs has reported operating such external cavity lasers to CW power levels in excess of 1 W.[16] These devices were mounted junction side up relative to the heat sink and thereby likely achieved a more uniform thermal profile in the laser.

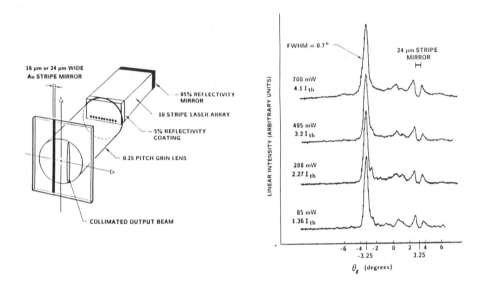

Fig. 9 External cavity self locked 10 emitter laser diode array emitting > 700 mw pulsed.

4. CONCLUSION

In conclusion, both high power partially coherent and coherent devices are available today. Partially coherent arrays emitting up to 5 W cw were recently announced as a commercial product while 75 W cw output has been demonstrated in the laboratory. Coherent single mode single stripe index guided lasers are available at 100 mw output powers at both 0.8 um and 1.3 um while coherent devices emitting up to 1 W cw are presently under development.

5. REFERENCES

1. D.R. Scifres, C. Lindstrom, R.D. Burnham, W. Streifer and T.L. Paoli. "Phase-locked (GaAl)As laser diode emitting 2.6 W cw from a single mirror", Elect. Lett. 19, 169, 1983.
2. D.F. Welch, B. Chan, W. Streifer and D.R. Scifres, "High-power, 8 W cw, single-quantum-well laser diode array", Elect. Lett. Vol.24, No.2, Jan 21, 1988, pp 113-115.

3. D.F. Welch, M. Cardinal, W. Streifer, D.R. Scifres and P.S. Cross, "High-brightness, high-efficiency, single-quantum-well laser diode array", Elect. Lett. Vol.23, No.23, Nov 5, 1987, pp 1240-1241.

4. M. Sakamoto et al, private communication.
M. Sakamoto, D.F. Welch, G.L. Harnagel, W. Streifer, H. Kung, and D.R. Scifres, "Ultrahigh power 30 W continuous-wave monolithic laser diode arrays", Appl. Phys. Lett 52(26), June 27, 1988 pp 220-221.

5. G.L. Harnagel, P.S. Cross, C.R. Lennon, M. DeVito, and D.R. Scifres, "Ultra-high-power quasi-cw monolithic laser diode arrays with high power conversion efficiency", Elect. Lett. Vol.23, No.14, July 2, 1987, 743.

6. P.S. Cross, G.L. Harnagel, W. Streifer, D.R. Scifres and D.F. Welch, "Ultrahigh-power semiconductor diode laser arrays", Science, Vol.237, Sept 1987, pp 1305-1309.

7. D.F. Welch et al, private communication.

8. D.F. Welch, P.S. Cross, D.R. Scifres, and W. Streifer, "Single-lobe 'Y' coupled laser diode arrays" Elect. Lett. Vol.23, No.6, March 1987, 270.

9. J.P. Donnelly, W.D. Goodhue, T.H. Windhorn, R.J. Bailey and S.A. Lambert, "Monolithic two-dimensional surface-emitting arrays of GaAs/AlGaAs diode lasers", Appl. Phys. Lett. 51(15),Oct 12, 1987, pp 1138 -1140.

10. J.J. Yang, M. Sergant, S.S. Ou, L. Eaton and W.W. Simmons, "Surface-emitting GaAlAs/GaAs linear laser arrays with etched mirrors", Appl. Phys. Lett. 49(18), Nov. 3, 1986, pp 1138-1139.

11. J. Puretz, R.K. DeFreez, R.A. Elliott, J. Orloff and R.L. Paoli, "300mW operation of a surface-emitting phase-locked array of diode lasers", Elect. Lett. Jan 29, 1987, Vol.23, No.3, pp 130-131.

12. D.R. Scifres, R.D. Burnham and W. Streifer, "Grating coupled GaAs/GaAlAs single heterostructure ring laser". Optics Commun. 18, 40 (1976).

13. G.A. Evans, N.W. Carlson, J.M. Hammer, M. Lurie, J.K. Butler, S.L. Palfrey, R. Amantea, L.A. Carr, F.Z. Hawrylo, E.A. James, C.J. Kaiser, J.B. Kirk and W.F. Reichert, "Coherent, monolithic two-dimensional (10x10) laser arrays using grating surface emission", Appl. Phys. Lett. 53(22) Nov. 28, 1988, pp 2123-2125.

14. K. Kojima, S. Noda, K. Mitsunaga, K Kyuma and K. Hamanaka, "Continuous wave operation of a surface-emitting AlGaAs/GaAs multiquantum well distributed Bragg reflector laser", Appl. Phys. Lett. 50(24) June 15, 1987, pp 1705 - 1707.

15. C.J. Chang-Hasnain, J. Berger, D.R. Scifres, W. Streifer, J.R. Whinnery and A. Dienes, "High Power with high efficiency in a narrow single-lobed beam from a diode laser array in an external cavity", Appl. Phys. Lett. 50(21), 1465, May 25, 1987.

16. W.f. Sharfin, J. Seppala, A. Mooradiam, B.A. Soltz, R.G. Walters, B.J. Vollner and K.J. Bystrom, "High-power, diffraction-limited, narrow-band, external cavity diode laser", 11th IEEE International Semiconductor Laser Conference, August 1988, Boston, MA.

SESSION 1

Novel Semiconductor Laser Structures and Processing

Chair
Chi-Shain Hong
Boeing Electronics High Technology Center

Invited Paper

Extremely low threshold InGaAsP DFB laser diode by the MOCVD/LPE

S.Kakimoto, K.Ikeda, H.Namizaki, W.Susaki and K.Shibayama

LSI R&D Laboratory, Mitsubishi Electric Corporation
4-1 Mizuhara, Itami, Hyogo 664, Japan

ABSTRACT

An extremely low threshold InGaAsP DFB laser diode has been developed by the MOCVD and LPE hybrid process. The threshold current of 3.1mA is the lowest value among InGaAsP laser diodes so far reported including those of the conventional Fabry Perot type. Using this low threshold DFB laser, 1 Gbit/s RZ zero bias modulation has been demonstrated.

1. INTRODUCTION

Much effort has been dedicated to lower the threshold current of laser diodes. Very low threshold laser diode plays an important role in reduction of the power consumption and it can be modulated at high speed without the bias current.

In AlGaAs laser diodes, ultra low threshold current lasers have been achieved appling quantum well structure[1-3]. Using such low threshold lasers, Gbit/s zero bias modulation has been demonstrated[3,4]. However, these lasers are so called short wavelength lasers and are not suitable for long distance and high bit rate optical communication systems.

In the practical long haul and high speed optical communication, so called long wavewlength, InGaAsP laser diodes are required. But the threshold currents of InGaAsP lasers are not small enough for zero bias modulation. For example, the lowest threshold current so far reported of the InGaAsP Fabry Perot type lasers is 4.5mA[5]. While, the lowest threshold current so far reported of the InGaAsP distributed feedback (DFB) lasers, 5.7mA[6], which is more suitable for long distance and high speed optical transmission systems.

We have developed an extremely low threshold InGaAsP DFB laser diode whose threshold current is 3.1mA. Optimization of the device parameters, such as the thickness of the active layer, the length of the device, the facet reflectivities and the depth of the grating, has been done to realize the low threshold, taking into account maintaining a stable single longitudinal mode operation. Moreover a metal organic chemical vapor deposition (MOCVD) technique was applied to control the thin active layer thickness accurately with good uniformity and preserve the corrugation very well, which could not be realized by liquid phase epitaxy (LPE). To fabricate a very low threshold current and stable single longitudinal mode laser, we made the cavity length short and the coupling coefficient (κ) large, since the internal absorption loss is reduced with the cavity length, and the larger κ is necessary for the shorter cavity length to achieve the stable single longitudinal mode operation.

Using this low threshold DFB laser, 1 Gbit/s RZ zero bias modulation was examined. The result showed a possibility of the high bit rate zero bias optical transmission.

2. DESIGN

The threshold current of a laser diode is expressed as follows.

$$I_{th} = (Wd/\beta\Gamma) \cdot (\alpha_{in}L + \alpha_m L) + WdJ_0 L \tag{1}$$

where α_{in} is the internal loss of the cavity, α_m is the mirror loss, β is the gain constant, J_0 is the current density for transparency, Γ is the optical confinement factor, W is the width of the active layer, d is the thickness of the active layer, and L is the length of the device.

Among these parameters, α, β and J_0 depend on the material of the laser and its crystal quality. Γ is determined by the thickness of the active layer and the difference of the refractive indices between the active layer and the cladding layer. α_m is determined by the reflevctivities of the facets of the laser and the length of the device in the case of the Fabry Perot laser, and is determined by the facet reflectivities and the product of the coupling constant κ and the length of the device L in the case of the DFB laser.

As seen in equ.(1), it is necessary for the reduction of the threshold current to lower $\alpha_{in}L$ and/or $\alpha_m L$. Assuming the front facet reflectivity, R_1, is 31% of that of the cleaved, the calculated relation between α_m and R_2 (the rear facet refractivity) is as shown in Fig.1, where $\kappa L=1.5$ in the case of DFB laser. As seen in this figure, the mirror loss α_m decreases as the rear facet reflectivity R_2 increases in both cases of the Fabry Perot laser and the DFB laser.

Figure 2 shows the calculated relation between the mirror loss α_m and κL. In this figure the relation between the threshold gain difference, $\Delta\alpha_{th}$, between the lowest threshold mode and the next lowest threshold mode of the DFB laser, which determines the stability of the single longitudinal mode operation, and κL is also shown, where R_1 and R_2 are assumed 31% and 95%, respectively. As seen in this figure, although α_m decreases as κL increases, the decreasing rate is little. For the increase of κL, it is necessary to fabricate higher grating. However it is difficult to obtain κ larger than 100cm^{-1} by the conventional method. So, we have to make L longer to increase κL. But if we make L longer, increases of $\alpha_{in}L$ and WdJ_0L in equ.(1) result in the increase of the threshold current.

Figure 3 shows the calculated relation between the threshold current and the length of the device L in the case of $\kappa=100$cm^{-1}. In the calculation, following parameters are used.

$W=1.5\mu$m, $d=0.1\mu$m, $\beta=0.17\mu$m^2/mA, $\Gamma=0.2$, $\alpha_{in}=20$cm^{-1}, $J_0=1.9\times 10^{-2}$mA/μm^3
$R_1=31\%$, $R_2=95\%$

As seen in this figure, the threshold current decreases as L decreases. However, if L decreases too much, the threshold gain difference also decreases as shown in Fig.2, and it becomes impossible to obtain the stable longitudinal mode operation. As the result, in the case of $\kappa=100$cm^{-1}, $L=150\mu$m($\kappa L=1.5$) is the optimal value for obtaining the low threshold and stable longitudinal mode DFB laser diode. In this condition a threshold current of about 3mA is expected from Fig.3.

3. STRUCTURE AND FABRICATION PROCEDURE

To fabricate the DFB laser, we used the MOCVD and LPE hybrid process. The MOCVD has an advantage of obtaining abrupt interface between the heterostrucures, preserving the grating during the crystal growth. While the LPE is suitable to embed the both side of the mesa structure.

The device investigated here is so called a p-substrate partially inverted buried heterostructure (PPIBH)[7] and its structure is shown in Fig.4. The fabrication procedure is as follows. At first p-InP buffer layer, 0.1μm undoped InGaAsP active layer ($\lambda g=1.3\mu$m) and n-InGaAsP guiding layer ($\lambda g=1.15\mu$m) are grown on a p-InP substrate by the first step MOCVD. Where λg denotes the corresponding bandgap energy. From equ.(1) the threshold current decreases as the thickness of the active layer decreases. However, if the active layer thickness decreases too much, the threshold current greatly increases because the optical confinement factor Γ decreases[8]. So we controlled the active layer thickness to be 0.1μ m.

After the first MOCVD a grating with the period of 2000 A and the height of 70nm is formed on the guiding layer. Then, by the second MOCVD n-InP cladding layer is grown on the grating. At this stage the wafer is selectively etched down to the buffer layer to fabricate the mesa structure. The width of the mesa at the active layer is about 1.5μ m.

Both sides of the mesa are buried with p-InP filling layer, n-InP current blocking layer and p-InP current blocking layer by the LPE. N-InP cladding layer and n-InGaAsP contact layer are grown successively by the LPE. During the LPE growth the tips of n-InP current blocking layer are separated from the former n-InP cladding layer by the diffusion of Zn from the surrounding p-InP filling layer and p-InP current blocking layer. So the leakage current is fully suppressed due to the very narrow leakage current paths and the relatively high resistance of the p-InP.

After the crystal growth, Cr/Au and Zn/Au are sputtered and evaporated on n- and p-side, respectively, and the alloying is done to make an ohmic contact. The wafer is cleaved into each chips with the length of 150μ m. The rear facet is coated with SiO_2 and α-Si. The reflectivity is estimated as 95%.

Fig.5 shows the scanning electron microscope photograph of the grating after the fabrication procedure. The grating is well preserved and its height is about 70nm. This good preservation of the grating is attributed to the MOCVD technique. In the case of the conventional LPE growth on the grating, its height reduces about half times the initial height.

The coupling constant κ estimated from the stop band width is about $100 cm^{-1}$ which is about twice the coupling constant obtained by the LPE.

4. CHARACTERISTICS

Figure 6 shows the light output power versus injection current of the device fabricate as explained in Sec.3 in c.w. condition at room temperature. The threshold current is as small as 3mA, which is the lowest value so far reported in InGaAsP lasers including those of the Fabry Perot type. In Sec.2 we calculated the threshold current of 3mA with the length of 150μ m and κ of $100 cm^{-1}$ not taking into account the leakage current. The measured threshold current is in good agreement with the predicted value, which implies that in PPIBH structure the leakage current is fully suppressed.

Figure 7 shows the lasing spectrum of the device at 5mW in c.w. condition. The laser oscillates in a single longitudinal mode and the side mode suppression ratio is 40dB.

5. ZERO BIAS MODULATION

In the case of the zero bias modulation of the laser diode, the delay time is a severe problem for a practical application. At high giga bit operation this delay time not only causes the reduction of the pulse width but also increases the jitter due to the pattern effect. In general the delay time less than 20% of the pulse width is required to suppress the bit error rate in a practical system. So, in giga bit rate transmission the delay time has to be suppressed less than 0.2nsec.

The delay time t_d of the laser diode in zero bias modulation is expressed as follows.

$$t_d = \tau_n \ln(I_p / (I_p - I_{th})) \qquad (2)$$

where τ_n is the carrier life time, I_p the pulse current, and I_{th} the threshold current. From equ.(2) the delay time t_d decreases with the increase of the pulse current I_p and with the decrease of the threshold current I_{th}. Assuming τ_n is 1.5nsec, we calculated the relation between the delay time and the pulse current for the two levels of the threshold current, 3mA and 20mA. The result is shown in Fig.8. In the case of I_{th} of 20mA, the delay time at I_p of 40mA which is compatible with logic-type drive current, is about 1nsec, which is too long for the giga bit rate transmission. While in the case of I_{th} of 3mA, the delay time at I_p of 40mA is 0.12nsec, which is short enough for the giga bit rate transmission. So an extremely low threshold current laser diode is a promising light source for the zero bias giga bit rate transmission.

Figure 9 shows the measured results of the pulse response at I_p of 40mA for the threshold currents of 3.1mA and 20mA. In the case of I_{th} of 3.1mA, the delay time is 0.18nsec. While in the case of I_{th} of 20mA, the delay time is 0.9nsec. These values are roughly coincide with the calculated values.

Figure 10 shows the output signal of the DFB laser with I_{th} of 3.1mA under 1 Gbit/sec RZ pseudo-random modulation with I_p of 40mA at zero bias level. Although a jitter due to the pattern effect is observed at the front of the signal, wide opened eye patterns are obtained. The amount of a jitter is about 80psec which might be allowable value for 1 Gbit/sec RZ modulation.

Figure 11 shows the lasing spectrum of the DFB laser with I_{th} of 3.1mA under 1 Gbit/sec RZ modulation at zero bias level. Although a small amount of chirp due to the fluctuation of the injected carrier concentration, the laser oscillates in the stable single longitudinal mode. The side mode suppression ratio is 37dB.

These results suggest the possibility of zero bias transmission of an extremely low threshold laser diode under giga bit rate transmission.

6.CONCLUSION

By optimizing the device parameters, such as the thickness of the active layer, the length of the device, the facet reflectivities and the depth of the grating, and appling the MOCVD technique to the fabrication of the DFB laser, an extremely low threshold of 3.1mA has been achieved in the InGaAsP laser diode.

Using this low threshold DFB laser diode, the possibility of giga bit rate zero bias transmission of the InGaAsP DFB laser has been demonstrated.

7.REFERENCE

1. H.Furuyama, A.Kurobe, S.Naritsuka, N.Sugiyama, Y.Kokubun and M.Nakamura, "Extremely low-threshold zinc-diffused mesa buried-hetero multiquantum-well lasers," Tech.dig.CLEO'87 Baltimore,MD,Paper TuE4
2. K.Y.Lau, N.Bar-Chaim, P.L.Derry and A.Yariv,"High-speed digital modulation of ultalow threshold (<1mA) GaAs single quantum well lasers without bias," Appl.Phys.Lett.51, 69-71 (1987)
3. K.Y.Lau, P.L.Derry and A.Yariv,"Ultimate limit in low threshold quantum well GaAlAs semiconductor lasers," Appl.Phys.Lett.52,88-90 (1988)
4. M.Nakamura, H.Furuyama and A.Kurobe,"1 Gbit/s automatic-power-control-free zero-bias modulation of very-low threshold MQW laser diodes," Electon.Lett.23,1352-1353 (1987)
5. D.Z.Tsang and Z.L.Liau,"Sinusoidal and digital high-speed modulation of p-type substrate mass-transported diode lasers," J.Lightwave Tech.LT-5,300-304 (1987)
6. Y.Itaya, H.Saito, G.Motosugi and Y.Tohmori,"Low threshold current GaInAsP/InP DFB lasers," IEEE J.Quantum Electron.QE-23,828-834 (1987)
7. A.Takemoto, Y.Sakakibara, Y.Nakajima, M.Fujiwara, S.Kakimoto, H.Namizaki and W.Susaki,"1.3μm InGaAsP distributed-feedback p-substrate partially inverted buried-heterostructure laser diode," Electron.Lett.23,546-547 (1987)
8. S.Tsuji, A.Ohishi, H.Nakamura, M.Hirao, N.Chinone and H.Matsumura,"Low threshold operation of 1.5-μm DFB laser diodes," J.Lightwave Tech.LT-5,822-826 (1987)

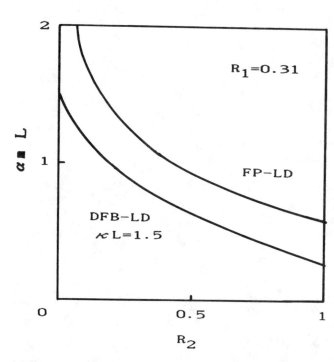

Fig.1 The mirror loss α_m versus the rear facet reflectivity R_2.

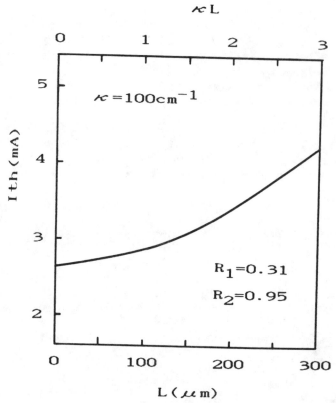

Fig.3 The threshold current I_{th} versus the length of the device L.

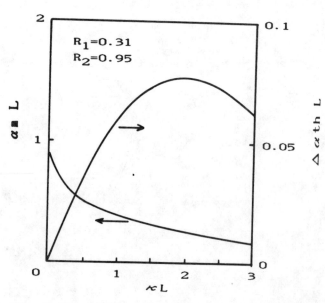

Fig.2 The mirror loss α_m, the threshold gain difference $\Delta\alpha_{th}$ versus the product of the coupling constant κ and the length of the device L.

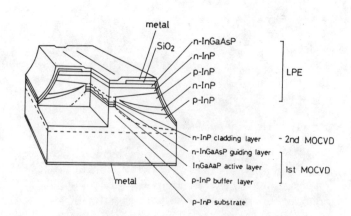

Fig.4 The schematic cross section of the DFB-PPIBH laser fabricated by the MOCVD and LPE hybrid process.

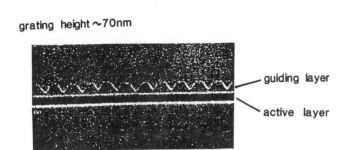

Fig.5 The scanning electron microscope photograph of the grating.

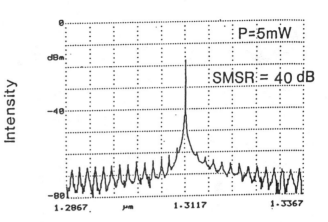

Fig.7 The lasing spectrum under c.w. condition.

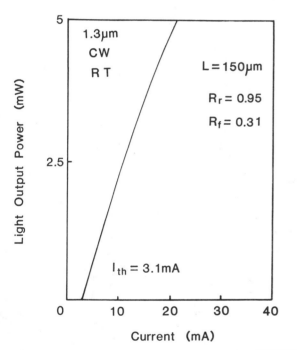

Fig.6 The light output power versus current.

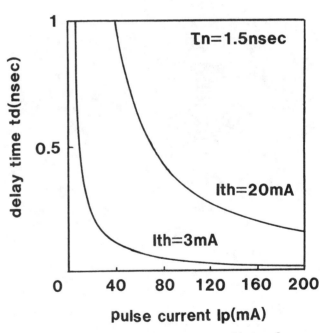

Fig.8 The delay time t_d versus the pulse current I_p.

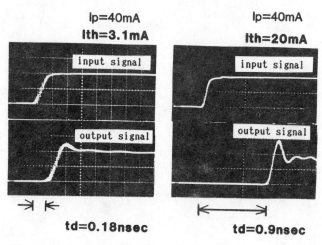

Fig.9 Pulse responses of laser diodes with threshold currents of 3.1mA and 20mA.

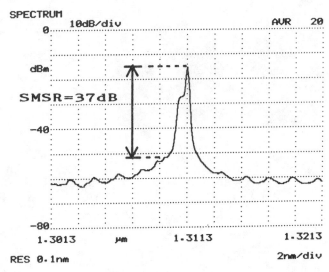

Fig.11 The lasing spectrum under 1Gbit/sec RZ zero bias modulation.

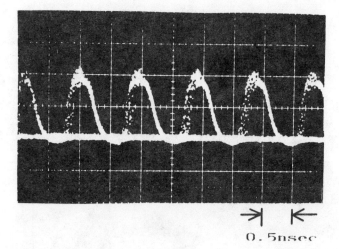

Fig.10 The output signal under 1 Gbit/sec RZ zero bias modulation.

Monolithic Four-Beam Semiconductor Laser Array with Built-in Monitoring Photodiodes

T. Yamaguchi, K. Yodoshi, K. Minakuchi, Y. Inoue, N. Tabuchi,
K. Komeda, H. Hamada. T. Niina

Semiconductor Research Center, SANYO Electric Co., Ltd.
1-18-13, Hashiridani, Hirakata, Osaka 573, Japan

ABSTRACT

A four-beam semiconductor laser was developed in which a monolithic array of four individually addressable GaAlAs high power lasers and four integrated Si photodiodes for monitoring the light output power of laser beams are housed in a single package. The main specifications are as follows; output power per beam, 40 mW; wavelength, 830 nm; and monitoring current at 30 mW, 100~200 µA. Thermal analysis by numerical simulation was carried out and compared to experimental values observed during simultaneous operation of the multiple elemental lasers. The operating lifetime is estimated to be more than 10,000 hrs at room temperature.

1. INTRODUCTION

The multi-beam semiconductor laser array is gaining much attention for high speed recording, realtime recording, and erasure. It can be used as a light source in a small-sized optical head in which multiple laser beams run along the same path. Furthermore it enables high speed recording by parallel processing of multiple tracks, or high speed erasure and recording function by focusing different laser beams on two successive spots on the same track.

Several reports have appeared concerning multi-beam semiconductor laser arrays that is, CDH-LOC laser arrays [1]-[2], CSP laser arrays [3], and PCW laser arrays, which have been developed for optical disk application. We previously reported on a three-beam semiconductor laser array [4] for real time recording and information erasing (over-write) in a magneto-optical disk system. In these devices, however, the optical output power was insufficient and the demand for higher output power and a larger number of laser beams is growing. In addition, the light output monitoring method for automatic power control (APC) is well-suited for practical application.

In this paper, we will report on a monolithic four beam semiconductor laser array which has high output power, can be individually addressed and has built-in monitoring photodiodes. The structure, fabrication process and basic characteristics of the device are described. Thermal characteristics during simultaneous operation of multiple lasers are also reported comparing with a numerical simulation based on heat flow analysis, followed by a discussion about optimizing device dimensions to decrease thermal crosstalk between the lasers. Finally, possible applications and future prospects of four-beam lasers are suggested.

2. STRUCTURE AND FABRICATION

2.1 Device structure

This laser is a unique device designed to emit four high output laser beams (each with a rated optical light output power of 30~40 mW) for various functions such as
reading, writing (recording), and erasing.

The structure of the device is shown schematically in Fig. 1. A GaAlAs semiconductor laser(LD) array chip and a Si PIN photodiode(PD) array are mounted in a single package. The laser chip has four elemental oscillating stripes integrated within it. The PIN photodiode array also has four elemental photo-sensing junctions integrated within it which correspond to four laser beams, and can measure output power from the rear facet of the laser chip. A unique "light-guide" is mounted between the laser chip and the PIN photodiodes for separate introduction of the laser beams with minimal crosstalk. The light-guide is not illustrated in Fig. 1 for simplicity. As shown in Fig. 1, this device has ten terminal leads, one for each laser (4) and photodiode (4) and two correspond to the common electrodes. The laser chip and the photodiode are electrically isolated to prevent possible mutual interferences.

One of the features of this laser is the incorporation of monitor diodes which provide a means to stabilize optical output power individually. By monitoring each element individually, stable output power can be obtained in spite of temperature changes or an unstable power supply voltage. This outstanding feature also helps to suppress light output instability arising from the thermal interaction of the lasers. This will be discussed later in detail.

A detailed cross sectional view of the laser chip is shown in Fig. 2. Four elemental lasers are integrated on a p-GaAs substrate. Each element is composed of an inner-stripe double heterostructure grown on a channeled substrate. The distance between each element is 100 µm and each laser is isolated electrically by etched grooves. The front and the rear facets are coated with Al_2O_3 and Al_2O/a-Si multi-layers respectively, by using the sputtering method. Reflectivity is asymmetrical, giving high output power from the front facets.

2.2 Fabrication process

The four-beam semiconductor laser is fabricated by liquid phase epitaxy (LPE). A conventional horizontal LPE system was improved for precise thickness control, and growth rate was decreased to about 50~100 Å/sec by accurately absorbing the super saturation of the growth melt for the active layer. The thickness of the active layer is controlled within a range of 500 to 600 Å, which enables a high output power of 60 mW. After LPE growth, a conventional laser chip fabrication process was carried out to make a laser chip 500 µm wide and 120 µm thick unless otherwise specified. A preliminary test was carried out for the cleaved bar and a successive series of four normally operating elements are selected for the final chip fabrication process. Reflectivity of the front and the rear facet are 8% and 70% respectively. The laser chip was mounted on a Si heat sink in a junction-up configuration as shown in Fig. 2. Fig. 3 shows the schematic structure of the "light-guide" that was aligned between the laser chip and the PIN photodiodes. The light-guide was fabricated by grooving the Si substrate and coating the inside of the groove with a highly reflective material. The laser chip, light guide and Si photodiodes are closely aligned for effective monitoring of the light output from the rear facet.

3. BASIC CHARACTERISTICS

3.1 Lasing characteristics

Fig. 4 shows typical light output-current characteristics (L-I characteristics) obtained by operating the four elemental lasers individually. The monitoring output currents of corresponding PIN photodiodes are also shown (L-Im characteristics). L-I characteristics and L-Im characteristics are marked in the figure as LD and PD, respectively. The horizontal scale designates the operating current of the lasers, and the monitoring output current of photodiodes. The vertical scale indicates the light output power of the laser both in L-I characteristics and L-Im characteristics.
As shown in Fig. 3, the L-I characteristics of the four lasers are very similar. Threshold currents range from 40 to 42 mA and operating currents at 30 mW are 75~80 mA. The monitoring currents change linearly with light output power, which indicates that the far-field pattern from the rear facet is stable in the range 0~40 mW and the output power from the rear facet is accurately proportional to that of the front facet.

Monitoring current, which ranges from 100 to 200 µA at 30 mW output power, is large enough to electrically feed-back to the driving circuit for automatic power control (APC). Optical crosstalk, which is leakage of light from a laser to a different monitoring photodiode, was also measured. Fig. 5 shows the monitoring output currents of the four photodiodes obtained when only laser 1 was operated. The monitoring currents of photodiodes 2,3 and 4 are less than 1.5% of the monitoring current of photodiode 1. As a result, optical crosstalk is confirmed to be small enough to prevent influence from other lasers through the monitoring circuit.

Stability of the near-field and far field pattern is an important requirement for the multi-beam laser. Fig. 6 shows a typical far-field pattern of an elemental laser in the device. Both in the vertical and horizontal directions, the far-field pattern are stable from 0 to 40 mW of output power. FWHM ranges from 28° to 30° ($\theta_\perp$) and from 9 to 11° ($\theta_\parallel$).

The oscillating wavelength is in the range of 830 ±1 nm, which is extremely uniform for the four lasers. Uniformity of the spectrum among the elements represents the uniformity of thermal dissipation as well as the homogeneity of the composition in LPE grown materials. In Table 1, basic specifications and other characteristics are summarized.

3.2 Thermal interaction between elemental lasers

In the multi-beam semiconductor laser, the thermal interaction between each element poses a problem during simultaneous operation of the multiple elements. We investigated the thermal interaction between two elements operating simultaneously by means of a pulse driving method. In this experiment elemental laser 2 is operated in automatic current control (ACC) mode of 80 mA which corresponds to 30 mW of output power, and element 1 is driven with a pulsed current of 80 mA peak value. Fig. 7 shows the light output of laser 2 (P_2) which changes with respect to the pulsed current of laser 1 (I_1). Reduction of the light output is considered to be caused from the thermal effect by the current I_1. The ratio of the light output reduction ΔP_2 to DC light output P_2, $\Delta P_2/P_2$, is about 3.6%. The temperature rise is estimated at 4°C, from the temperature dependency of L-1 characteristics measured in laser 2. In the same manner, the thermal interaction between laser 1 and 3, 1 and 4, are found to be 2% and 1% respectively. Fluctuations are a hindrance to practical application. There are two driving methods to reduce this function. One is the automatic power control (APC) method, in which I_2 is controlled to maintain P_2 constant by the feed-back signal of the monitoring photodiode. Fig. 8 shows the waveform of P_2 observed under the same conditions as Fig. 7 except that laser 2 was operated in APC mode. In this case, reduction of P_2 is rapidly restored by the APC circuit, though fluctuations remained because of the slow response of the APC circuit. Fluctuation is reduced to 2.6%, which shows the effectiveness of APC operation by the monitoring photodiode. The other method to suppress the fluctuation is the DC bias method, in which a constant DC current just below the threshold is sent to laser 1. For pulse driving of laser 1 at 30 mW, the current pulse of the operating current (Iop) minus threshold current (Ith) added to the bias current is enough. Therefore the temperature fluctuation affecting laser 2 is reduced. Fig. 9 shows the relationship between fluctuation of light output P_2 and pulse current I, in two cases, that is, with and without DC biasing I_1. It was found that fluctuation can be reduced clearly by means of the DC bias method.

A change in oscillation wavelength by the thermal interaction from the other elements is also observed. We found the spectrum shift of laser 2 to be about 3 nm with laser 1 driving at 30 mW. This problem is now under study.

4. THERMAL ANALYSIS OF THE MULTI-BEAM LASER

4.1 Simulation of the temperature rise distribution

As described in the preceding section, thermal crosstalk (thermal interaction between two elemental lasers) is an important problem which needs to be analyzed for stable operation of the device. In this section we describe a numerical simulation of the temperature rise distribution and compare the results with experimentally observed thermal crosstalk. In our analysis, the model as shown in Fig. 10 is used. The heat source embedding the laser chip are assumed at the position of laser stripes. As described before by Joyce et al[5], the basic solution of Laplace's equation for temperature T_i is represented by a two-dimensional Fourier series as follows:

$$T_i(x,y) = \beta_{i0}(1-\gamma_{i0}y) + \sum \beta_n [\cosh(k_n y) - \gamma_{in}\sinh(k_n y)]\cos(k_n x) \cdots\cdots(1)$$

where ß, γ are undetermined coefficients. Suffix i denotes the order of the layer numbered from the heat source. Evaluation of ß, γ and kn are carried out under the following conditions: no heat escapes from the lateral faces and top surface of the device, continuity of temperature and normal heat flow at the interface. A heat generation J are introduced as heat flow per unit area having a width A at the junction position. After determination of ß, γ temperature distribution was numerically simulated by using Eq. (1). The summation is carried out with n=1~200. Fig. 11 shows temperature distribution when laser 1 is operated at a light output of 30 mW. Electric power applied to laser 1 minus light output is used as the heat source. The temperature rise from room temperature is indicated by the isothermal curves drawn in the cross section of the laser chip and Si heat sink system. As shown in Fig. 11, the temperature rise is about 4° C at the position of laser 2, which agrees well with the value 4°C obtained experimentally as described before. Temperature distribution along the active layer was also simulated as shown in Fig. 12. The temperature rise at laser 3 and 4 positions (x = 200 µm, 300 µm) also agree with the experimental value. Good agreement of simulation with experiment results suggests that heat flow at the interface of the laser chip and the Si heat sink is extremely smooth. This is because heat flow simulation is carried out without any thermal-resistive layer between them such as a low-conductive metalized region. It was found that beam spacing can be reduced to approximately 50 µm without a severe temperature rise caused by the nearest element as shown in Fig. 12.

4.2 Optimization of device dimensions from the standpoint of thermal crosstalk

Device dimensions related to thermal crosstalk are thickness and cavity length of the laser chip. It is clear that heat dissipation increases by thinning the chip. But the possibility of layer damage and handling difficult limit thinning. We consider the practical limit of chip thickness to be approximately 60 μm. Temperature distribution was numerically simulated for a 60 μm thick chip. Fig. 13 shows the simulated results. It was found that temperature rise is much reduced compared to conditions shown in Fig. 11. The simulated results were confirmed experimentally by using a laser chip that was 60 μm thick. Fig. 14 shows the light output, ΔP_2, observed in the same manner as described before, for the chip. Compared to the results in Fig. 7, it is obvious that thinning is very effective for reducing thermal crosstalk between two elements.

Cavity length also affects the thermal parameters of a device. As is well known, operating current density J_{op} is given by the following equation:

$$J_{op} = \{\alpha_i + (1/L)\ln(1/R)\}\{(d/\beta\Gamma) + P_0(\beta/h\nu)(1/A\eta_i)\cdot\ln(1/R)\} + dJ_0 \cdots\cdots (2)$$

where L and A are the cavity length and the stripe width respectively. Other parameters are constant and are determined by the structure of the device and physical constants. From Eq. (2), We surmise that the heat emission rate from the stripe, which is approximately proportional to current density, decreases as cavity length is extended. To determine optimum cavity length, we fabricated devices with cavity lengths longer than 250 μm and compared them with operating current density at 30 mW. We call these devices long cavity lasers in this paper. Fig. 15 shows L-J characteristics obtained by these lasers. As shown in Fig. 15, the operating current density decreases by extending the cavity length and it was found that the reduction ratio is much larger from 250 μm to 350 μm than from 350 μm to 400 μm. Therefore we have tested the 400-μm cavity length device as a representative of the long cavity lasers. Heat generation rate for the 400-μm long cavity laser is estimated at 140 mW with the experimental value of the operation current density at 30 mW. Fig. 16 shows the simulated temperature distribution, and we found that the temperature rise at the laser 2 position is 3.0°C, which is much smaller than the temperature rise for a 250-μm cavity laser as shown in Fig. 11. Variation in the light output power of laser 2 is maintained at 2.2% which is much smaller than those of the 250-μm cavity laser.

5. RELIABILITY

Each of the elemental lasers integrated in the chip is an extremely reliable high-power laser. We have confirmed their reliability by continuous operation under accelerated conditions. A large number of devices are tested by selecting one of the four elements for the reliability test. The samples were operated in an APC mode of 40 mW at 50°C for more than 3000 hrs and operating currents were maintained at nearly constant. By this test a high-reliability equivalent of over 30,000 hrs at room temperature under high output power was estimated for each element. However, the four-beam laser must be operated under extremely severe operating conditions, that is, all of the elemental lasers should be operated simultaneously at high output power. Therefore the junction temperature during simultaneous operation of the lasers must be estimated. Fig. 17 shows simulation of temperature rise distribution during simultaneous operation at an output power of 40 mW. The device parameters are a cavity length of 250 μm and a chip thickness of 60 μm. As shown in Fig. 17, the isothermal temperature curves become denser near the elemental stripes and the temperature rise of the lasers is estimated to be approximately 23°C. This temperature rise is approximately 6°C higher than that of single-laser operation. Therefore the lifetime of the device when all four elements operate simultaneously is nearly half of that for single-laser operation, assuming that the activation energy Ea related to degradation is 0.7 eV. We expect that the lifetime of the four-beam laser is more than 15,000 hrs at room temperature with simultaneous operation of all four lasers at 40 mW. An experimental aging test was carried out and stable operation for longer than 1,000 hrs was confirmed for the 4 lasers at 40 mW and 50°C, that is, the lifetime at room temperature is estimated to be longer than 10,000 hrs.

6. APPLICATIONS AND FUTURE PROSPECTS

Several kinds of multi-beam semiconductor lasers have been developed and experimentally applied to mainly optical disk system. The outstanding features of our four-beam laser have broadened the application field for the multi-beam laser. In the field of optical disk memory systems, a high speed recording by simultaneous processing of closely spaced parallel tracks, or real time recording and erasure (over-write) with successive processing of erasure and recording by separate beams are the most useful applications. OA equipment other than optical disk memory, such as laser beam printers are also interesting fields for multi-beam lasers. The main subjects for multi-beam lasers are to increase output power; shorten wavelength; and to increase the number of beams. By developing these technologies, the multi-beam laser is expected to come into widespread use in the future as an important component in optoelectronics devices.

REFERENCES

1) D.B. Carlin, J.P. Bendnaz, C.J. Kaiser, J.C. Connolly, and M.G. Harvey, Appl. Opt . Vol. 23, Nov. 15, 3994 (1984); "Erratum" Dec. 15, 4613 (1984)

2) D. Botez, J.C. Connolly, D.B. Gillbert, M.G. Harvey and M. Ettenberg, Appl. Phys. Lett., vol. 41, 1040 (1982)

3) D.B. Carlin, B. Goldstein, J.P. Bendnaz, M.G. Harvey and N.A. Dinkel, IEEE J. Quantum Electronics, vol. QE-23, No. 5, 476 (1987)

4) SPIE Optical Engineering Reports No.40/APRIL 5A (1987)

5) W.B. Joyce and R.W. Dixon, J. Appl. Phys. vol. 46, No. 2, 855 (1975)

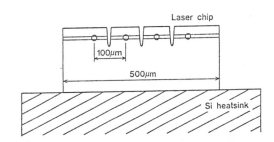

Fig. 2   Schematic cross sectional view of the laser chip.

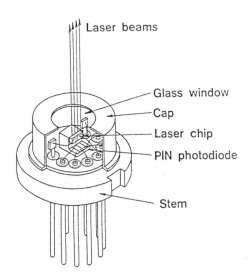

Fig. 1   Schematic structure of the four-beam semiconductor laser.

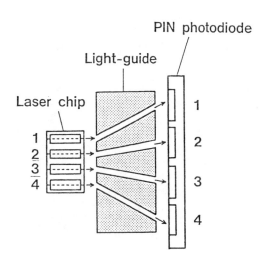

Fig. 3   Schematic structure of the light-guide.

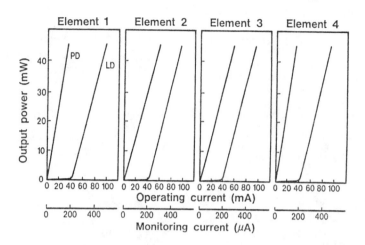

Fig. 4 Typical light output-current characteristics.

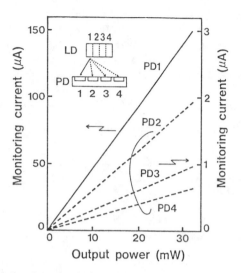

Fig. 5 Monitoring output currents of the four photodiodes obtained when only laser 1 is operated.

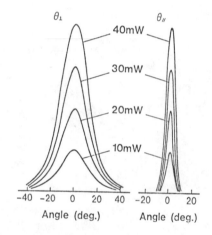

Fig. 6 Typical far-field pattern of an elemental laser in the four-beam laser.

Table 1 Specifications of the four-beam laser.

Parameter		Symbol	Typ.	Unit
Wavelength		λ	830	nm
Threshold current		I_{th}	40	mA
Operating current		I_{op}	80	mA
Operating voltage		V_{op}	1.85	V
Output power		P_o	30	mW
Beam divergence	Parallel	$\theta_{//}$	10	deg.
	Perpendicular	$\theta_\perp$	30	deg.
Monitoring current	Element 1,4	$I_{m1,4}$	100	μA
	Element 2,3	$I_{m2,3}$	200	μA

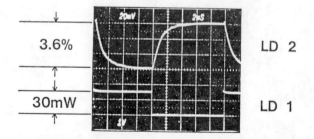

Fig. 7 Variation of laser 2's light output in ACC operation, when laser 1 is driven in the pulse operation.

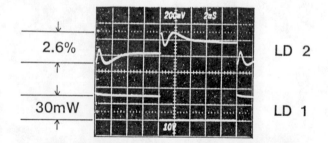

Fig. 8 Variation of laser 2's light output in APC operation, when laser 1 is driven in the pulse operation.

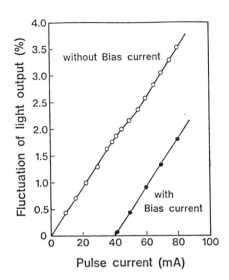

Fig. 9 Relationship between fluctuation of laser 2's light output and pulse current of laser 1.

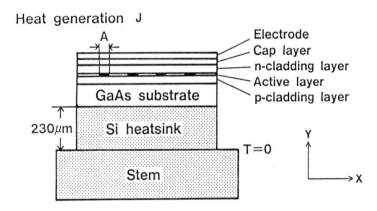

Fig. 10 Model used for the thermal analysis.

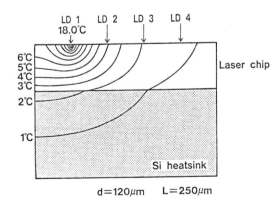

Fig. 11 Simulated temperature distribution when laser 1 is operated at 30 mW light output.

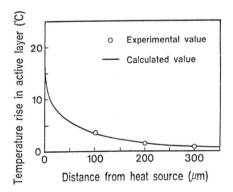

Fig. 12 Simulated temperature distribution along the active layer.

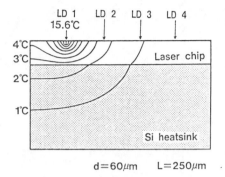

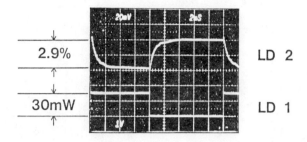

Fig. 13 Temperature distribution when laser 1 is operated at 30 mW light output by using 60 μm thick laser chip and 250 μm long cavity.

Fig. 14 Variation of laser 2's light output in ACC operation, when laser 1 is driven in the pulse operation by using 60 μm thick laser chip.

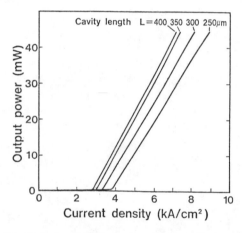

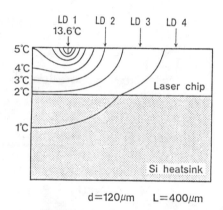

Fig. 15 Relationship between the light output and the current density for devices of various cavity length.

Fig. 16 Simulated temperature distribution when laser 1 is operated at 30 mW light output by using 120 μm thick laser chip and 400 μm long cavity.

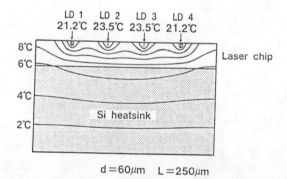

Fig. 17 Simulated temperature distribution when four lasers are simultaneously operated at 40 mW light output by using 60 μm thick laser chip and 250 μm long cavity.

Invited Paper

FOCUSED-ION-BEAM MICROMACHINED DIODE LASER MIRRORS

R. K. DeFreez, J. Puretz, R. A. Elliott, G. A. Crow, H. Ximen,
D. J. Bossert, G. A. Wilson, and J. Orloff

Oregon Graduate Center, Dept. of Applied Physics and Elec. Eng.
19600 N.W. Von Neumann Dr., Beaverton, OR 97006-1999

ABSTRACT

Focused-ion-beam micromachining is a new technique for forming optical quality surfaces in semiconductor laser materials. It exploits the precise, computer controlled, maskless, sputter-etching afforded by a beam of 15 - 25 keV Ga^+ ions focused to a 50 to 250 nm spot to fabricate features in semiconductor laser dice and wafers. Diode laser output mirrors of quality comparable to that of cleaved facets have been fabricated. Focused-ion-beam micromachined (FIBM) single stripe coupled cavity lasers have demonstrated widely and continuously tunable single mode operation. As much as 80 mW of pulsed tunable single longitudinal mode optical power has been achieved with FIBM coupled cavity phase-locked arrays of AlGaAs semiconductor lasers. Hundreds of milliwatts of pulsed optical power has been observed from surface-emitting phase-locked arrays with FIBM turning and oscillator mirrors. The use of vector scanning of the ion beam to produce arbitrary surface contours, such as linear and curved turning mirrors and micron pitch gratings with various profiles, has been demonstrated. Recent results from elevated temperature aging tests suggest that FIBM does not cause significant damage to transverse junction stripe laser diodes and that it can be a promising tool for fabrication of etched mirrors for optoelectronic integrated circuits.

Continuing research includes work on the fabrication of (i) monolithic dual micromachined coupled cavity single frequency lasers with wavelength separations continuously variable from 0 to 600 GHz, (ii) linear and parabolic turning mirrors for two-dimensionally coherent surface emitting arrays of lasers, (iii) total-internal-reflection mirrors to route light in the plane of the wafer, (iv) single wavelength micromachined coupled cavity lasers tunable at high frequencies, (v) a methanometer with a continuously tunable micromachined coupled cavity InGaAs/InP optical source, (vi) curved laser mirrors, and (vii) submicron, arbitrarily profiled, diffraction gratings for distributed feedback and distributed Bragg reflector lasers.

1. INTRODUCTION

The past few years has seen the beginning development of a promising new technique for forming microoptical surfaces in semiconductor materials[1-5]. This technique, focused-ion-beam micromachining (FIBM), makes use of a tightly focused beam of 15 to 25 keV Ga^+ ions derived by field evaporation from a liquid gallium "point" source[6]. The beam of ions emitted by the liquid metal source is apertured and focused in an ion-optical column which, depending on the design, can provide a focal spot ranging from 50 to 250 nm[7-10]. Current densities of the order of 1 A/cm^2 are readily achieved.

The focused beam of ions can be deflected under computer control over areas approaching 1 mm² with a precision comparable to or smaller than the spot size. This allows the removal of material by sputter-etching to form submicron features with optically smooth surfaces. A significant advantage of FIBM is that it is a completely maskless process and no photolithography, wet chemistry, or other processing is required so that mounted and partially packaged devices can be modified without fear of adverse interactions with heatsink or packaging materials.

The ability to deflect the ion beam under computer control provides added flexibility for producing features with arbitrary surface profiles. For simple shapes this is not so important since the ion beam can be raster scanned at a uniform rate over a field to remove a thin laminar layer over the entire field and adjusting subsequent fields scanned to form the topography desired. For example a V-shaped groove can be formed by rastering the ion beam over a sequence of successively narrower rectangles on a common center. For more complex shapes it is useful to be able to control the beam dwell time at each pixel of the field of view. Topographical features such as the sinusoidal gratings described below can be micromachined using this *vector scanning* method[5,11].

Section 2 is a description of semiconductor lasers with FIBM output mirrors including a discussion of their operating characteristics and an evaluation of the optical quality of the micromachined mirrors as determined from lasing threshold and differential efficiency measurements and aging tests. The next section is devoted to micromachined coupled-cavity (MC^2) semiconductor lasers and their slow and high speed tuning characteristics. Following this, Section 4, details the fabrication and properties of surface emitting phase-locked arrays of diode formed by FIBM oscillator and turning mirrors. Micromachined diffraction gratings suitable for distributed Bragg reflector (DBR) surface emitting two-dimensional arrays of diode lasers are also discussed in Section 4. A brief discussion placing FIBM in context with other microfabrication techniques and outlining work in progress and plans for further studies concludes the paper in Section 5.

2. FOCUSED-ION-BEAM MICROMACHINED DIODE LASER MIRRORS

We reported earlier on the focused-ion-beam micromachining of output mirrors on AlGaAs V-channel-substrate inner-stripe diode lasers[1]. These were standard commercial devices (Misubishi ML-4102) which had the original cleaved facet mirror passivated with an Al_2O_3 coating. The micromachined mirrors were formed by raster scanning a 300 pA beam of 20 keV Ga^+ ions in a rectangular pattern overlapping the output end of the device. The beam direction was approximately normal to the top, non-optical surface with the new optical quality mirror surface being formed parallel to the scanning beam. The micromachined devices had lasing thresholds which were essentially unchanged from those with cleaved facet mirrors. The differential efficiency was degraded by about 20%.

In more recent work similar experiments were performed on transverse junction stripe (TJS) lasers some of which had not been passivated[12,13]. Figure 1 is a scanning electron micrograph of a TJS laser with a micromachined output mirror. The optical properties of these lasers were identical within measurement error as shown by the optical power versus drive current curves in Figure 2. The electrical characteristics, as shown in the Log I versus V curves of Figure 3, are similar to the unmodified devices except for a small leakage current of less than 100 μA. The leakage current is probably due to redeposition of a small amount of gallium on the mirror surface during the micromachining process. Although these devices were not so treated, it has been shown[2] that rinsing the diode assembly in dilute HCl after micromachining removes redeposited gallium and improves the diode electrical characteristics.

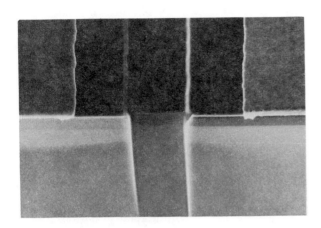

Figure 1. Micromachined TJS diode laser mirror.

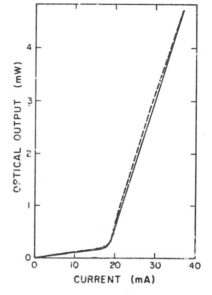

Figure 2. Light versus current characteristics of the laser shown in Figure 1.

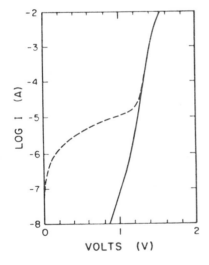

Figure 3. Current versus voltage characteristics of the laser shown in Figure 1.

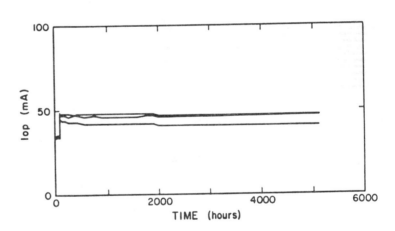

Figure 4. Operating current required to maintain optical output of 4 mW versus time for 3 micromachined TJS lasers. Heatsink temperature 55°C.

It is clear from the SEM micrograph in Figure 1 that the micromachined surface is smooth with no apparent surface roughness. The fact that the FIBM mirror performs as well optically as the cleaved facet mirror testifies further to the excellent surface quality. It is not known from this evidence whether the micromachining process introduces invisible defects in the surface which might degrade the mirror in long term operation. Figure 4 shows a plot of operating current versus time for 3 FIBM

TJS lasers operating at 4 mW cw at a temperature of 55°C. The facets of these samples were passivated with half-wavelength Al_2O_3 films to prevent facet oxidation, a condition which complicates the micromachining process somewhat since the sputter rate of the film is nearly an order of magnitude slower than the underlying semiconductor material. After these devices were aged for 100 h the micromachined mirrors were formed as described above and the surface repassivated. The increased operating current needed to maintain 4 mW optical output following micromachining may be due to complications arising from the presence of the oxide film or to misalignment of the mirror normal and the optic axis of the laser. All three devices have continued to operate stably for more than 5000 hours.

3. MICROMACHINED COUPLED-CAVITY LASERS

Coupled-cavity diode lasers are of interest primarily because of their electronic tuning capability. The use of a focused ion beam to fabricate micromachined-coupled-cavity (MC^2) lasers adds flexibility since both the position and width of the coupling groove can be controlled to a high degree of precision. Figure 5 is an SEM micrograph of an MC^2 laser fabricated from a commercially available diode laser (Mitsubishi ML-4102). Slow speed tuning of an MC^2 laser of this type over 30Å discretely and 3Å continuously was reported earlier[2]. Our more recent work has been concerned with the high speed tuning characteristics of MC^2 lasers and with the monolithic fabrication of two such devices on a single die.

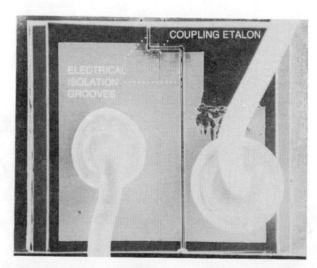

Figure 5. SEM micrograph of MC^2 diode laser.

An experimental setup designed to study high speed mode switching of MC^2 lasers is shown in Figure 6. Light from the laser was focused onto the input slit of a 0.25 meter grating spectrometer. The spectrometer was used in first order to minimize temporal spreading due to path length differences[14] yet obtain adequate spectral resolution to separate the longitudinal modes of the diode laser. The exit slit of the spectrometer was removed so that the entire spectral range of the MC^2 laser could be imaged along the length of the entrance slit of a Hamamatsu C1587 Streak Camera. When used in this way the streak camera generates a wavelength versus time plot. Figure 7 is a halftone reproduction of observed tuning between two adjacent longitudinal modes separated by about 3Å. The time of tuning here is about 300 ps.

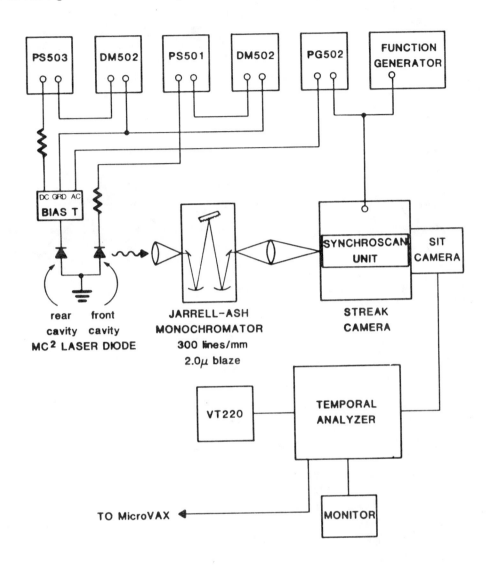

Figure 6. Schematic of the experiment to measure high speed tuning of the MC^2 laser.

The construction of monolithic-dual-micromachined-coupled-cavity ($MDMC^2$) diode lasers is illustrated in Figure 8. The die on which the device was fabricated was not designed specifically for this purpose but was cleaved from a wafer produced by Xerox PARC. This material had been proton implanted to define 10 emitter arrays of gain-guided lasers and metallized in the conventional manner. In the micrograph the vertical lines and the long horizontal lines are shallow micromachined grooves to provide electrical isolation. The short horizontal lines are the optical coupling grooves of the two MC^2 lasers. The center 8 emitters of the 10 emitter array have been isolated and are not driven. In experiments on one $MDMC^2$ laser we were able to tune the two devices to maintain a continuously variable difference frequency between the two lasers over a range of 0 to 600 GHz.

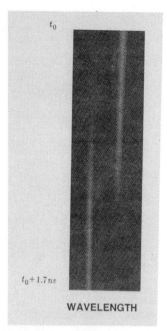

Figure 7. Halftone reproduction of streak camera record of high speed tuning.

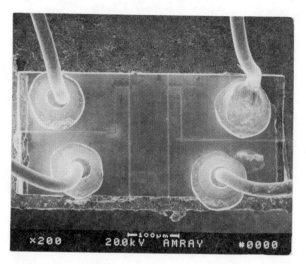

Figure 8. SEM micrograph of MDMC² diode laser.

4. SURFACE EMITTING COHERENT ARRAYS OF DIODE LASERS

The possibility of forming a coherent two-dimensional array of diode lasers has led to the investigation of ways making semiconductor lasers which emit normal to the plane of the wafer. Three types of surface-emitting lasers have been constructed. One has a short oscillator cavity perpendicular to the wafer plane[15] and the other two have oscillator cavities in the plane of the wafer with emission normal to the surface being accomplished with a turning mirror[4,16] or a distributed Bragg reflector grating[17]. We earlier reported construction and operation of a surface-emitting phase-locked array of diode lasers with FIBM turning and oscillator mirrors[4]. 330 mW of optical power was emitted at the turning mirror of this 10 emitter array. The oscillator and turning mirrors were micromachined simultaneously by rastering the ion beam over a sequence of rectangles of decreasing width aligned along one edge. The decrease in width and the ion dose applied in each of the rectangular rasters was calculated so as to produce a 45° surface for the turning mirror facing a vertical surface for the oscillator output mirror.

Our more recent and current work on FIBM has been concerned with improving the quality of the micromachined surfaces by techniques designed to reduce redeposition of sputtered material and with developing methods of forming more complex surfaces. Figure 9 shows a cross section of an ideal turning/oscillator mirror combination. The short vertical sections through the active layer and optical waveguide serves as the oscillator mirror providing feedback to the cavity. The parabolic sections deflect the emitted radiation perpendicular to the wafer surface and provide some degree of collimation. Some of the light emitted from the one output mirror also impinges on the other oscillator mirror and should promote coherence between the opposed lasers. This longitudinal coupling together with evanescent coupling between emitters in the lateral direction could then provide two-dimensional coherence.

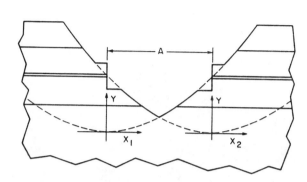

Figure 9. Schematic of ideal turning mirror/ oscillator mirror structure.

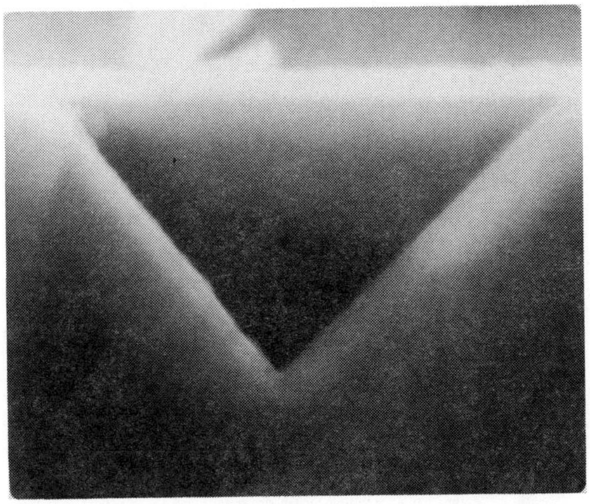

Figure 10. SEM micrograph of micromachined V groove.

Figure 10 is a cross section through a micromachined groove designed to have opposed 45° walls. In this case the sample was tilted so the beam struck the surface at ≈ 45° and was rastered over a sequence of rectangles of increasing width. The beam direction was parallel to the right hand surface. Some redeposition of gallium rich material is evident on the left hand surface. The left wall is at 42° from the surface normal and the right at 48°. An attempt to form a parabolic groove is shown in Figure 11. In this case vector scanning of the beam was used with the beam scanned at a constant rate in the direction perpendicular to the figure and with a deflecting voltage that varied as

$$V(t) \propto (2t/T)^{1/2}, \; 0 \leq t \leq T/2;$$
$$V(t) \propto [2-(2-2t/T)^{1/2}], \; T/2 \leq t \leq T$$

across the figure with T being the time taken to scan entirely across the groove.

We have initiated some preliminary work directed to making diffraction gratings such as might be used for distributed feedback lasers or as distributed Bragg reflectors for surface emitting lasers. The FIB workstation which has been used for most of our micromachining experiments has an ion gun which produces a focused beam with diameter 250 nm. This is clearly too large to make even 2000Å period second order gratings. We can however demonstrate some of the possibilities as illustrated in Figures 12 and 13. Here we see in Figure 12 a sinusoidal grating generated by deflecting the beam at a constant rate along the lines of the grating and with a deflecting voltage varying as the inverse cosine of time across the grating. The period of this grating is 2.2 μm[11]. Figure 13 was formed in the same way except the total ion dose was roughly double that used in the prior figure. Here an interesting effect due to "self-focusing" of the beam caused by deflections from the ever steepening surfaces as the micromachining progresses has yielded a profile which looks like sine-squared behaviour. If the inverse cosine time dependence is used in two orthogonal directions a two-dimensional grating as displayed in Figure 14 is generated. The grating period is 1.25 μm in each direction.

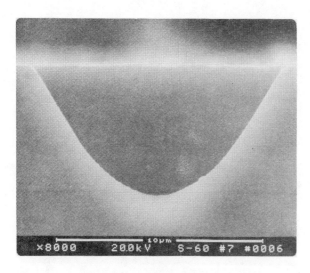

Figure 11. SEM micrograph of micromachined parabolic groove.

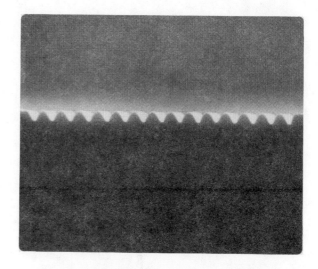

Figure 12. SEM micrograph of micromachined sinusoidal grating.

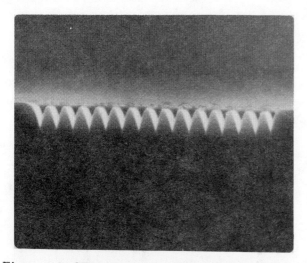

Figure 13. SEM micrograph of micromachined sine-squared grating.

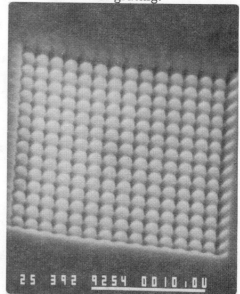

Figure 14. SEM micrograph of micromachined two-dimensional grating.

In order to make gratings with line spacings small enough to be useful for DBR or DFB applications a higher resolution ion system is required. FEI Co. has recently introduced a two lens ion column with a focused beam diameter of 500Å into its product line. The 2500Å period grating displayed in Figure 15 was produced on one of these new systems.

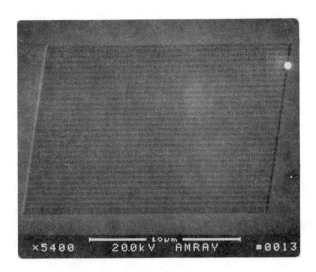

Figure 15. 2500Å period micromachined grating.

5. DISCUSSION

In the foregoing sections we have described some of the devices and structures which have been fabricated by FIBM. The surfaces formed by this method have been shown to be of excellent optical quality and it has been shown that even quite complex topographical features can be generated. Many of the devices have been formed on commercial or preprocessed laser dice which illustrates one of the advantages FIBM has over other means of etching small features in semiconductor materials. The fact that it is a completely maskless process makes it a versatile tool for modifying devices. The ability to observe the micromachining in situ, while not yet perfected, also allows one to intervene as a desired feature is being formed to correct errors and fine tune the process. The major disadvantage of FIBM is that it is inherently a serial process and the time required to form features typical of those described here is measured in minutes to tens of minutes. It is thus definitely not a volume production process but can be very useful for making small numbers of specialized devices.

Our current work includes continuing the effort to produce oscillator/turning mirrors and arbitrarily profiled DBR gratings for two-dimensionally coherent surface-emitting arrays of diode lasers. This involves perfecting the micromachining techniques and the control software for generating grating structures and either V or parabolic grooves with vertical sections to both couple the lasers longitudinally and emit light normal to the surface as described above. Further work on high speed tuning of MC^2 lasers and monolithic dual micromachined coupled cavity lasers for producing two stable single wavelength lasers separated by a variable frequency in the GHz range is also in progress. Another project involves developing an MC^2 InGaAs/InP laser which can be tuned to a methane absorption line and used as the source in a DIAL methanometer for detecting natural gas leaks. We have also begun exploring the use of the FIB system to make curved diode laser mirrors and total-internal-reflection mirrors to direct light from one optical waveguide to another in the plane of the wafer.

6. ACKNOWLEDGEMENT

This work was supported in part by the Innovative Science and Technology Office of the Strategic Defense Initiative Organization, Gas Research Institute, Tektronix, Hughes Research Laboratories, Boeing High Technology Center, David Sarnoff Research Center, AT&T Bell Laboratories, Xerox PARC, and Mitsubishi Electric Corp.

The authors thank Alice Reinheimer for her technical assistance.

References

1. J. Puretz, R. K. DeFreez, R. A. Elliott, and J. Orloff, "Focused-ion-beam micromachined AlGaAs semiconductor laser mirrors," *Electron. Lett.*, vol. 22, pp. 700-702, 19 June 1986.
2. R. K. DeFreez, J. Puretz, R. A. Elliott, J. Orloff, and L. W. Swanson, "CW operation of widely and continuously tunable micromachined-coupled-cavity diode lasers," *Electron. Lett.*, vol. 22, pp. 919-921, 14 August 1986.
3. R. K. DeFreez, J. Puretz, R. A. Elliott, J. Orloff, and T. L. Paoli, "Focussed-ion-beam micromachined coupled-cavity and surface-emitting arrays of diode lasers," *Technical Digest of CLEO '87*, pp. 134-135, Baltimore, Maryland, 26 April to 1 May 1987. Paper WG3
4. J. Puretz, R. K. DeFreez, R. A. Elliott, J. Orloff, and T. L. Paoli, "300 mW operation of a surface-emitting phase-locked array of diode lasers," *Electron. Lett.*, vol. 23, pp. 130-131, 29 January, 1987.
5. R. A. Elliott, R. K. DeFreez, J. Puretz, J. Orloff, and G. A. Crow, "Focused-ion-beam micromachining of diode laser mirrors," *Proceedings of the SPIE Symposium on Communications Networking in Dense Electromagnetic Environments*, vol. 876, pp. 114-120, 14-15 January 1988.
6. L. W. Swanson, G. A. Schwind, A. E. Bell, and J. E. Brady, "Emission characteristics of gallium and bismuth liquid metal field ion sources," *J. Vac. Sci. Technol.*, vol. 16, pp. 1864-1867, November/December 1979.
7. J. Orloff and L. W. Swanson, "Optical column design with liquid metal ion sources," *J. Vac. Sci. Technol.*, vol. 19, pp. 1149-1152, Nov./Dec. 1981.
8. J. Orloff and J. Whitney, "Design of a new, two lens ion gun for micromachining," *Proceedings SPIE Symposium on Electron, X-Ray and Ion Beam Technology: Submicrometer Lithographies VII*, vol. 923, pp. 121-129, 1988.
9. J. Orloff, "An optimized two lens optical column for use with a liquid metal ion source," *Microcircuit Engineering*, vol. 6, pp. 327-332, 1987.
10. J. Orloff, "Optical design approaches for use with liquid metal ion sources," *J. Vac. Sci. Tech. B*, vol. 5, pp. 175-177, 1987.
11. G. Crow, J. Puretz, J. Orloff, R. K. DeFreez, and R. A. Elliott, "The use of vector scanning for producing arbitrary surface contours with a focused ion beam," *J. Vac. Sci. Technol. B*, vol. 6, pp. 1605-1607, September/October 1988.
12. R. K. DeFreez, J. Puretz, J. Orloff, R. A. Elliott, H. Namba, E. Omura, and H. Namizaki, "Operating characteristics and elevated temperature lifetests of focussed ion beam micromachined transverse junction stripe lasers," *Appl. Phys. Lett.*, vol. 53, pp. 1153-1155, 26 September 1988.

13. R. A. Elliott, R. K. DeFreez, J. Puretz, J. Orloff, H. Namba, E. Omura, and H. Namizaki, "Performance and lifetests of focused ion beam micromachined diode lasers," *Proceedings of IEEE LEOS Annual Meeting*, pp. 34-36, Santa Clara, California, 2-4 November 1988.

14. N. H. Schiller and R. R. Alfano, "Picosecond characteristics of a spectrograph measured by a streak camera/video readout system," *Opt. Comm.*, vol. 35, pp. 451-454, December 1980.

15. K. Iga, S. Ishikawa, S. Ohkouchi, and T. Nishimura, "Room temperature pulsed oscillation of GaAlAs/GaAs surface emitting junction laser," *IEEE J. Quantum Electron.*, vol. QE-21, pp. 663-668, June 1985.

16. J. N. Walpole and Z. L. Liau, "Monolithic two-dimensional arrays of high-power GaInAsP/InP surface-emitting diode lasers," *Appl. Phys. Lett.*, vol. 48, pp. 1636-1638, 16 June 1986.

17. G. A. Evans, J. M. Hammer, N. W. Carlson, F. R. Elia, E. A. James, and J. B. Kirk, "Surface-emitting second order distributed Bragg reflector laser with dynamic wavelength stabilization and far-field angle of $0.25°$," *Appl. Phys. Lett*, vol. 49, pp. 314-315, 11 August 1986.

Invited Paper

Laser-patterned desorption of GaAs in an inverted metalorganic chemical vapor deposition reactor

J. E. Epler, D. W. Treat, H. F. Chung, and T. L. Paoli

Xerox Palo Alto Research Center
3333 Coyote Hill Rd. Palo Alto, CA 94304

ABSTRACT

A new laser-assisted processing technique for thinning or removing GaAs and AlGaAs quantum well (QW) layers during epitaxial growth is demonstrated. In the particular application reported here, epitaxial growth of an optoelectronic device structure is interrupted while the QW active layer is locally heated with superimposed Ar+ and Nd:YAG laser beams. The evaporation rate of the GaAs or AlGaAs is greatly increased by the optically induced heating, resulting in a local thinning of the QW. After exposure, epitaxial growth is resumed, burying the patterned QW within the crystal. Transmission electron microscopy and photoluminescence are used to characterize the spatial variation of the energy bandgap. Broad area and high power laser diodes are fabricated from the modified region of the wafer. As expected, the wavelength of operation varies from laser to laser, consistent with the spatial variation in the energy bandgap.

1. INTRODUCTION

The development of laser-assisted semiconductor processing has resulted in a wide range of patterning techniques[1-4]. Most of these processes can be used either in a crystal growth chamber or in an auxiliary chamber connected by a loadlock to the growth chamber. In such a system, epitaxial growth can be interrupted, processing can be done on selected layers of a structure, and growth resumed without exposing the sample to a contaminating ambient. An important goal of in situ laser assisted processing is to perform all the major patterning steps of device processing within the reactor itself (or in the subsidiary chamber). This "clean-room in a reactor" concept has several advantages over standard assembly line techniques. Firstly, true three dimensional device structures unattainable by standard etch and regrowth can be constructed. As described below, three dimensional patterning enables new forms of optoelectronic devices. Secondly, the reactor environment is far less contaminating than even the most advanced clean room. The elimination of oxygen, acid and solvent exposure (and the reduction in operator handling) increases the yield and reliability of device fabrication. Thirdly, there are inherent economic advantages of an integrated growth/processing system. By automating and combining the various patterning steps, one can reduce the number of man-hours required for device fabrication.

One of the most important and applicable patterning processes is the laser patterned etching of a semiconductor layer. Typically this is accomplished using either a halogen bearing gas[5-7] or an aqueous etchant[8]. In the case of a gaseous ambient, which is more appropriate for in situ processing, the laser may serve to dissociate either the gas phase or adsorbed etchant. In addition, photogenerated electron-hole pairs and thermal energy often play a central role in accelerating the etching process. The complexity of the process is one of several factors that hinders the application of laser assisted etching in commercial production. Another difficulty is that the gaseous etchants pose a contamination hazard to ultra clean crystal growth reactors. For example, Cl bearing gases react in a polymerization process with metalorganic (MO) gases to yield complex organic molecules. Also, residual etchants on the substrate surface may complicate regrowth over the patterned layer.

In this paper we describe a laser patterned etching process that requires no etchants or reactor-incompatible ambient gases. In this technique, an intense laser beam is used to thermally etch GaAs by locally increasing the evaporation rate. Selected areas of GaAs quantum wells (QW) are thinned within the ultraclean environment of the metal-organic chemical vapor deposition (MOCVD) reactor. This laser patterned desorption (LPD) process could also be applied to MBE, vapor phase epitaxy, or any growth technique that has a transparent ambient. At present, LPD is limited to a relatively slow evaporation rate to prevent the thermal creation of defects in the material. Consequently it is presently practised only on a quantum layer scale. However, quantum layers are of great importance in advanced optoelectronic devices and many applications for this technique are possible. In this work, we use LPD to locally etch the QW active layer within a GaAs-AlGaAs laser structure. Consistent with the quantum size effect[12], the thinned QW results in a spatially patterned energy bandgap of the crystal. Broad area and high power laser diodes fabricated from the wafers exhibit emission wavelengths that vary with location on a diode bar. Also discussed is a four-element, four-wavelength bar of high power lasers diodes that is a prototype wavelength-multiplexing communication source.

2. MATERIALS GROWTH AND CHARACTERIZATION

The GaAs-AlGaAs heterostructures described in this work are grown by MOCVD in an inverted chimney chamber operated at atmospheric pressure as described previously[9,10]. This reactor has consistently produced high quality device material with good uniformity and excellent surface morphology. A schematic of the laser-assisted growth chamber is shown in Fig. 1. The 40 mm diameter GaAs substrate faces downward and is held against the lip of the quartz cup holder by the weight of the graphite susceptor. The susceptor is inductively heated with an external RF coil. Dual gas inlets are located near the bottom of the all-quartz tube and the gases are exhausted out of the top. The bottom of the reactor chamber is a quartz window through which the cw Ar+ and Nd:YAG laser beams are introduced. The inverted design is used primarily to avoid the wall deposits that normally inhibit optical access. For the data described herein, the Ar+ laser is operated in the TEM_{00} mode, single line at 514.5 nm with a power output of 2.4 W. The Nd:YAG beam is multi-mode with a 5.0 W output. The lasers are aligned to coincide on the surface of the sample to provide maximum increase in the surface temperature. Similar effects have been observed (although not yet fully characterized) using only the Nd:YAG laser and will be presented elsewhere. We believe that LPD is a purely thermal process and the experimental results are not attributed to the combination of visible and infrared radiation.

2.1. Experimental procedure

The epitaxial layers are grown at the optimum temperature of 800 °C and include (in order of growth) a Se-doped GaAs buffer layer (0.3 μm), a Se-doped $Al_{0.8}Ga_{0.2}As$ lower confining layer (1.0 μm), an undoped $Al_{0.4}Ga_{0.6}As$ waveguide layer (0.6 μm), and a GaAs quantum-well (13.6 nm). At this point in the growth, the metalorganic sources are vented and a 1% arsine/hydrogen mixture is introduced into the chamber. The substrate temperature is increased to 825 °C and the combined laser beams are applied to the surface. The laser spot is slightly "vibrated" by the galvanometer-controlled turning mirror to spatially average any nonuniformity in the optical intensity. For 90 s, GaAs is desorbed from the surface at a greatly enhanced rate within the laser heated spot. We estimate a temperature rise of 200 °C (to ~1030 °C) based upon the published data of Kojima, et al[11]. The data of Ref. 11 was obtained in a molecular beam epitaxy chamber with an impinging arsenic flux. Since the presence of the gaseous ambient will affect the evaporation rate, we are conducting experiments to determine independently the spot temperature. Neglible thinning of the QW occurs in the field outside of the laser heated region during this time. After the desired desorption is completed, the substrate temperature is returned to 800 °C and the growth is resumed. The remaining layers are another $Al_{0.4}Ga_{0.6}As$ waveguide layer (0.6 μm), a Mg-doped $Al_{0.8}Ga_{0.2}As$ upper confining layer (0.9 μm), and a Mg-doped GaAs cap layer.

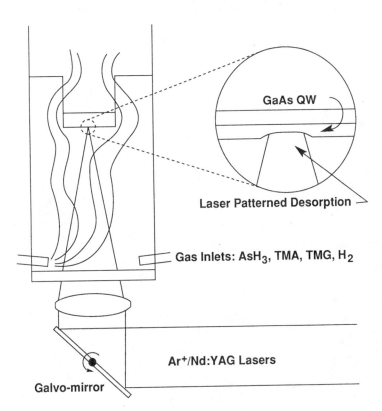

Fig. 1. Schematic representation of the upflow chimney reactor with an in situ Ar+ laser beam. The upward flow of the gas mixture prevents wall deposits on the bottom half of the tube. The laser beam is scanned with the galvanometer-controlled turning mirror.

2.2. Materials characterization

The direct measurement of the thickness of the QW layer requires the resolution of transmission electron microscopy (TEM). To obtain a series of images as shown in Fig. 2, the sample is carefully profiled with photoluminescence (PL) and is cleaved at four parallel planes through the laser spot center. Each rectangular section is further cleaved to yield a chip with a clean corner. Then, corner incidence[13] TEM is used to image the waveguide regions. These cross sections provide an accurate determination of the thickness of the crystal layers. The corner of each of the four samples is towards the right, practically coincident with the edge of the image. As discussed in Ref. 13, the vertical bands in the micrograph are the Fresnel fringes formed by the transmitted electrons. In Fig. 2(a), near the center of the laser spot, the GaAs QW has been thinned to 7.4 nm during the 90 s exposure. At this location in the beam profile, 6.2 nm of GaAs has been desorbed at a rate of 1 monolayer per 4 s. During the evaporation the products are carried away from the heated area by the flowing arsine/hydrogen ambient. The arsine provides an effective arsenic overpressure to prevent the formation of Ga droplets. Presumably consistent with the thermal profile, the QW thickness is decreased to (b) 8.5 nm at 0.7 mm from spot center, (c) 11.3 nm at a distance of 1.3 mm. Relatively far from the heated region in (d), the QW thickness is 13.6 nm. This thickness is representative of the region unilluminated by the lasers. The absence of any disruption at the GaAs-AlGaAs interfaces is one indication that the desorption process has not damaged the crystal. Note that the TEM magnification is nearly constant between micrographs so that the apparent increase in waveguide size is mainly a result of the thicker QW.

Thinning of the QW's as shown in Fig. 2(a), 2(b) and 2(c) substantially increases the electron and hole energy levels because of the well-known quantum size effect[12]. As a result, the energy bandgap of the crystal is locally increased. We spatially profile the energy bandgap through the laser desorbed area with low level, room temperature PL. The sample is excited over a 3-mm spot by a 150 mW stationary Ar+ laser beam. The resulting luminescence is profiled with high spatial resolution by adjusting the optical setup to collect light only over a region with 100-µm diameter. The wafer is translated relative to the laser beam to access different areas.

In Fig. 3, spectra from four positions along the LPD region of the wafer are shown. Fig. 3(a) is the spectrum obtained near the center of the laser spot. The emission maximum at 792 nm approximately corresponds to the 7.4 nm GaAs QW of Fig. 2(a). Fig. 3(b) and 3(c), drawn with a lighter line, are 0.9 and 1.1 mm from the spot center and exhibit peaks at 805 and 819 nm, respectively. Although these spectra correspond to the region where the thickness of the QW is graded, the PL intensities are fairly constant and do not indicate any degradation of crystal quality. In Fig. 3(d), the PL spectrum of the field (5 mm from the laser spot) is shown. The emission peak of 832 nm corresponds to the QW thickness of 13.6 nm. The exhibited range in the energy bandgap (~80 meV) is routinely obtainable with this process. As more extensive studies are made this type of data can be used to accurately determine the QW size from the measured PL peak.

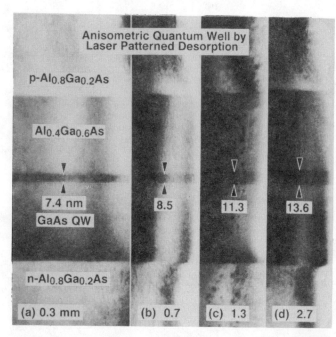

Fig. 2. The transmission electron microscope image taken at four positions along the laser desorbed region of the sample. The quantum well thickness and distance from the spot center are respectively: (a) 7.4 nm, 0.3 mm; (b) 8.5 nm, 0.7 mm; (c) 11.3 nm, 1.3 mm; and (d) 13.6 nm, 2.7 mm. The desorption has occured at a maximum rate of 1 monolayer per 4 s.

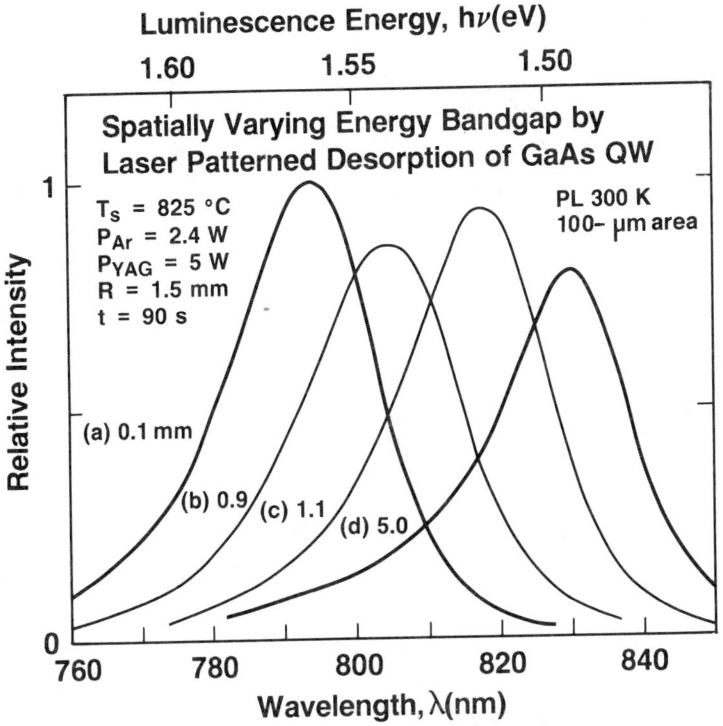

Fig. 3. The photoluminescence spectra taken at four positions along the laser patterned wafer. The emission maxima and the distance from the spot center are respectively: (a) 792 nm, 0.1 mm; (b) 805 nm, 0.9 mm; (c) 819 nm, 1.1 mm; and (d) 831 nm, 5.0 mm. The reasonably constant amplitude of the luminescence is a good indication that no significant crystal damage is introduced by the laser patterned desorption process.

3. DEVICE FABRICATION

3.1. Broad area lasers

To demonstrate the quality of the LPD material for device, the wafer is processed in standard fashion into broad area laser bars. The bars are ~1 cm long with shallow saw cuts to electrically isolate neighboring devices. Each individual broad area laser on the bar is 250 µm long and 250 µm wide. The threshold current and emission wavelength as a function of position on the bar are shown in Fig. 4. Data points are drawn for every other laser diode. Including the data points not shown, several individually addressable wavelengths can be obtained from each half of the bar. Consistent with the PL data, the emission wavelength varies from 792 nm in the center of the laser spot to 830 nm in the field, with the graded regions lasing at intermediate wavelengths. The threshold current density varies from 500 A/cm^2 in the field to 480 A/cm^2 in the center of the laser spot. The threshold current density is lowest at the laser spot center because the 13.6 nm QW in the field is thicker than optimum. In fact, this type of data is very useful when studying the variation of threshold current with QW thickness. The 480 A/cm^2 is still rather high for a GaAs QW laser but the structure and growth conditions are not yet optimized for low threshold current density. Approximately four bars are obtained from each wafer and all exhibit consistent characteristics. As the bar position moves further than 1 mm from the laser spot center, however, the total wavelength shift decreases sharply. The L-I curves (not shown) are very similar to normal broad area devices and do not exhibit any unusual features. The differential efficiency varies from wafer to wafer but 50% is a representative value.

The emission spectra exhibited by four of the devices from one bar are shown in Fig. 5. The injection current for each device is 300 mA (pulsed) and only every other longitudinal mode is drawn to simplify the drafting of the figure. Also, the data has been scaled to give an approximately constant amplitude. The devices in Fig. 5(a) and Fig. 5(d) operate with a single set of longitudinal modes across the device. However, lasers fabricated from the regions with graded QW's show a greater tendency to operate with two sets of modes with different center wavelengths. The spatial variation of the wavelength shift within a broad area device corresponds to the gradient in energy bandgap. (For the spectral measurements one set of modes is spatially filtered since the device junction is oriented perpendicular to the slits of the spectrometer.) For commercial applications this characteristic would be eliminated partly by the formation of more localized stripes and/or by "terracing" the intensity of the laser beam to reduce the gradient within a device. In any case, the wide spectral separation of the individually addressable lasers suggests the potential application of these devices as wavelength multiplexed communication sources.

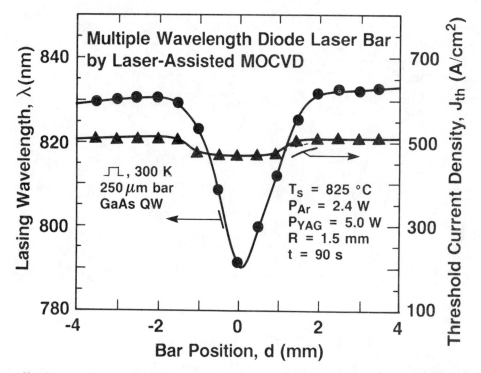

Fig. 4. The lasing wavelength and threshold current density as a function of position along the wafer. The decrease in the lasing wavelength corresponds to the thinning of the quantum well. The devices from the graded region of the wafer commonly display more than one set of longitudinal modes.

We have also patterned the active layers of wafers with AlGaAs QW's. The experimental conditions are similar to that described above, except that an $Al_xGa_{1-x}As$ (x~0.12) QW is grown and desorbed for 85 s. As one might expect, the desorption proceeds at a slower rate for Al containing alloys because of the more refractory nature of AlAs. In Fig. 6 the emission wavelength and threshold current are given for a single QW bar of broad area lasers. Once again the wavelength shift is consistent with a thinned QW, but in this case the shift in energy bandgap, 40 meV, is less even though the conditions for laser exposure are similar. We estimate that the initial QW thickness is approximately 9 nm. Based upon the broad area results from numerous similar short wavelength structures, it is reasonable to conclude that the increase in threshold current is due to the overly thin (~6 nm) QW near the laser spot center and the expected difficulty of approaching the short wavelength limit of the GaAs-AlGaAs system. Thus, the threshold current densities are still quite good given the operating wavelength and are consistent with a generally high crystal quality.

3.2. Multiple wavelength SuperArray.

A more useful form of laser diode is the high power gain-guided array[13] in which proton bombardment[14] is used to pattern the current injection into the active region. Typically ten stripes on 10-μm centers provide a 500 mW output capability. By combining this form of device with a laser patterned wafer, we can monolithically fabricate a multiple wavelength

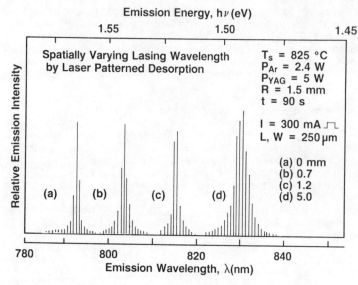

Fig. 5. The emission spectra of four broad area lasers along one bar. The drive current of each device is 300 mA (pulsed). The spectra have been scaled to correct for the varying threshold current.

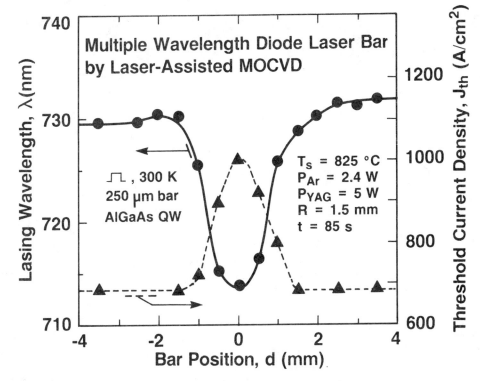

Fig. 6. The lasing wavelength and threshold current density as a function of position along the wafer with an AlGaAs quantum well. The decrease in the lasing wavelength is associated with the thinning of the quantum well. The increase in the threshold current is attributed to the overly thin quantum well.

array of arrays. A schematic of this SuperArray chip is depicted in Fig. 7. Each laser is 100-μm wide and contains ten array elements. The devices are on 500-μm centers and are individually addressable. Since they are attached to the copper heatsink junction side up, only pulsed operation is reported here.

In Fig. 8, the light versus current curves are shown for each device from one SuperArray chip. The differential efficiencies are ~35% and the maximum power output per wavelength is well over 200 mW (pulsed). The devices have a high reflection back facet coating and a half-wavelength Al_2O_3 coating on the front facet. Consistent with the data of Fig. 4, the device with the shortest wavelength (Fig. 8(a)) has the lowest threshold (90 mA). As the operating wavelength is increased from (a) 806 nm to (d) 835 nm, the threshold current increases to the field value of 120 mA. Considering the broad area threshold current density of ~500 A/cm^2, these characteristics compare favorably with commercially available 10-stripe laser arrays.

Emission spectra of the four lasers are shown in Fig. 9. Note that the four outputs are well separated spectrally and therefore could be used as independent channels in a free space communication link. Because the devices are gain-guided, there are multiple longitudinal modes present throughout the operating range of 0.1 to 1.7 A. Each laser is internally phase locked and exhibits a single symmetric spatial mode near threshold. As the current is increased, multiple array modes lase. These characteristics are all consistent with the expected behaviour of a gain-guided array.

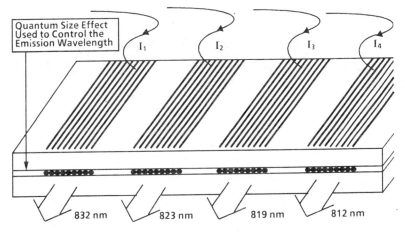

Fig. 7. A schematic depiction of a four-element multiple-wavelength SuperArray. The devices are individually addressable.

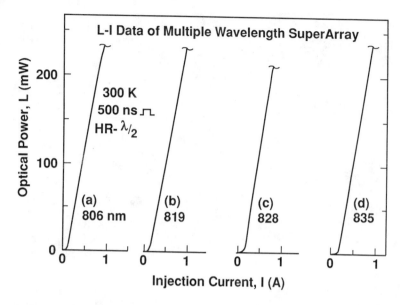

Fig. 8. Optical power versus injection current (L-I) of a four-wavelength. The devices are limited to pulsed operation because of the junction-side-up bonding.

Presently under study is the effect of the gradient in the QW thickness upon device performance, especially those devices lasing at intermediate wavelengths. The graded QW introduces an anisotropy in the physical characteristics within the array. For example, injected carriers will tend to move laterally to the region with the lowest energy bandgap. This shift in carrier population will result in an increased temperature rise on the long wavelength side and, accordingly, a variation in the index of refraction. Also, there is an inherent tendency for lasing to occur at slightly longer wavelengths on the side of the array where the QW is thickest. Spectrally resolved measurements of the near-field indicate that near threshold the array is well behaved and fully coupled. However, at injection currents greater than $1.5 \times I_{th}$, spatial modes that are localized at the long wavelength end of the array begin to lase. Because of the anisotropy in the temperature and gain profile, these modes are shifted to longer wavelength. Similarly, at even higher currents, localized short wavelength modes appear on the opposite edge of the array. Thus the coherence of the laser is degraded along with the quality of the far-field pattern. Several improvements are needed for a commercially acceptable device. These improvements could include reducing the width of the array to lessen the extent of the energy shift, terracing the laser intensity to reduce gradients within a device, adjusting the intensity to yield equal wavelength separations between each array on the chip, and implementing an index-guided structure to permit single mode operation at each of the four wavelengths.

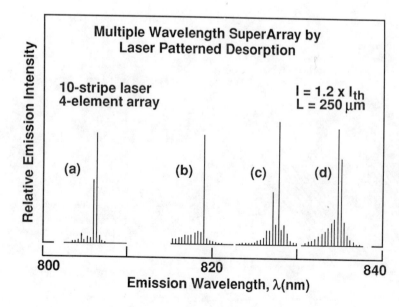

Fig. 9. Emission spectra of the SuperArray. The spectra are typical of a gain-guided 10-stripe laser.

4. CONCLUSIONS

In conclusion, a new in situ laser patterning technique is demonstrated that is capable of thinning QW layers within optoelectronic device structures. The technique is used to spatially modify the energy bandgap of the crystal in a controlled manner. Multiple-wavelength broad area laser bars and high power diode lasers are monolithically fabricated. The results do not indicate any compromise in crystal quality. Device applications for such a technique include the fabrication of multiple-wavelength lasers for wavelength multiplexed communications, continuously tunable spectroscopic sources, and unique forms of multiple-wavelength detectors. Future efforts will be directed at improving the general device performance and broadening the scope of applications.

5. ACKNOWLEDGEMENTS

The authors wish to thank G. Anderson and F. Ponce for the TEM micrographs and W. Mosby, R. Donaldson, S. Nelson, F. Endicott, and E. Taggart for technical assistance. Helpful discussions with N. Connell, R. Bringans, P. D. Dapkus and N. Holonyak, Jr. are gratefully acknowledged. This work is supported in part by the Defense Advanced Research Projects Agency (J. D. Murphy).

6. REFERENCES

1. R. M. Osgood, Jr., Ann. Rev. Phys. Chem. 34, 77 (1983).
2. D. J. Ehrlich, J. G. Black, M. Rothschild, and S. W. Pang, J. Vac. Sci. Technol. B 6 (3), 895 (1988).
3. F. Michelli and I. W. Boyd, Optics and Laser Tech. 18, 313 (1986). Part 2: ibid 19, 19 (1987). Part 3: ibid 19, 75 (1987).
4. F. A. Houle, SPIE Vol. 459 "Laser Assisted Deposition, Etching, and Doping", 110 (1984).
5. D. J. Ehrlich, R. M. Osgood, Jr., and T. F. Deutsch, IEEE Journ. Quantum Electron. QE-16, 1233 (1980).
6. A. W. Tucker and M. Birnbaum, IEEE Electron Device Letters, EDL-4, 39 (1983).
7. M. Takai, J. Tokuda, H. Nakai, K. Gamo, and S. Namba, Mat. Res. Soc. Symp. Proc. 29, 211 (1984).
8. D. J. Ehrlich, R. M. Osgood, Jr., and T. F. Deutsch, Appl. Phys. Lett. 38, 1018 (1981).
9. J. E. Epler, H. F. Chung, D. W. Treat, and T. L. Paoli, Appl. Phys. Lett. 52, 1499 (1988).
10. J. E. Epler, D. W. Treat, H. F. Chung, T. Tjoe, and T. L. Paoli. "In situ laser patterned desorption of GaAs quantum wells for monolithic multiple wave-length diode lasers", Appl. Phys. Lett. 54, to be published March 1989.
11. T. Kojima, N. J. Kawai, T. Nakagawa, K. Ohta, T. Sakamoto, and M. Kawashima, Appl. Phys. Lett. 47, 286 (1985).
12. J. R. Schrieffer, Phys. Rev. 97, 641 (1955). For a discussion of quantum well lasers see: N. Holonyak, Jr., R. M. Kolbas, R. D. Dupuis, and P. D. Dapkus, IEEE J. Quantum Electron. QE-16, 170 (1980).
13. R. D. Burnham, D. R. Scifres, and W. Streifer, Appl. Phys, Lett. 41, 228 (1982).
14. J. C. Dyment, J. C. North, and L. A. D'Asaro, J. Appl. Phys. 44, 207 (1973).

MONOLITHICALLY INTEGRATED TWO-DIMENSIONAL ARRAYS OF OPTOELECTRONIC THRESHOLD DEVICES FOR NEURAL NETWORK APPLICATIONS

J. H. Kim, S. H. Lin*, J. Katz, and D. Psaltis*

Jet Propulsion Laboratory, Photonic Devices Group
California Institute of Technology, Pasadena, CA 91109

* Department of Electrical Engineering, California Institute of Technology, Pasadena, CA 91125

ABSTRACT

We report on the design, fabrication, and testing of a 10x10 monolithic integrated two-dimensional array of AlGaAs optoelectronic threshold elements (optical neurons) for neural network applications. The array has dimensions of 5x5 mm^2 and the neuron has dimensions of 250x250 μm^2. Each neuron consists of a light emitting diode (LED) driven by a double-heterojunction bipolar transistor, which is driven by the output of a double-heterojunction phototransistor. We demonstrated the partial functional operation of 2-D array of optical neurons by independently characterizing each device on the integrated circuit. DC current gain of 30 was obtained at the collector current density of 1.0×10^3 A-cm^{-2} with the emitter area of 3.5×10^{-5} cm^2 in a single transistor without spacer layers. The output power densities of the light emitting diodes were about 1.0×10^2 W-cm^{-2} at a current of 20 mA. However, the overall integrated structure showed the semiconductor controlled rectifier characteristics with the breakover voltage of 75 V, the holding current of 10 mA at the holding voltage of 25 V, and the reverse breakdown voltage of 60 V. This is attributed to the parasitic p-n-p transistor that exists due to the sharing of the same n-AlGaAs collector between the transistors and LED.

1. INTRODUCTION

The optical implementation of computing systems, whose structure and function are motivated by natural intelligence system, would be a unique way to optical computing and neural network models for computation. Electronic interconnects are becoming the bottleneck in the realization of neural networks and other globally interconnected systems. The heat dissipation and interconnection delay are also serious design performance limiting factors. One possible solution is to use free space optical interconnects as implemented, for example, in volume holograms recorded in photorefractive crystals. With optics it is possible to have large arrays of processing elements communicating with one another without wire interconnections.

The optical implementation of a neural network consists of two basic components: neurons and interconnections. The neuron is an optical nonlinear processing element (e.g. , threshold unit) that can be implemented by a single switching device. The practical neural computer may require millions of neurons operating in parallel. Each neuron accepts inputs from other neurons and produces a single output that is connected to many other neurons, typically several thousands. Hence the number of interconnections in a network is much larger than the number of neurons. While this massive connectivity is relatively difficult to achieve electronically, optics is practically suitable for realization of interconnects. This fact provides the main motivation for considering optical implementation of neural networks.

Several emerging optical technologies have been considered for the realization of neural networks: spatial light modulators (SLMs), integrated optoelectronics, and arrays of nonlinear optical switches. SLMs have been investigated primarily for optical image processing. However, practically useful devices are not yet available except for laboratory experiments. The arrays of nonlinear optical switches are intended either for optical communications or digital optical computing. The major problem with these arrays is the high power required to switch each element and the sensitivity of their operation parameters to environmental conditions. One of the most promising implementation technology may be optoelectronics [1, 2]. The optoelectronic approach to simulating an array of neurons involves monolithic integration of two-dimensional (2-D) arrays of photodetectors and light sources on a single chip. The output of each detector is connected to the corresponding light source via a saturating amplifier or an appropriate analog circuit that performs the required nonlinear mapping. The only electrical connection would be the power and the global bias to optoelectronic integrated circuits (OEICs).

We have developed optoelectronic threshold elements (optical neurons) by using optoelectronic integrated circuits (OEICs). In this paper, we first report on a 10x10 monolithic integrated 2-D array of optical neurons. In the future, the fabricated 2-D arrays will be utilized to demonstrate basic neural network operation (e.g., flip-flops and associative memories) in conjunction with the volume holographic optical element (VHOE), which specifies free-space interconnects between the optical neurons as shown in Fig. 1.

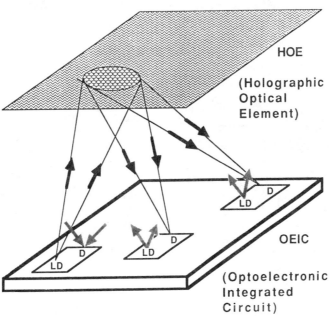

Figure 1.   Schematic free space optical interconnects implemented through holographic optical elements.

2. OPTOELECTRONIC THRESHOLD ELEMENTS ('OPTICAL NEURONS')

Each optical neuron consists of a light emitting diode (LED) driven by a double heterojunction bipolar transistor (DHBT), which is in turn driven by the output of a double heterojunction phototransistor (DHPT). The feasibility of this integrated structure has been demonstrated by Katz et al. [3], who integrated a DHBT and an injection laser on a single GaAs substrate. Fig. 2(a) shows the fabricated 10x10 2-D array of optical neurons. The array has dimensions of 5x5 mm^2 and each neuron has dimensions of 250x250 µm^2. The light-emitting area of the LED has dimensions of 8x8 µm^2. The light-detecting area of the DHPT has dimensions of 50x130 µm^2. Fig. 2(b) shows the internal organization of each neuron array. The neurons labeled with the same character are connected in parallel in the same group whereas the neurons labeled with different characters are electrically independent from one another. Blank neurons are not connected in order to eliminate the undesired signals generated due to the shift-invariant property of the hologram.

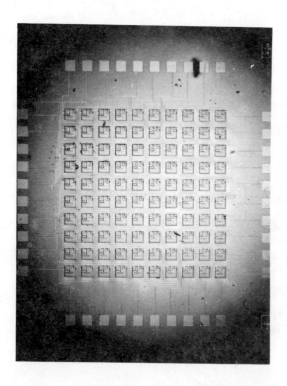

A		A		C	C	B			B
	A		A	C	C		B	B	
A		A		D	D	B			B
	A		A	D	D		B	B	
E		E		E		E	L	L	
E		E		E		E	L	L	N
F			F			F	K	K	M
G		G		G		G	K	K	
H			H			H	J	J	J
I		I		I		I	J	J	J

(A) (B)

Figure 2. Two-dimensional optical neurons: (a) 10x10 fabricated array; (b) internal organization of each neuron array.

3. FABRICATION OF OPTOELECTRONIC THRESHOLD ELEMENTS

Several 10x10 2-D arrays of optical neurons have been fabricated on GaAs substrates as shown in Fig. 2(a). The single optical neuron and its equivalent circuit are shown in Fig. 3(a) and (b), respectively. The cross-sectional structure of each neuron is shown in Fig. 4. Double heterojunction (DH) structures were epitaxially grown on (100) Cr-doped semi-insulating GaAs substrates ($\approx 5 \times 10^7$ Ω-cm) by both metalorganic chemical vapor deposition (MOCVD) and molecular beam epitaxy (MBE). For initial characterization of discrete devices, epitaxial layers grown by liquid phase epitaxy (LPE) were also utilized. According to doping profile measurements by a electro-chemical cell, DH layers consist of: Si-doped (2×10^{18} cm^{-3}) n-GaAs buffer layer, 0.5 µm; Si-doped (5×10^{16}-2×10^{17} cm^{-3}) n-Al$_{0.3}$Ga$_{0.7}$As collector (or lower cladding) layer 1.0-1.5 µm; undoped GaAs spacer layer, 100 Å; Zn-doped (2×10^{17}-10^{19} cm^{-3}) p-GaAs base (or active) layer, 0.1-0.3 µm; undoped GaAs spacer layer, 100 Å; Si-doped (5×10^{17} cm^{-3}) n-Al$_{0.3}$Ga$_{0.7}$As emitter (or upper cladding) layer, 1.0 µm; and Si-doped (2×10^{18} cm^{-3}) n-GaAs cap layer, 0.2 µm.

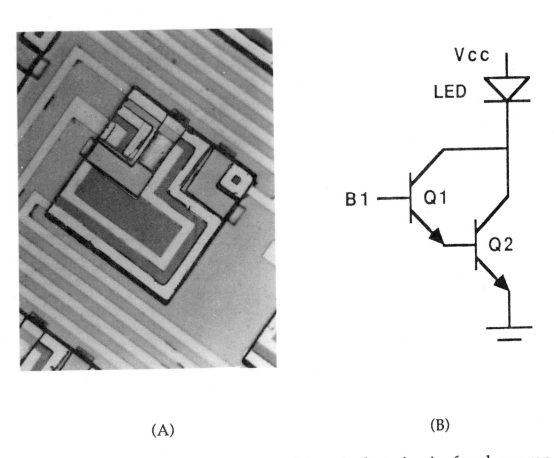

(A) (B)

Figure 3. (a) Single optical neuron; (b) equivalent circuit of each neuron.

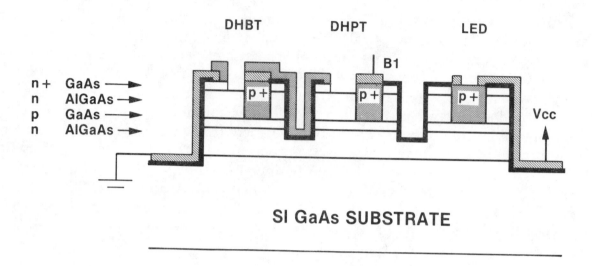

Figure. 4 Cross-sectional structure of each neuron.

The thickness of the base layer is designed as a compromise between high current gain for the transports and adequate photoresponse of the phototransistor. In structures fabricated with two-steps of epitaxial growth, these parameters could be separately optimized. Since the emitter injection efficiency is enhanced by the large band gap discontinuities which effectively block the injection of carriers into the emitter, the current gain is independent of the doping ratio of the emitter and base layers. Therefore, the emitter can be lightly doped to reduce the emitter-base junction capacitance and the base can be heavily doped to minimize the spreading resistance and contact resistance of the base layer. This reduces the amount of crowding and effectively eliminates possible punch-through at the reverse-biased collector-base junction. The collector buffer layer may be heavily doped so that the collector resistance can be reduced without affecting device performance.

The array fabrication procedure is as follows. Following the standard post-growth wafer cleaning procedure, the first nonselective etching of GaAs/AlGaAs DH layer into the semi-insulating GaAs substrate was performed for isolation between the individual neuron cells. The etching solution of $H_3PO_4:H_2O_2:CH_3COOH$ was used to minimize undercut. (The maximum undercut allowance is 5 μm in our design). The second nonselective chemical etching was performed for device isolation between DHBT, DHPT, and LED in each neuron. The wafer was aligned to the etching mask along the [0$\bar{1}$1] direction to get the required mesa structure for subsequent step coverage of metalization. Following the etching steps, a 1500 Å silicon nitride layer was deposited at 680°C by thermal chemical vapor deposition system, and then the regions to be Zn-diffused were opened by plasma etching of Si_3N_4. Zinc was diffused selectively at 650°C for 45 min down the p-GaAs base layer using $ZnAs_2$ source by the standard sealed ampoule technique. The photosensitive areas of DHPTs were then opened by plasma etching of a Si_3N_4 layer. Cr/Au were evaporated for p-type ohmic contact and interconnection lines. For n-type ohmic contact, Au-Ge/Au were deposited and alloyed at 380°C. The initial on-chip device characterization was performed on the probe station.

4. RESULTS AND DISCUSSIONS

We fabricated 2-D array of 10x10 monolithic integrated optoelectronic threshold elements (optical neurons) for neural network applications. Discrete devices in neuron were independently tested. DC current gain of 30 has been obtained in a double heterojunction bipolar transistor (DHBT) grown by LPE as shown in Fig. 5(a). The collector current density was 1.0×10^3 A-cm^{-2} and the emitter area was 3.5×10^{-5} cm^2. However, most of DHBTs grown by MBE had a lower gain (as shown in Fig. 5(b). The main reasons for the low gain may be attributed to: (1) displacement of the emitter-base junction from the AlGaAs/GaAs heterointerface due to Be (or Zn) out-diffusion during growth and subsequent high temperature device processing (e. g. , selective zinc diffusion at 650°C); (2) leakage currents through the p^+-n heterojunction of DHBT. This leakage current may be reduced by optimizing the Zn-diffusion process; (3) unoptimized device parameters (e. g. , thickness and doping concentration of the base layer); (4) no spacer layers in LPE-grown DHBTs between the emitter and the base layers and between the base and the collector layers. The double-heterojunction phototransistor (DHPT) responded to light signal even without removing the GaAs cap layer. The power densities of light emitting diodes were about 1.0×10^2 W-cm^{-2} at a current of 20 mA. Figure 6 shows LED light emitted from the neurons in the "J"-group (see Fig. 2b).

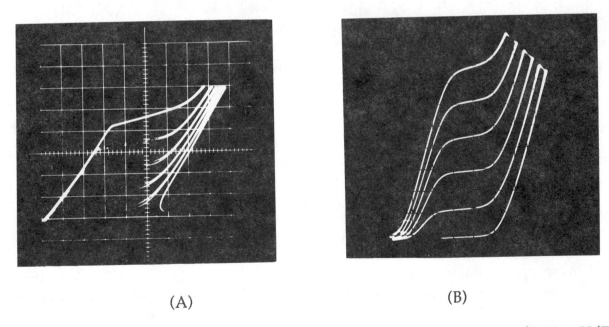

(A) (B)

Figure 5. Current-voltage characteristics of: (a) LPE-grown DHBT at 5 mA/DIV, 1 V/DIV, and 0. 2 mA/STEP; (b) MBE-grown DHBT at 0. 1 mA/DIV, 0. 2 V/DIV and 0. 2 mA/STEP.

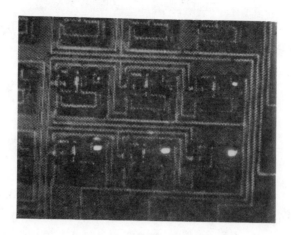

Figure 6.   LED light emitted from the neurons in the "J"-group.

The doping profile is very sensitive to the growth temperature. In particular, the inevitable Be or Zn out-diffusion during growth may shift the emitter-base junction into the AlGaAs layer. Therefore, the growth temperature should be chosen to optimize the tradeoff between prevention of the junction shift and high epitaxial layer quality. The spacer layer with optimized thickness would solve this problem by properly placing the emitter-base junction at the heterointerface. In addition, zinc-diffusion front should be controlled so that it would be located within the AlGaAs collector layer. Since the built-in potential of an AlGaAs homojunction is larger than that of an AlGaAs/GaAs heterojunction, the leakage current through the p^+-n homojunction is expected to be smaller than that through the p^+-n heterojunction.

When the integrated structure was tested, p-n-p-n characteristics were observed. The forward breakdown voltage was 75 V with the holding voltage and current at 25 V and 10 mA, respectively. The reverse breakdown voltage was observed at 60 V. The I-V characteristics are shown in Fig. 7(a). By increasing the base current (either electrically or by light illumination), the forward breakdown voltage decreased gradually from 75 V and eventually diminished showing a typical diode characteristics. This device also responded to light very sensitively in the same way as applying the base current. This is manifested in Fig. 7(b), in which the breakover voltage was reduced to 35 V when the p-n-p-n was subjected to external light illumination. Light was emitted from the device in the forward breakdown mode, implying the carriers were recombining in the low bandgap GaAs layer.

Careful inspection of the integrated LED with Darlington transistor pair revealed that the SCR was present in the device due to the parasitic p-n-p transistor, which was coupled to the n-p-n DHBT in the same way that a p-n-p and an n-p-n transistors were coupled in the SCR. The anode was the Zn-diffused area in the original LED region, while the cathode was the original emitter (ground). Darlington transistor pair were effectively shorted so that the phototransistor practically played no role in the SCR switching behavior because its base-emitte junction was shorted. When the SCR switched in the forward mode, the sum of the common base gain of each transistor in the SCR equaled to one ($\alpha_{npn}+\alpha_{pnp}=1$), causing the originally reverse-biased n-p junction to become forward-biased. This occurred at 75 V, suggesting a high breakdown voltage for this originally reverse-biased n-p junction, thus a quite lightly doped collector. The parasitic p-n-p transistor existed because the LED and the transistor pair shared the same collector layer. Since the p-n-p transistor has an effective base layer width of at least the separation between the LED and the DHPT, which is 20 µm, extremely low gain should have been expected for this parasitic p-n-p transistor, implying a very small value of α_{pnp}. This parasitic p-n-p transistor will be eliminated in future devices by isolating all the devices electrically and then employing metalization to connect them as required. An alternative may be to degrade the gain of the parasitic p-n-p transistor by separating the LED and the Darlington transistor pair farther apart. However, the latter approach may require a rather large chip area which is not suitable for large arrays.

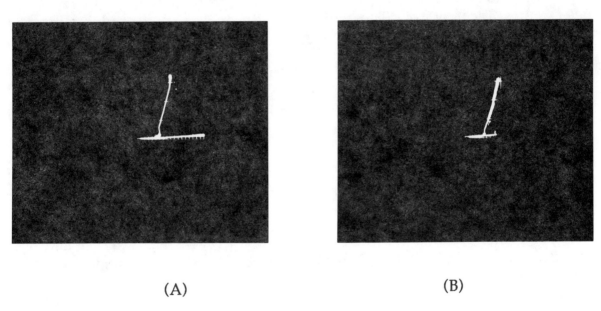

(A)　　　　　　　　　　　　　　(B)

Figure 7.　Current-voltage characteristics of the overall integrated structure: (a) without light; (b) with light, both at 5 mA/DIV, 20 V/DIV, and no base current.

5. SUMMARY AND CONCLUSIONS

We have developed optoelectronic integrated circuits (OEIC) implementing two-dimensional array of optical neurons for neural network applications. Each neuron consists of a phototransistor, a saturating amplifier, and a light source (LED), with each device independently characterized and its functional operation demonstrated. However, when the integrated structure was tested, the Darlington transistor pair was coupled to the LED by the parasitic p-n-p transistor. As a result, SCR characteristics were obtained. (This mode of operation may be useful for optical switching because of the infinite gain of a switching compared with the finite gain of Darlington pair transistors). In future OEIC, the parasitic transistor will be eliminated by electrically isolating all devices in the neuron. The complete device will be utilized in an experimental setup in which the neurons are interconnected through free space via holographic optical elements, thus serving as building blocks in more compact realizations of optical neural computation. The work on the complete optical implementation is under current investigation and will be reported elsewhere.

ACKNOWLEDGMENT

The work described in this paper was carried out by the Jet Propulsion Laboratory, California Institute of Technology, and was jointly sponsored by the Defense Advanced Research Project Agency, and the Strategic Defense Initiative Organization, Innovative Science and Technology Center through an agreement with the National Aeronautics and Space Administration. This work was performed as part of the JPL Center for Space Microelectronics Technology. The work at Caltech was sponsored by the Defense Advanced Research Project Agency.

REFERENCES

[1] D. Psaltis, "Optical Realizations of Neural Network Models," Proc. of IEEE FJCC conference, Dallas, Texas, Nov. 1986.

[2] D. Psaltis and N. Farhat, "Optical Information Processing Based on an Associative Memory Model of Neural Nets with Thresholding and Feedback," Opt. Lett., 10, 98, 1985.

[3] J. Katz, N. Bar-Chaim, P. C. Chen, S. Margalit, I. Ury, D. Wilt, M. Yust, and A. Yariv, "A Monolithic Integration of GaAs/AlGaAs Bipolar Transistor and Heterostructure Laser," Appl. Phys. Lett. 37, 211, 1980.

LASER DIODE TECHNOLOGY AND APPLICATIONS

Volume 1043

SESSION 2

High Power Semiconductor Lasers

Chair
Dan Botez
TRW Space and Technology Group

Invited Paper

High Power Single Mode Laser Diodes

David F. Welch, W. Streifer, D. R. Scifres
Spectra Diode Laboratories
80 Rose Orchard way, San Jose, Ca 95134

Many of the growing number of applications of laser diodes are demanding high power diffraction limited sources. For such applications real refractive index guided laser diodes have been used. For the past few years the highest power available commercially from an index guided single mode diode has been 30 mW cw. Recently several manufacturers have introduced single mode diode lasers which emit much higher powers rated reliably at 100 mW.

Single stripe diodes are designed to operate in the lowest transverse mode. Due to the stability of the refractive index step in semiconductor lasers the aperture size is limited to less than 5 um. As the diode is driven to higher powers the index step changes from localized thermal variations and charge variations in the active layer. The change in the index of refraction results in the diode operating in modes other than the fundamental transverse mode. Below this power level the lowest order transverse mode propagates emitting a single gaussian beam.

The maximum output power out of a laser diode is limited by catastrophic degradation and/or thermal dissipation. Laser diodes fabricated from GaInAsP are limited by thermal dissipation when operated under cw conditions[1]. GaAlAs diodes have historically been limited by catastrophic degradation of the mirror facet until recently where development of non-absorbing mirrors[2-4] has lead to higher catastrophic power levels. By raising the catastrophic damage level of the facets the cw output power of the diodes has become limited by thermal dissipation. Further increases in the total efficiency of AlGaAs laser diodes has reduced the thermal dissipation, and as a result even higher output powers have been achieved. The maximum output power from a GaInAsP index guided laser diode has been 200 mW[1] while that of GaAlAs index guided diodes have reached 500 mW.

Two of the possible degradation modes of laser diodes result from either optically induced damage at the facet or thermally induced recombination centers in the bulk. Optical facet damage as a function of time is related to the catastrophic damage threshold of the laser. The higher maximum output power the laser can operate at, the less susceptible the laser is to degradation of the facet. Typically, facet damage results in sudden failure of the diode when operated under constant output power conditions. Thermally induced degradation is a result of the total efficiency and the output power of the diode. Thermally limited operation of AlGaAs diodes occurs above 500 mW output while that for GaInAsP diodes have been reported at 200 mW. From these considerations, we believe that the reliability of AlGaAs diodes should be as good or better than that of GaInAsP laser diodes. As will be discussed below, the expected lifetime of AlGaAs diodes operated at 100 mW and 35°C is greater than 10,000 hrs., where a 50% increase in operating current is considered to be failure.

In figure 1 the characteristics of an index guided laser diode similar to the SDL-5410 is presented. The threshold current of the laser is 16 mA and the differential efficiency is 87%. With a series resistance of 2.5 ohms, the total power conversion efficiency is greater than 60%. This is the highest reported conversion of electrical to optical power for any optical system. The maximum output power from the 5 um aperture is 500 mW, the highest brightness for any laser diode reported.

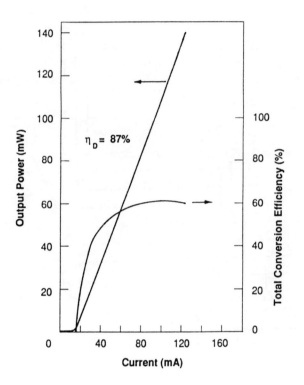
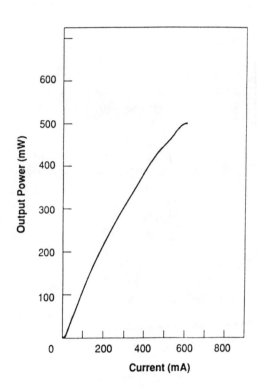

Figure 1
Light output as a function of input current
for a single stripe AlGaAs laser diode.

The spectral characteristics of the index guided laser diode are shown in figure 2. The diode radiates in the lowest transverse mode up to powers of 180 mW. The far field pattern is single lobed with divergence of 8° x 22° parallel and perpendicular to the p-n junction respectively. Single longitudinal behavior is also maintained over this operating range. Characteristic of this particular index guided laser is the large range over which longitudinal mode stability is maintained. The diode operates on a particular longitudinal mode over an operating range of 70 mW.

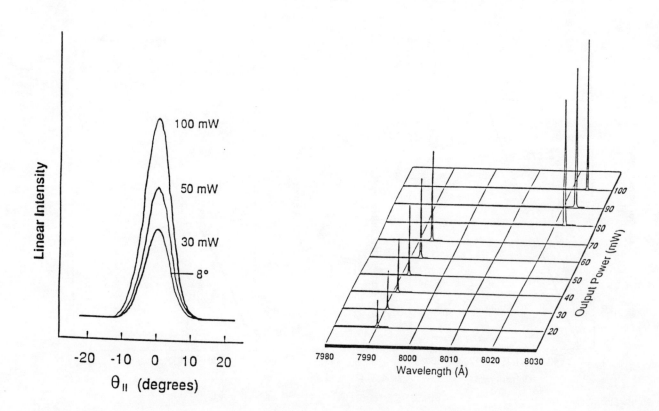

Figure 2
Transverse and longitudinal modal characteristics
of single stripe laser diode.

The linewidth of the longitudinal mode has been measured to be as narrow as 1.5 MHz at an output power of 50 mW[5], as shown in figure 3. The linewidth is linear with inverse power and does not show a linewidth floor, while the intercept at infinite power is 380 kHz.

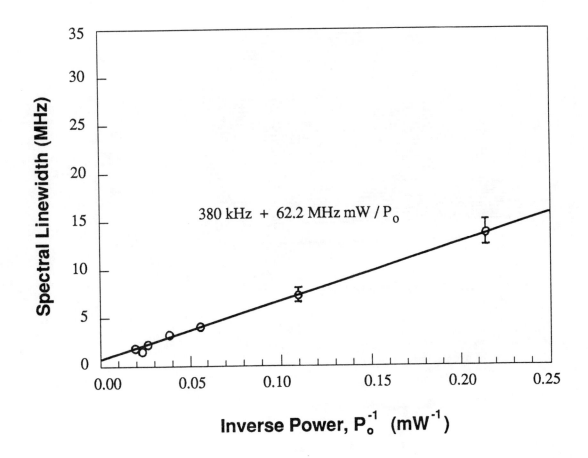

Figure 3
Spectral linewidth as a function of inverse output power for a single stripe laser diode.

Other characteristics include a RMS phase front error better than 1/20 of a wavelength (figure 4) as measured by interference in the far field with a controlled gaussian beam. The modulation response of the laser diode has also been measured, and is shown in figure 5. At an output power of 70 mW the 3dB bandwidth is greater than 4 GHz.

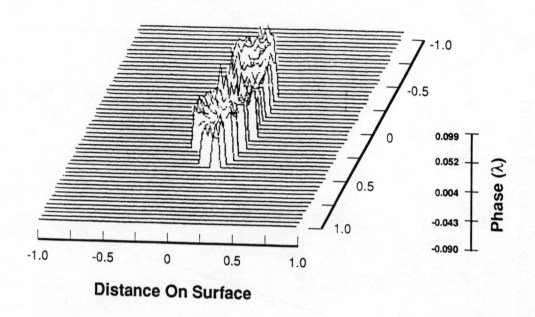

Figure 4
Phase error measurement of the far field
radiation pattern of a single stripe laser diode.

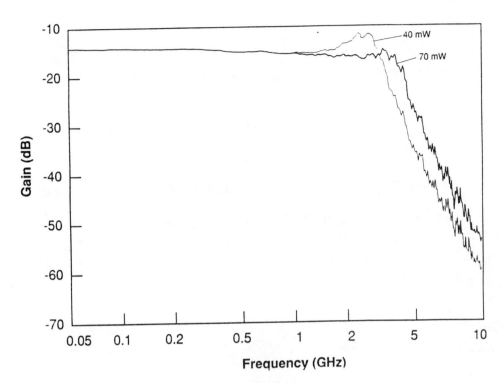

Figure 5
Frequency response of a single stripe laser diode operating at 40 and 70 mW.

In conclusion, AlGaAs single stripe index guided lasers have been fabricated which emit over 500 mW from a 4 um aperture, with a total conversion efficiency of greater than 60%. Single longitudinal and transverse mode output is maintained to 180 mW. The spectral linewidth has been measured to be as low as 1.5 MHz at 50 mW output. These sources are suited for applications which require diffraction limited optics such as space communications, optical recording, and fiber amplifiers.

The authors would like to acknowledge the asistance of T. Tally, P. Tally, M. Cardinal, O. Calderon, and S. Ogarrio from Spectra Diode Labs, R. D. Esman from the Naval Research Laboratories for the linewidth and modulation response measurements, and J. Abshire from NASA for the phase front measurements.

References

1) S. Oshiba, A Matoba, M. Kawahara, Y. Kawai, Journ. of Quant. Electr., QE-23(6), 738-743, 1987.

2) D. F. Welch, W. Streifer, R. Thornton, T. Paoli, Electr. Letts., 23(10), 525-526, 1987.

3) J. Ungar, N. Bar-Chaim, I. Ury, Electr. Lett., 22, 279-280, 1986.

4) H. Nakashima, S. Semura, T. Ohta, T. Kuroda, Jpn. J. Appl. Phys., 24, L647-L649, 1985.

5) R. D. Esman, L. Goldberg, Electr. Lett., 24(22), 1393-1395, 1988.

Quantum Well Ridge Waveguide Lasers Optimised for High Power Single Spatial Mode Applications.

D. R. Daniel, D. Buckley and B. Garrett

STC Defence Systems, Optical Devices Division, Brixham Road, Paignton, Devon, TQ4 7BE, England

ABSTRACT

High power, single spatial mode (AlGa)As/GaAs quantum well lasers have been fabricated which combine very high power operation with a low threshold current.

Optimisation of the performance of these lasers has been aided by modelling the electron-photon interaction (hole-burning) at high drive levels.

Single element ridge waveguide lasers have been fabricated using a combination of wet and dry etching techniques. These structures combine a high continuous wave burn-off power density of 9.0 MW/cm^2 (non facet-coated) with a high single spatial mode purity. Single spatial mode powers in excess of 128mW have been measured on non-coated devices.

Performance improvements have been obtained by facet coating giving zero-order mode powers of 175mW, burn-off power levels in excess of 300 mW and slope efficiencies of 0.84mW/mA.

1. INTRODUCTION

High power single spatial mode lasers operating in the 790nm - 860nm wavelength range have a number of important applications including optical disc data storage/retrieval, integrated opto-electronics, printing and free space communications.

To date many device structures in the (AlGa)As/GaAs system have been reported yielding high output powers in a fundamental spatial mode. Channelled substrate type lasers have been demonstrated to operate to 60mW in a single spatial mode (ref.1, 2)˙ Goldstein et. al. (ref.3) achieved 170mW (cw) in a single spatial mode and 190mW (cw) maximum power with this type of device. Various other structures have achieved 80mW(cw) in a single spatial mode (ref.4, 5, 6). Some of these lasers employ non-absorbing mirrors fabricated by various means (ref.1, 5).

More recently quantum well active layers have been used in ridge-type waveguide structures in order to lower the threshold current to around 5mA (ref. 7) but with reduced output power capability. Harder et. al.(ref. 8) employed a similar SQW-GRINSCH structure and ridge guide and increased the output power to 35mW in a single spatial mode whilst obtaining a threshold current of 9mA. Garrett et al (ref. 9) achieved in excess of 56mW in a single spatial mode with a new type of quantum well laser (DQW-SCH) which also maintained a low threshold current of 10mA.

This paper describes results on DQW-SCH lasers with improved power performance. Single spatial mode operation to an output power in excess of 175mW ex-facet is demonstrated together with maximum output power of 310mW.

2. DESIGN AND MODELLING

2.1 Chip Structure

The structure chosen to fulfil the requirement for high power in a single spatial mode is shown in Fig. 1. This is a metal clad ridge waveguide (MC-RWG) fabricated from a planar Double-Quantum-Well Separate Confinement Heterostructure (DQW-SCH) grown by Metal Organic Chemical Vapour Deposition (MOCVD). Undoped GaAs quantum wells are incorporated into an $Al_xGa_{1-x}As$ central waveguide (CWG) region which is in turn sandwiched between cladding layers of $Al_yGa_{1-y}As$ of higher Al content. The quantum well active region enables enhanced optical-to electrical power conversion and reduced absorption losses compared with double heterostructure lasers.

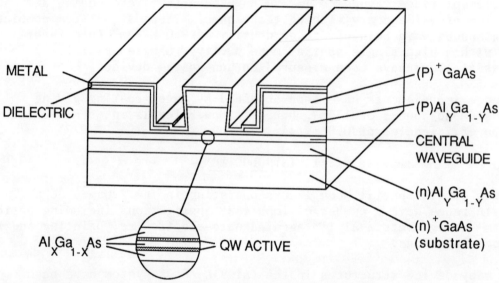

FIG.1. METAL-CLAD RIDGE-WAVEGUIDE (MC-RWG)

2.2 Laser Modelling

The waveguide and lateral mode stability above threshold were modelled employing comprehensive computer programmes reported in detail elsewhere (ref.10, 11, 12).

The above threshold analysis was based on the work of Hakki (ref. 13). The mode stability was assessed by taking into account carrier induced index and gain profile perturbations at high photon densities (hole-burning) and carrier diffusion and the optical distributions in the perturbed waveguide. An iterative technique was used to achieve consistency between the optical and carrier distributions in the plane of the layers.

The qualitative analysis has aided the optimisation of the MC-RWG shown in Fig. 1 for high power in a single spatial mode.

3.0 GROWTH AND FABRICATION

The DQW-SCH structure is grown on a 2" diameter GaAs substrate (n doped - $1 \times 10^{18} cm^{-3}$) by MOCVD using an in-house designed reactor cell capable of taking up to three 2" wafers. The system operates at atmospheric pressure and employs a linear fast-switching gas manifold situated close to the inlet of the reactor cell. Trimethyl-gallium [$(CH_3)_3Ga$] and Trimethyl-aluminium [$(CH_3)_3Al$] are used as group III sources with Arsine (AsH_3) providing the group V source. The n-and p-dopants are hydrogen selenide (H_2Se) and Di-ethyl zinc [$(C_2H_5)_2Zn$] respectively.

The DWQ-SCH were grown at a temperature of 760°C with the exception of the highly doped capping layer which was grown at 650°C. A more comprehensive description of the growth process is contained elsewhere (ref. 14).

After growth, the wafers exhibit a specular surface finish, free of any striations or topographical features.

Wafer fabrication begins with the formation of the ridge waveguide. Standard photolithographic techniques are employed to define the double channel pattern in AZ1470 photoresist. A two stage wet chemical process is used to remove the semiconductor exposed by the windows in the resist such that precise ridge dimensions demanded by the model are accurately achieved. Plasma deposition of a dielectric film (oxy-nitride) follows and this is subsequently patterned using a combination of photolithography and dry etching to accurately define the current injection region parallel to and straddling the ridges.

Thinning of the n-substrate to facilitate accurate and stress free cleaving is then achieved by chemo-mechanically polishing the wafer to a thickness of 100 microns.

Metallisations are applied to the wafer by electron-beam evaporation. Ti/Pt/Au is used to form a Schottky contact to the p+ capping layer of the ridge and Ge/Ni/Au provides an ohmic contact to the n-side of the wafer.

From the fully processed wafers, bars are cleaved off with a sample being diced to produce uncoated chips for assessment. The remaining bars are mounted in a jig for facet coating. Antireflective ($\lambda/4$) coatings are applied to the front and reflective coatings to the rear facets of the bars. They are then diced before being mounted into stud packages for assessment.

4. CHARACTERISATION

4.1 Wafer Uniformity

The uniformity of the planar DQW-SCH structures is clearly of key importance if a valid comparison between modelled and empirical results is to be made. Therefore, to assess the uniformity of material characteristics over a full 2" wafer, a grown slice was fabricated into conventional oxide stripe lasers which were then assessed for their lasing parameters. A total of 215 non-coated laser chips (150μm stripe x 500μm cavity) were taken from evenly distributed positions around the wafer with their locations recorded to enable spatial trends to be investigated.

Threshold current densities as low as 320A/cm^2 were achieved under narrow pulsed conditions (50ns, 10kHz).

Wavelength is a particularly sensitive indicator of layer thickness and composition variations. Fig. 2 shows the excellent uniformity achieved over a full 2" wafer with only marginal trends apparent and no chip failures. The mean wavelength was 808.3nm with a standard deviation of 1.46nm. These results represent the accumulation of performance variations due to growth, processing, cleaving and measurement.

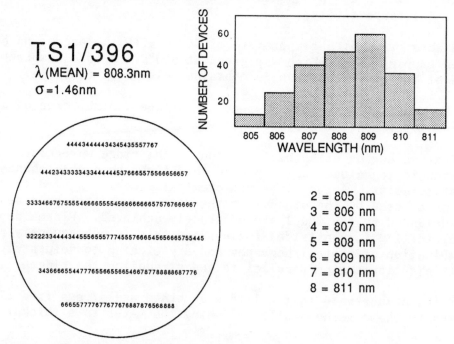

Fig. 2. Wavelength uniformity of DQW-SCH over 2" wafer.

4.2 MC-RWG Laser Performance

4.2.1 Non-coated Chip Assessment

Preliminary testing of non-coated MC-RWG devices was performed to evaluate performance limits at room temperature. Initial results indicated that their burn-off powers, at which catastrophic facet damage occurs, were significantly higher than conventional DH lasers, the highest CW burn off power measured on a double-quantum well device was 45W/mm which translates to a burn off power density of 9MW/cm^2 assuming a perpendicular near-field width of 0.5µm (inferred from far field measurements). This is significantly higher than conventional DH structures.

The lasers were found to emit radiation in a single lobed far-field pattern at output powers up to 128mW (Fig. 3) before side lobes started to appear, indicating the onset of higher order lateral modes. Threshold currents as low as 16mA have been recorded on some devices although they were not optimised for low threshold.

Incremental slopes of 0.5 - 0.6 mW/mA per facet were recorded on typical devices.

4.2.2 Facet-coated Device Performance

MC-RWG laser chips with AR and reflector facet coatings were mounted on coaxial-stud assemblies for assessment. The results indicate a significant increase in maximum single spatial mode power, burn off power and incremental slope compared with non-coated chips.

Fig. 4 shows the light/current (L/I) characteristic of a facet coated DQW-SCH laser. The burn-off power of this facet-coated device is in excess of 310mW at a drive current of approximately ten times the threshold current of 55mA.

Incremental slope efficiencies at 100mW output power were typically 0.75mW/mA though values of 0.84mW/mA have been obtained.

The far field radiation pattern parallel to the junction was found to be single lobed up to an output power of 175mW (Fig. 5). The corresponding full width half maximum (FWHM) of the envelope is approximately 7 degrees and was free of any discernable side lobes. This is believed to be the highest zero-order output power achieved on a single element device.

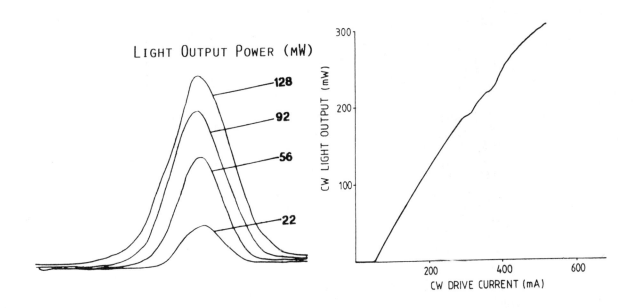

FIG. 3. PARALLEL FAR FIELD PATTERN OF UNCOATED MC-RWG LASER

FIG. 4. LIGHT OUTPUT vs DRIVE CURRENT FOR HIGH POWER SINGLE SPATIAL MODE LASER

Furthermore, investigation of the spectral properties of the laser showed that the devices can emit in a single longitudinal mode up to the point where the parallel far-field becomes unstable. Fig. 6 shows the spectra of a typical device operating at 150mW at a constant temperature of 25°C.

This compares very favourably with the 170mW zero-order output power achieved by Goldstein et. al. (ref. 3), the highest reported value to date for a single element device.

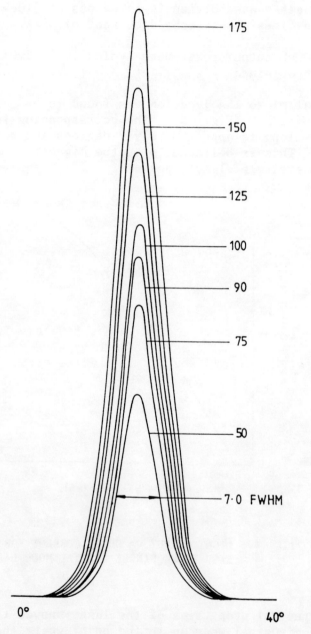

FIG. 5. PARALLEL FAR FIELD PATTERN FOR FACET COATED MC-RWG LASER

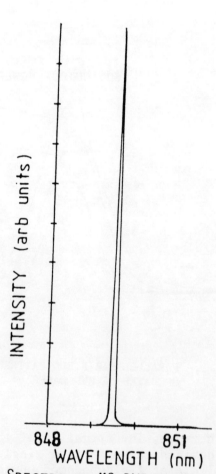

FIG. 6. SPECTRA OF MC-RWG SSM LASER OPERATING AT 150mW

5. CONCLUSIONS

MC-RWG lasers have been fabricated from (AlGa)As DQW-SCH structures grown by MOCVD which exhibit high continuous wave (CW) output powers (175mW) in a single spatial mode, believed to be the highest recorded on a single element device. Burn off powers of 310mW have been achieved on facet-coated devices optimised for high power in a zero-order lateral mode.

Non-coated devices show CW burn-off power densities of $9MW/cm^2$, a state-of-the-art result. Threshold currents as low as 16mA have been recorded on devices despite not having been optimised for low threshold.

Theoretical modelling has been used to provide a qualitative analysis of the MC-RWG structure enabling optimisation for high power in a single spatial mode.

6. ACKNOWLEDGEMENTS

The authors wish to thank Dr. D. R. Wight (RSRE) and Dr. R. S. Butlin (STC) for their support and encouragement. Thanks are also extended to Mr. R. K. Simpson and Mr. S. L. Dewhirst for the preparation of devices and Dr. M. W. Jones for the MOCVD growth of the epi-structures.

"This work has been supported and sponsored by the Procurement Executive, Ministry of Defence (Royal Signals and Radar Establishment)".

7. REFERENCES

Yamamoto S., Hayashi K., Kayakawa T., Miyanchi N., Yano S., Hijikata T., "High optical power on operation in visible spectral range by window V-channelled substrate inner stripe lasers" Appl. Phys. Letts. 42(5), (1983). pp 406 - 408.

2. Fu R.J., Hwang C. J., Wang C. S., Lalevic B.,
"Single mode, high power GaAlAs/GaAs lasers"
Appl. Phys. Letts. 45(7), (1984), pp 716-718.

3. Goldstein B., Ettenberg M., Dinkel N. A., Butler J. K.,
Appl. Phys. Letts., 47(7), (1985), pp 655-657.

4. Endo K., Kawano K., Veno M., Nido M., Kuwamura Y., Furuse T., Sakuma I. "High-power buried coarctate mesa-structure AlGaAs lasers".
Electronics letts., 20 (18), (1984), pp 728-729.

5. Ungar J., Bar-Chain N., Vry I.,
"High-power GaAlAs window lasers".
Electronics letts., 22 (5), (1986), pp 279-280.

6. Nakatsuka S., Ono Y., Kajimura T.,
"A new self-aligned structure for (GaAl)As high power lasers with selectively grown light absorbing GaAs layers fabricated by MOCVD".
Jap. J. Appl. Phys., 25 (6), (1980) pp L498-L500

7. Wada O., Sanada T., Kuno M., Fujii T.,
    "Very low threshold current ridge waveguide (AlGa)As/GaAs single quantum well lasers",
    Electronics Letts., 21 (22), (1985), pp 1025-1026

8. Harder C., Buchmann P., Meier M.,
    "High-power ridge-waveguide AlGaAs GRIN-SCH laser diode",
    Electronics Letts., 22(20), (1986), pp 1081-1082.

9. Garrett B., Glew R.W.,
    "Low-threshold, high power zero-order lateral mode DQW-SCH metal clad ridge waveguide (AlGa)As/GaAs lasers",
    Electronics Letts., 23(8), (1987), pp 371-373

10. Garrett B., Whiteaway J. E. A.,
    "Optimisation of four- and five-layer AlGaAs/Ga large optical cavity lasers for high power, low threshold current density operation"
    IEE Proc. Pt. J., 133 (5), (1986), pp319-326

11. Whiteaway J. E. A., Thompson G. H. B., Goodwin A. R.,
    "Mode stability in real index guided semiconductor laser arrays".
    Electronics Letts. 21(25/26), (1085), pp 1194-1195.

12. Garrett B., Whiteaway J. E. A.,
    "Self stabilisaion of the fundamental lateral mode in index guided semiconductor lasers".
    IEE Proc. Pt. J., 134(1), (1987), pp11-15

13. Hakki B. W.,
    "GaAs double heterojunction lasing behaviour along the junction plane".
    J. Appl. Phys., 46 (1), (1975), pp 292-302.

14. Jones M. W., Daniel D. R., Buckley D., Ridge M., Watts D., Butlin R. S.,
    "Uniform high power, pulsed and CW GaAs/GaAlAs lasers produced from 2" AP-MOCVD reactor".
    "2nd European Workshop on MOCVD", St. Andrews, Scotland, June 1988

Invited Paper

Monolithic Two-Dimensional Arrays of Diode Lasers

W.W. Simmons, E. Anderson, L. Eaton, L. Heflinger, J. Huang, M. Jansen, , S.S. Ou, M. Sergant, J.Z. Wilcox, J.J. Yang

TRW Space & Technology Group
One Space Park
Redondo Beach, Ca. 90278

Abstract

Two rows of surface-emitting (ten-element each), linear arrays were coherently locked to an external master oscillator. Tuneable operation was achieved over a greater than 40 A wavelength range, and coherence was confirmed by far-field interference.

* Work sponsored by the Air Force

Summary

Injection locking of discrete edge emitting semiconductor diode lasers to an external master oscillator (MO) has been successfully demonstrated for single stripe devices[1], linear arrays[2,3] and broad area lasers[4]. In this paper we report the coherent operation of an injection-locked monolithic array of coupled resonators.

The coupled resonator concept features monolithic linear arrays (10 elements each), vertical and 45 degree outcoupling micromirrors for vertical emission[5], and interconnecting optical waveguides. Coherence across the device at a single wavelength is achieved by external injection locking.

Figure 1 shows a top view of the architecture, which consists of 10 surface emitting unit cells (each one comprising a ten element linear array), and one "driver" unit which couples the two rows of devices. The dimensions are illustrated in the lower insert.

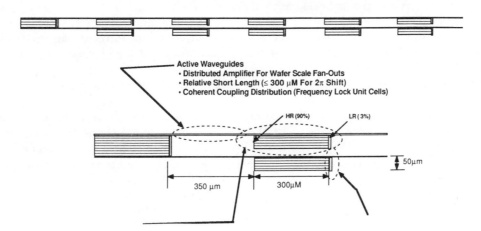

Figure 1-   Top View of TRW Monolithic Surface Emitting Array Architecture

A schematic diagram showing the transverse and lateral unit cell dimensions, and the device geometry (growth layers) are shown in Figure 2. The figure illustrates surface-emitting linear arrays of both epi-up and epi-down configurations. The latter offer superior thermal management, and have been successfully fabricated. Nevertheless, results reported herein are for the epi-up configuration only.

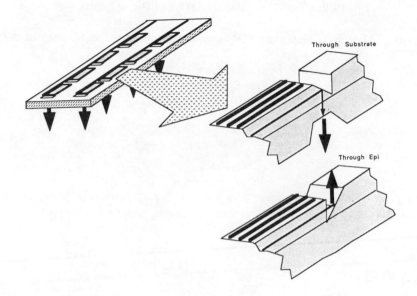

Figure 2- Transverse and Lateral Device Geometry

Each unit cell has 10 stripes, 3 um wide and 300 um long. The device transverse structure is a double quantum well-separate confinement heterostructure (DQW-SCH) grown by metal organic chemical vapor deposition (MOCVD). The 90^0 cavity mirrors of the unit cells are coated with a 3% low reflectivity (LR) facet, and a 90% high reflectivity (HR) coating. this choice provides an enhanced injection locking bandwidth (relative to uncoated mirrors) and single-ended emission, without a substantial efficiency penalty in operation.

The optical waveguides between adjacent unit cells couple them coherently and efficiently. External injection locking results in tuning over a significant wavelength band (> 40 A). Individual waveguide current bias control permits signal amplification without significant phase lock degradation. External injection locking forces strong phase coherence across the array. The design is amenable to relatively simple aperture filling through the use of external optics. The planar wafer geometry provides efficient diode operation and output coupling, and simple heat removal through a back-plane submount. Finally, this array architecture is robust (light continues to propagate through degraded unit cells)

Device uniformity is achieved by using reproducibly uniform material growth, and fabrication techniques which are compatible with the monolithic integration on the wafer. We have developed MOCVD material growth techniques which result in very uniform material, as well as dry-etching technologies (reactive ion-etching and ion-milling), used for defining waveguide structures, and 45 degree outcoupling micromirrors and vertical laser facets with an optical quality comparable to that of cleaved devices.
Figure 3 shows a close-up view of a TRW fabricated and packaged 2-D array.

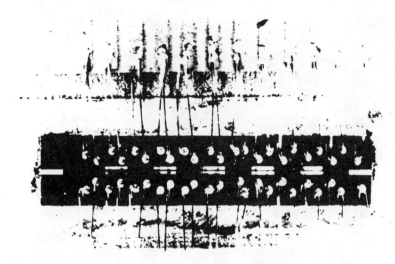

Figure 3- Top View of Fabricated TRW 2x5 Array

2-D arrays were operated under CW conditions at -30^0 C. Figure 4 a, b, and c shows P-I curves, a near-field and a far-field of such an array under CW operation. Single devices were injection locked as shown in Figure 4d, while Figure 4e shows interference between devices 1 and 4 in a row of 4 self-locked devices operating under CW conditions.

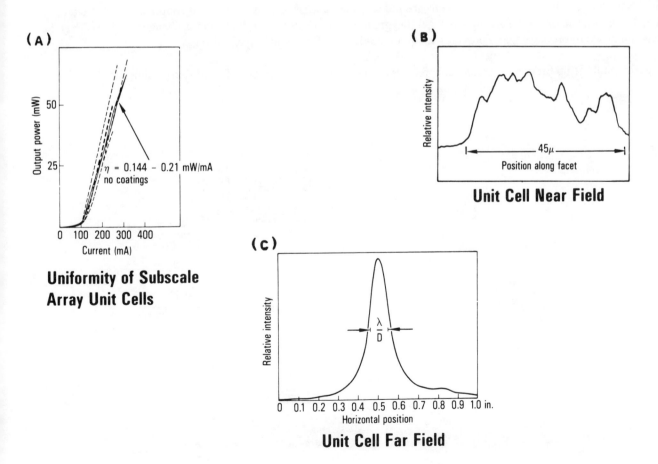

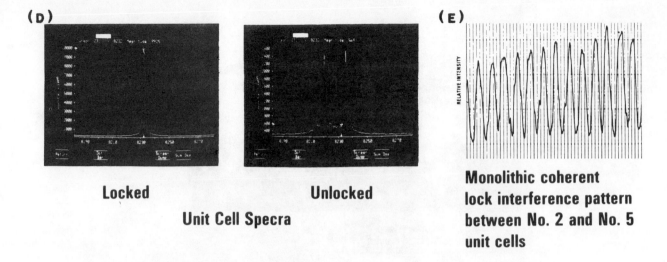

Figure 4- Results for CW-Operated Monolithic Surface-Emitting Array
    a- P-I Curves
    b- Array Near-Field Profile
    c- Array Far-Field Profile
    d- Injection Locked Operation (Spectra)
    e- Interference Pattern between Devices 1 and 4 in a Self-Locked Row of Four Devices

The ridge waveguides which couple the unit cells are index-guided and provide strong lateral confinement. The edge cladding depth of .25 um provides strong index guiding greater than the carrier-induced index changes, it allows only the fundamental mode to propagate, and provides adequate modal gain for signal amplification.

The experimental set-up for demonstrating coherent operation under injection locked conditions is illustrated in Figure 5.

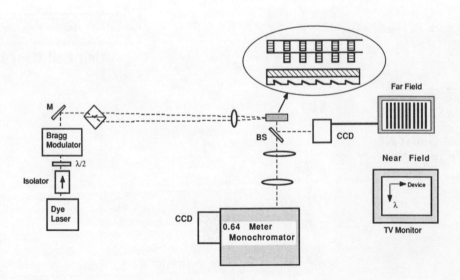

Figure 5- Experimental Arrangement for Injection Locking

2x5 arrays were injection locked from an external master oscillator (M.O.) under pulsed operation. The M.O. was a commercial dye laser. An isolator and half-wave plate were used to minimize reflections back into the M.O.. A Bragg modulator was used to synchronize the dye laser and slave laser pulses. A cube beam-splitter was used to split the M.O. beam in two, and to inject each beam into one of the rows of devices. The spectral output was monitored with the monochromator, while far-fields were measured directly with a CCD camera.

The TRW 2-D 2x5 array exhibits spectral coherence under both free-running, and injection locked conditions, as illustrated by the free-running and injection locked array spectra of Figure 6.

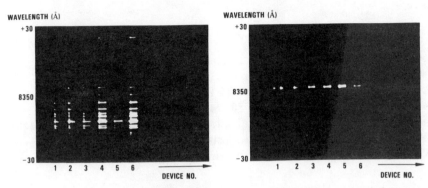

Figure 6
- a- Free-Running Spectrum of 2x5 Surface Emitting Array
- b- Injection Locked Spectrum of 2x5 Surface Emitting Array

The injection locked 2x5 array can be tuned over a greater than 40 Å spectral range, while maintaining phase lock. The injected power from the dye laser is 2 mW, and the array output is 100-200 mW. The high transparency of the quantum well material results in system robustness. Light continues to propagate through turned-off unit cells, and coherent lock is maintained under both free-running and injection locked conditions.

Fringe visibilities in excess of 60% have been achieved for single rows of unit cells, as illustrated in figure 7. The fringe width is approximately 1.6x the theoretical value predicted for a coherent array of light sources.

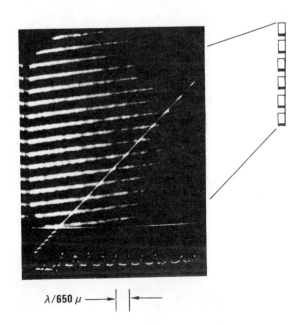

Figure 7-

Far-Field Interference Pattern for a 1x6 Row of Unit Cells

In conclusion, we have demonstrated a coherent, monolithic, robust, two-dimensional array of diode lasers. The free running array is spectrally coherent, and it is phase coherent under injection locking from an external master oscillator. The injected 2-D array is tunable over a 50 A spectral range. Far-field fringe visibilities in excess of 60% were achieved.

References

1. S. Kobayashi and T. Kimura, IEEE J. Quantum Electron., **QE-17** (5) 681 (1981)
2. J.P. Hohimer, A. Owyoung, and G.R. Hadley, Appl. Phys. Lett., **47** (12), 1244 (1985)
3. L. Goldberg and J.F. Weller, Appl. Phys. Lett., **50** (24), 1713 (1987)
4. G.L. Abbas, S. Yang, V.W.S. Chan and J.G. Fujimoto, IEEE J. Quantum Electron., **24** (4), 609 (1988)
5. J.J. Yang, M. Jansen and M. Sergant, Electronics Letters **22** (8) 438 (1986), and J.J. Yang, M. Sergant, M. Jansen, S.S. Ou, L. Eaton, and W. W. Simmons, Appl. Phys Lett. **49** (18), 1138 (1986)

Invited Paper

Long-life GaAlAs high-power lasers with nonabsorbing mirrors

Hirokazu Shimizu

Matsushita Electronics Corporation, Electronics Research Laboratory
Takatsuki, Osaka 569, Japan

ABSTRACT

We report long-life GaAlAs lasers showing fundamental-mode high-power operations, which have been developed by providing current blocked nonabsorbing mirror (NAM) regions in the conventional buried twin ridge substrate (BTRS) structure. Suppression of the mirror degradation due to local heating for the NAM and use of the loss-guide mechanism for the BTRS structure are the main cause of the excellent operations. For the fabrication, use of a substrate having a mesa on it and a hybrid epitaxial technique of LPE and MOCVD is an essential point. As a result we have obtained the stable fundamental spatial mode operations up to 120 mW and the maximum output power of 300 mW under a CW operation. Degradation has been insignificant for 6000 hours under the output power of 100 mW and the temperature of 50°C.

1. INTRODUCTION

GaAlAs laser diodes with the output power up to 40 mW are being used for wide applications such as audiodisk and optical disk memory systems. In recent years, there has appeared an increasing demand for devices operating reliably at powers in excess of 50 mW for applications such as space communications, optical recording, and SHG light sources with blue coherent light. For such applications, use of the fundamental-spatial-mode oscillation is of crucial importance for attaining precice beam definition.

We have already developed a high-power GaAlAs laser designated as buried twin ridge substrate (BTRS) laser, in which the maximum output power of 200 mW was obtained by using a thin active layer and inner stripe for current confinement.[1] Under high output power more than 50 mW, however, the conventional structure lasers have a disadvantage of impractically short lifetime, which is caused by mirror facet degradation due to the optical absorption around the facets. Another disadvantage of the conventional lasers is that the maximum available output power is determined by the catastrophic degradation of the mirrors. In order to prevent the mirror degradation especially due to the local heating by optical absorption, an effective approach of so called window structure[2,3] or nonabsorbing mirrors (NAM)[4,5,6] structure has been utilized. However, a disadvantage of the conventional NAM-type devices is poor lateral mode control, which results in lateral mode deformation limiting the maximun output power of fundamental mode to a value less than 80 mW. Furthermore few reliability data have been reported for such lasers.

In this paper we describe long-life GaAlAs lasers showing a reliable fundamental-mode high-power operations, which have been obtained by applying the NAM approach to the conventional BTRS structure. The high power operation has been attained by using the structure having current-blocked NAM in order to suppress the mirror degradation due to local heating. The stable fundamental-mode is obtained by using the BTRS structure which provides index guiding in the nonabsorbing mirror regions. The optical guide layer adjacent to the active layer also permits the suppression of the coupling loss between the active layer and the NAM region. Starting with a substrate having a mesa on it for the laser fabrication is a key point for providing easily the current-blocking operation. On the other hand, use of a hybrid epitaxial technique of LPE and MOCVD is also of crucial importance for obtaining sufficiently good quality layers of the NAM above the current-blocked regions.

2. BASIC CONCEPT OF NAM-BTRS LASER

The schematic structure of the NAM-BTRS laser is shown in Fig.1. This laser is developed with the aim of attaining strong suppression of the mirror degradation and high stabilization of the spatial mode on the basis of the following basic concepts.

2.1. Suppression of the mirror degradation

The most important factor limiting the output power in the GaAlAs laser is the catastrophic optical damage (COD) at the mirror facets. The main cause of the COD is the local heating due to the optical absorption at the facets.[7,8] From this viewpoint, the COD is prevented by forming nonabsorbing mirrors for suppressing the local heating due to the absorption of the laser light. The nonabsorbing mirrors are obtained by removing the active layer from the regions around both facets of the large optical cavity which consists of the

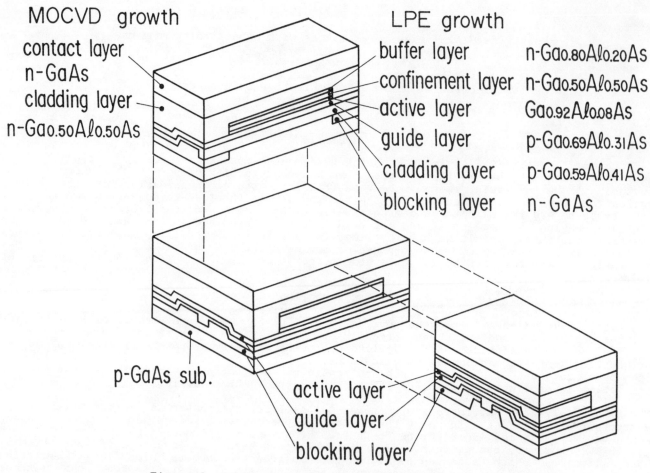

Figure 1. Schematic structure of a NAM-BTRS laser

active layer and the optical guide layer, as shown in Fig.1. The diffraction loss which may occur in the NAM region is suppressed by providing the guide layer which does not absorb the laser light.

Now the current flow in the NAM region is another cause of the local heating. In order to prevent this heating, the current flow is suppressed by providing the current-blocking layer in the NAM region. Thus the local heating is strongly suppressed by providing the current-blocking region as well as the NAM region.

2.2. Stabilization of the spatial mode

The fundamental spatial mode in high power operations is stabilized by the use of the BTRS structure. Twin ridges, which are formed on the current blocking layer, allow the formation of an excellently uniform thin active layer and the guide layer under the liquid phase epitaxial growth. The channel between two ridges well stabilizes the lateral mode in both inner and NAM regions owing to the loss guide mechanism.

3. DESIGN CONSIDERATIONS

3.1. Structure parameters

At the position where the catastrophic mirror degradation has been well suppressed by the NAM structure, the power saturation due to the junction temperature rise is now an important factor limiting the ouput power. This rise is caused by the flow of the operation current. In order to suppress the junction temperature rise, therefore, the operating current must be designed to be as low as possible. We determine structure parameters so as to attain low threshold current and high efficiency. The inner LOC section consists of p-$Ga_{0.59}Al_{0.41}As$ clad layer, p-$Ga_{0.69}Al_{0.31}As$ guide layer, undoped $Ga_{0.92}Al_{0.08}As$ active layer, n-$Ga_{0.50}Al_{0.50}As$ confinement layer, n-$Ga_{0.80}Al_{0.20}As$ buffer layer, and n-$Ga_{0.50}Al_{0.50}As$ clad layer for 830 nm wavelength lasers. The low AlAs content buffer layer is inserted into a region between high AlAs content layers to secure low resistivity. The AlAs mole fractions and the thicknesses of these layers are determined so as to obtain the minimum threshold current. The thicknesses determined for 830 nm wavelength lasers are listed in Table 1. The lengths of the NAM region and of the inner region are chosen to be 25 µm and 200 µm, respectively, and the channel width to be 7 µm.

Table 1. Thickness of each layer

Layer	Thickness (µm)
Optical guide layer	0.15
Active layer	0.06
Confinement layer	0.45
Buffer layer	0.05

3.2. MOCVD growth for layer formation

A process for obtaining the NAM contains a step of growing GaAlAs layers on a GaAlAs layer of relatively high AlAs content. It is found that the LPE technique is not useful for this step. Here the MOCVD technique is used as a powerful method for forming good quality layers consisting the NAM.

4. FABRICATION

The device fabrication process shown in Fig.2 involves the following sequential steps.
(a) A rectangular mesa is formed on a (100) surface of a p-GaAs substrate.
(b) An n-GaAs current blocking layer is grown on the substrate with the above mesa by the LPE growth.
(c) Two ridges are formed by chemical etching in parallel to the mesa under a ridge height such that the channel between the ridges reaches the mesa on the substrate.
(d) A lower clad layer, a guide layer, an active layer, a confinement layer, and a buffer layer are successively grown by the second LPE growth.
(e) The epitaxial layers are etched down to the guide layer near the facets.
(f) A top clad layer and a contact layer are grown by the MOCVD growth.

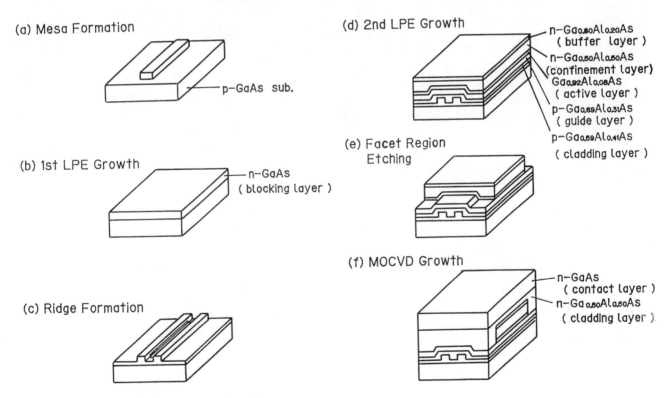

Figure 2. Schematic diagram of fabrication process

After the lasers are cleaved to a length of 250 µm, the mirror facets are coated to produce reflectivities of 4% and 96% for the front and rear facets, respectively. The diodes is mounted junction-side down on a silicon submount.

A longitudinal cross section of a typical NAM-BTRS laser thus fabricated is depicted in the scanning electron micrograph (SEM) of Fig.3.

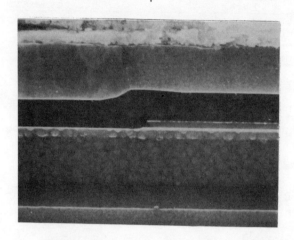

Figure 3. SEM cross-section of a NAM-BTRS laser

5. CHARACTERISTICS AND RELIABILITY

The light output power versus current characteristics under CW and 100-ns pulsed operations are shown in Fig. 4. We successfuly achieved high power output over 300 mW under CW operation and over 1200 mW under pulsed operation. The maximum output power is found to be determined simply by the Joule heating under both CW and pulsed operations. The threshold current and the external quantum efficiency are 40 mA and 51%, respectively.

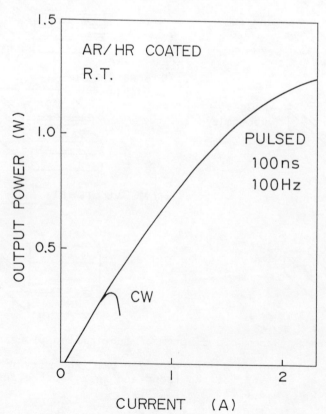

Figure 4. Light output power vs. current characteristics of a NAM-BTRS laser

The typical far-field patterns of the laser are shown in Fig.5. Fundamental spatial mode operation is observed up to 120 mW. The beam divergence angles parallel and perpendicular to the junction plane are 12° and 24°, respectively.

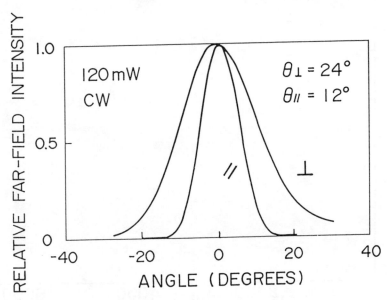

Figure 5. Far-field patterns of a NAM-BTRS laser

The reliability of the 830 nm NAM-BTRS lasers were examined at the power of 100 mW and an ambient temperature of 50°C. The aging test results of the NAM-BTRS lasers in a short time range are shown in Fig.6 together with those of the conventional BTRS lasers without nonabsorbing mirrors for comparison. As is clearly seen, the new NAM lasers show very stable operations, although the conventional lasers fail in very short times. Figure 7 shows the lifetest results of the NAM-BTRS lasers in a long time range. Even after 6000 hours, the lasers show no obvious degradation. These results indicate that the current blocked nonabsorbing mirrors are very effective in suppressing the mirror facet degradation.

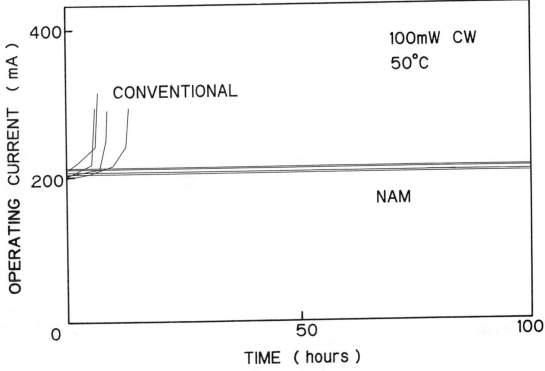

Figure 6. Lifetest results of the NAM-BTRS lasers and the conventional BTRS lasers

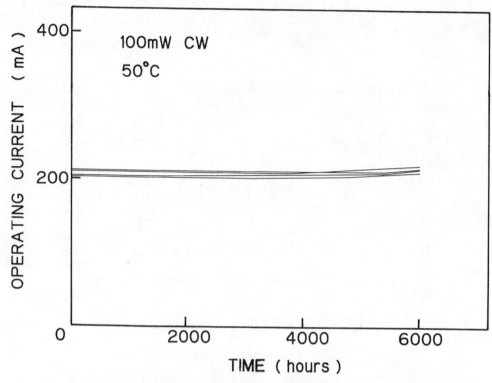

Figure 7. Lifetest results of the NAM-BTRS lasers

6. CONCLUSION

The long-life operation at high output power has been demonstrated in the BTRS lasers with nonabsorbing mirrors, which were grown by LPE and MOCVD hybrid method. The lasers have exhibited the stable fundamental spatial mode up to 120 mW and the maximum output power of 300 mW under a CW operation. No significant degradation has been observed for 6000 hours under the output power 100 mW and the temperature 50°C.

7. ACKNOWLEDGMENT

The author wishes to thank Dr. Teramoto, Dr. Kano, and Dr. Takeshima for their helpful discussions and continuous encouragement.

8. REFERENCES

1. K.Hamada, M.Wada, H.Shimizu,M.Kume,F.Susa,T.Shibutani,N.Yoshikawa,K.Itoh,G.Kano, and I.teramoto, "A 0.2W CW laser with buried twin ridge substrate structure," IEEE J. Quantum Electron.,vol.QE-21,pp.623-628,1985.
2. H.Yonezu,M.Ueno,T.Kamejima, and I.Hayashi,"An AlGaAs window structure laser," IEEE J.Quantum Electron.,vol.QE-15,pp.775-781,1979.
3. H.Kumabe,T.Tanaka,S.Nita,Y.Seiwa,T.Sogo,and S.Takamiya,"15mW single mode CW operation of crank structure TJS laser diodes at high temperature," Jpn.J.Appl.Phys., Suppl.21-1, pp.347-351,1982.
4. H.Blauvelt,S.Margalit,and A.Yariv,"Large optical Cavity AlGaAs buried heterostructure window lasers,"Appl.Phys.Lett.,vol.40,pp.1029-1031,1982.
5. D.Botez and J.C.Connolly, "Nonabsorbing-mirror (NAM) CDH-LOC diode lasers," Electron.Lett.,vol.20,pp.530-532,1984.
6. J.Unger, N.Bar-chaim, and I.Ury, "High-power GaAlAs window lasers," Electron.Lett.,vol22,pp.279-280,1986.
7. C.H.Henry,P.M.Petroff,R.A.Logan, and F.R.Merritt,"Catastrophic damage of $Al_x Ga_{1-x} As$ double-heterostructure laser material," J.Appl.Phys.vol.50,pp.3721-3732, 1979.
8. R.W.H.Engelmann and D.Kerps,"CW facet damage power of DH lasers based on thermal runaway model,"Proceedings of the 8th IEEE International Semiconductor Laser Conference,Ottawa 1982,pp.26-27.

Transverse Mode Controlled Wide-Single-Stripe Lasers by Loading Modal Filters

K. Ikeda, K. Shigihara, T. Aoyagi, S. Hinata, Y. Nagai, N. Kaneno,
Y. Mihashi, Y. Seiwa and W. Susaki

Optoelectronic and Microwave Devices R&D Laboratory,
Mitsubishi Electric Corporation
4-1 Mizuhara, Itami, Hyogo JAPAN 664

ABSTRACT

Two kinds of modal filter for high power diode lasers with a wide stripe have been examined. The first one is a partially narrow region formed in the active region. Flared-SBA(self-aligned bent active layer) laser in which the active layer flares the width from the narrow filter region to the wide output facet oscillates in a fundamental transverse mode under cw condition up to the output power of 64mW. The second one is a partial coating at the output facet of lasers. By applying it to an SBA laser whose stripe width is 150μm, the laser oscillates in a single lobed far-field pattern up to 300mW, whose divergent angle is as narrow as 1.7° in FAHM(full angle at half maximum) under cw conditions.

1. Introduction

When higher power is desired, cross section of the lasing mode should be enlarged at the output facet of the laser diode, because maximum power density is limited by catastrophic optical damage(COD). We would classify approaches reported previously into three categories. The first has a relatively narrow active region where only fundamental transverse mode can propagate. By using a thinner active layer, cross section area of the fundamental mode is enlarged. Generally, the maximum output power may reach approximately one hundred mW at the present stage. When the non-absorbing mirror(NAM) structure is combined, the maximum power is as high as 300mW[1]. The second type is phase-locked laser array, in which the individual stripe width, interval among the stripes, and gain distribution for individual stripe regions have been studied to control the super modes into the lowest order one[2]. In almost all of these array lasers, realizing both output power and the fundamental super-mode seems to require much more precise fabrication technique[3,4]. Output power of two- to three-hundred mW in the fundamental super mode under cw condition is considered best in the record at present. The third approach is broad or wide-stripe lasers including unstable resonator. In such lasers, it seems to be important to control gain or loss, which is dependent on mode order.

We also have investigated phase-locked laser arrays especially on their super mode control[4-6]. And in our previous paper[7], we pointed out that much more prompt progress should be required in precise fabrication technology to realize a stable fundamental super mode oscillation even at higher power than several hundred mW. In this paper, we demonstrate some of our progresses on wide-stripe high power lasers, which belong to the third category. The main efforts in the work is to accept present fabrication technique and accuracy. Then, we get narrow single lobed far-field pattern at 300mW CW operations.

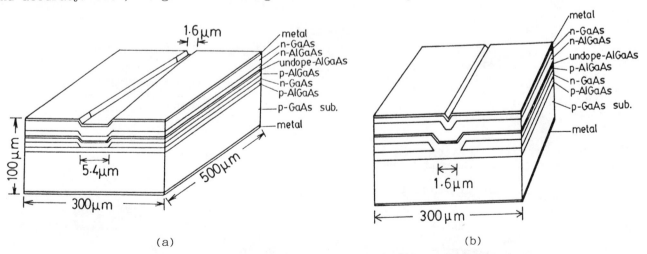

Fig. 1 F-SBA laser chip(a) and C-SBA laser chip(b). Each chip is solderd on Si-dsubmount in junction-down configuration.

2. Modal Filter in Stripe

Our first interest in the transverse mode control on a wide-stripe laser is a flared stripe laser, in which the active region width at output facet is wide, while the width at the center portion or at the rear facet is as narrow as the only fundamental mode can pass through. This idea was at first realized in BH type laser by welch et al.[8].

Figure 1 shows our Flared-SBA(self-aligned bent active layer) laser chip[9] and the conventional SBA laser chip. Here, we call them as F-SBA and C-SBA. These lasers have an index-guiding mechanism similarly to the BH type. According to our calculation, cutoff condition of 1st. order mode corresponds to the active region width of $1.4\mu m$ in case of the C-SBA lasers. However, even when the width is $1.6\mu m$, 1st. order mode has not oscillated experimentally because of remarkable scattering loss at side wall of the active layer.

Figure 2 shows the far-field patterns of the F-SBA laser at various power levels obtained at CW condition. Single fundamental transverse mode oscillation is reconfirmed at every power level up to 64mW at room temperature cw operation. The c-SBA laser having active region width of about $1.5\mu m$ without any wide portion can emit at most 30mW. On the other hand, c-SBA lasers having wide active region in excess of $1.6\mu m$ without any narrow portions oscillates in no fundamental mode. Then the narrow part in the F-SBA laser can be understood to play a role of modal filter in the waveguide.

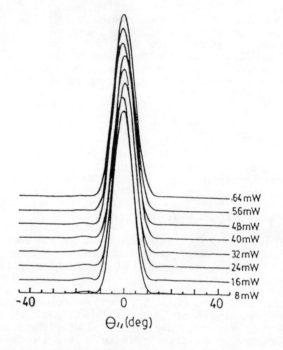

Fig. 2 Far-field patterns for parallel direction to the junction plane obtained at various power levels in the F-SBA laser.

3. Modal Filter at Output Facet

Many approaches have been tried to control transverse mode of not only laser arrays but also wide-stripe lasers into a fundamental mode. Almost all of them propose some kinds of gain profile modification in the stripe. However, changing the gain distribution brings temperature and/or index profile change. Then we employ a modal filter at the facet.

Concept

Our idea of modal filter is that reflection for desired fundamental mode is higher whereas lower for undesired higher order mode. This idea might have a physically similar background to the well-known unstable resonator in the field of high power gas-laser. J.Wittke et al.[10] and C.Ninagawa et al.[11] already tried experimentally similar structures at 1977 and 1979, although power levels examined was much lower level as compared with this work. Recently A.K.Chan et al.[12] discussed theoretically on reflection profiles at facet.

Mode Selectability

We have at first investigated theoretically optimum width of high reflective region. Here, stripe width is supposed to be $150\mu m$. In this case, 98 modes can propagate through the active region. It is supposed that only a part of the facet whose width of $2B\mu m$ has non-zero reflection, and reflection of the remaining region is zero. Relative modal reflectivity for each mode has been calculated as shown in Fig. 3. Since high reflection region is located at the center of the stripe, the fundamental mode has always the highest reflection. Second highest mode is not always 1st or 2nd mode. Reflection of second highest mode against the fundamental mode is illustrated in Fig. 4. As can be seen in the figure, when the width, 2B, is approximately $40-60\mu m$, second highest mode has approximately 60-70% of the reflection of the fundamental transverse mode. This corresponds to threshold gain difference of $4cm^{-1}$.

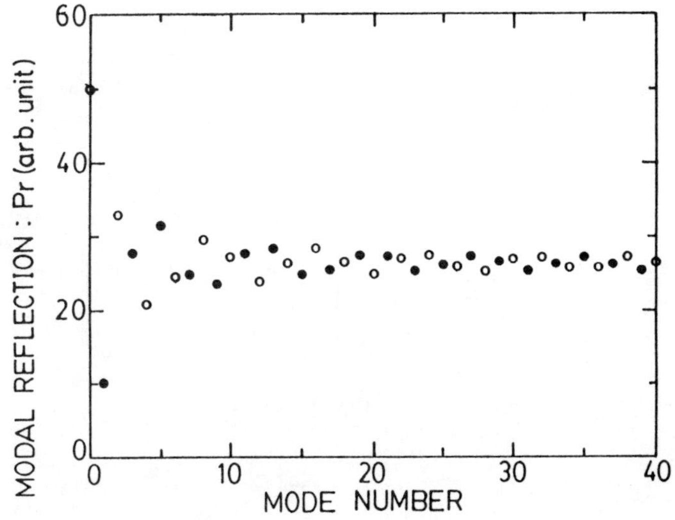

Fig. 3 Calculated modal reflection of each mode for an SBA laser with the stripe width of 150μm.

Fig. 4 Relative modal reflection of the second highest mode as a function of the partially coated width, 2B.

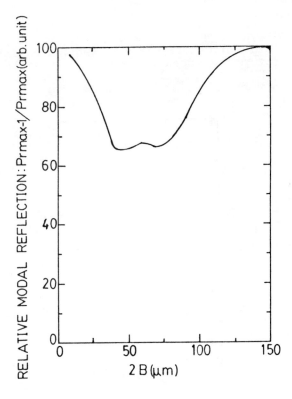

Experiment

Figure 5 illustrates our laser diode chip examined, in which width of the active region is 150μm. The SBA laser configuration is employed. The active layer consists of so-called single quantum well(SQW) which is grown by low-pressure MOCVD, then the laser has SCH-SQW structure. The well width is approximately 100Å. Cavity length (L) is made to be 500μm by taking threshold current density and thermal resistance into accounts[13]. Reflection of the rear facet is 98% by a-Si/SiO$_2$ multi-layer coating. On the front facet, anti-reflecting coating by using Al$_2$O$_3$ was made as the first step, subsequently a partial coating process has been added.

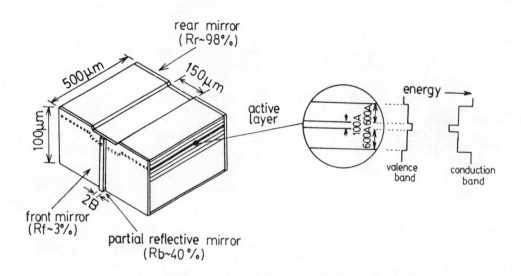

Fig. 5 Illustration of the examined wide-stripe SBA laser having a partial coating.

Figure 6 represents a typical output power(P) vs. current(I) characteristic and far-field patterns(FFPs) for fabricated lasers without partial coating obtained in room temperature cw operation. One can see that the threshold is approximately 0.6-0.7A and that FFP for parallel to the junction plane has many peaks whose full-angle at half-maximum(FAHM) is 19.4degree. This result suggests that the wide stripe laser without any mode selection mechanisms exhibits multiple higher order mode oscillation.

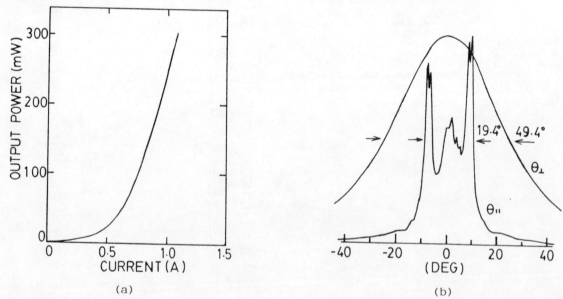

Fig. 6 A typical output power(p) vs. current(I) characteristic(a) and FFPs(b) measured on a wide-stripe SBA laser without the partial coating.

A typical FFP for parallel direction to the junction plane obtained on samples after partial coating is demonstrated in Fig. 7. In this case, width of the partial coating is 22μm. As can be seen in the figure, divergent angle in FAHM is 1.7° even when output power is 300mW in cw operation. Such narrow far-field angle like this means that the wave front is almost flat and that oscillating mode is almost single fundamental mode.

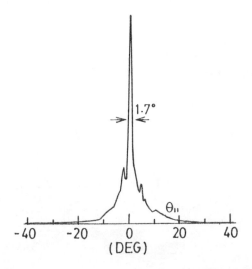

Fig. 7   A typical FFP obtained in the wide-stripe SBA laser with a partial coating (2B=22μm).

Figure 8 shows another FFPs observed in lasers having wider partial coating width of 34μm. The divergent angle at higher power level(300mW) becomes wider(3.7°) in spite of as narrow as 0.7° at lower power (50mW). The divergent angle of 0.7° in FAHM does not correspond to the diffraction limit from 150μm waveguide and is slightly wide. When wider partial coatings were employed, the FFPs were not only improved but also defective at lower power. Inhomogeneities of layers or spatial hole burnings may prevent lasers from single transverse mode oscillation.

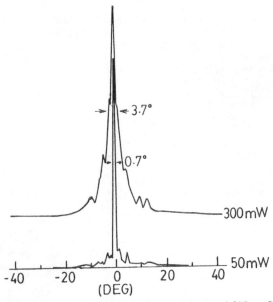

Fig. 8   FFP obtained for the partial coating width of 34μm.

Comparison with Calculation

Figure 9 shows power distribution of the fundamental mode calculated by using a simple model in which the mode propagates in waveguide whose width is 150μm and diffracts at every slit whose width is 2B(20μm). Here, separation between the slits corresponds to 2L(1000μm) and number of slits is 100. Although there are some ripple on the curve, curve looks like a Gaussian. This result suggests that mode propagating in the active region has not an eigenmode of the waveguide but slit-limited narrow mode.

As reflectivity at output facet has spatial distribution, at least, intensity profile of the output beam must be deformed. These phenomena might give some reasonable explanation on low level satellite peaks in FFPs as shown in Figs. 7 and 8.

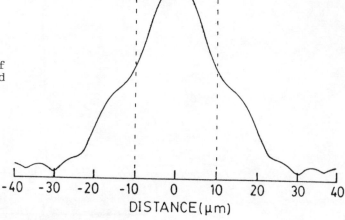

Fig. 9 Optical power distribution of the fundamental mode calculated by a slit model.

4. Conclusion

We have demonstrated two types of modal-filter-loaded high power diode lasers. A narrow region formed in an active waveguide of the F-SBA laser has an obvious effect as the modal filter applicable to inside of a laser chip. Partial coating on the output facet of the laser has clear mode selection effects as modal filter. One could expect to get higher power in the fundamental transverse mode by employing both the filters to one chip.

The high power laser diodes applied by these kinds of modal filters will become important key devices in the fields of the end-pumping for solid-state laser and some other applications.

References

1) H. Naito, M. Kume, K. Hamada, H. Shimizu and G. Kano, "High Reliable CW Operation of 100mW GaAlAs Buried Twin Ridge Substrate Lasers with Nonabsorbing-Mirrors", 11th IEEE Int'l Semiconductor Laser Conf. (held at Boston, U.S.A., Sept. 1988), L-2, p.p. 150-151.
2) D. Botez, L.J. Mawst, P. Hayashida, G. Peterson and T.J. Roth, "High-Power diffraction-Limited beam Operation from Phase-Locked Diode-Laser Array of Closely Spaced "Leaky" Waveguides (Antiguides)", Appl. Phys. Lett., vol. 53, (1988), p.p. 464-466.
3) E.M. Garmire, "Tolerances for Phase Locking of Semiconductor Laser Arrays", Proceedings of SPIE vol. 893, High Power Laser Diodes and Applications (1988) p.p. 91-99
4) Y. Seiwa, S. Hinata, T. Aoyagi, T. Kadowaki, N. Kaneno, and K. Ikeda, "Achiving a Stable Fundamental Supermode in Phased-Array Lasers up to High Power", Tech. Digest, CLEO'86, TUM5, 1986.
5) J. Ohsawa, S. Hinata, T. Aoyagi, T. Kadowaki, N. Kaneno, K. Ikeda and W. Susaki, "Triple-Stripe Phase-Locked Diode Lasers Emitting 100mW CW with Single-Lobed Far-Field Patterns", Elec. Lett., vol. 21 (1985), p.p. 779-780.
6) N. Kaneno, T. Kadowaki, J. ohsawa, T. Aoyagi, S. Hinata, K. Ikeda and W. Susaki, "Phased Array of AlGaAs Multistripe Index-Guided Lasers", Elec. Lett., vol. 21 (1985), p.p. 780-781.
7) K. Ikeda, H. Kumabe, H. Namizaki and W. Susaki, "High Power Diode Laser Research in Mitsubishi Electric", Proc. of SPIE vol. 893, High Power Laser Diodes and Applications (1988), p.p. 79-83.
8) D.F. Welch, P.S. Cross, D.R. Scifres, W. Streifer, and R.D. Burnham, "High Power, AlGaAs Buried Heterostructure Lasers with Flared Waveguides", Appl. Phys. Lett., vol. 50, (1987), p.p. 233-235.
9) K. Shigihara, T. Aoyagi, S. Hinata, Y. Nagai, Y. Mihashi, Y. Seiwa, K. Ikeda and W. Susaki, "High Power and Fundamental Mode Oscillating Flared SBA Lasers", Elec. Lett., vol. 24 (1988), p. 1182.
10) J. Wittke and I. Ladany, "Lateral Mode Selection in Semiconductor Injection Lasers", J. Appl. Phys., vol. 48, (1977), p.p. 3122-3124.
11) C. Ninagawa, Y. Miyazaki and Y. Akao, "Mirror Reflectivity Dependence of Transverse-Modes in Semiconductor Lasers", JPN. J. Appl. Phys., vol. 18, (1979), p.p. 967-974.
12) A.K. Chan, H.F. Taylor and C.P. Lai, "Designs for High Power, Single Mode Operation in Broad Stripe Semiconductor Lasers", Proc. of SPIE vol. 893, High power Laser Diodes and Applications (1988), p.p. 38-45.
13) T. Aoyagi, S. Hinata, K. Shigihara, Y. Seiwa, K. Ikeda and W. Susaki, "High Power Operation of Long-Cavity Phase-Locked Laser Array2, Elec. Lett., vol. 22, (1987), p.p. 1396-1397.

Fundamental Lateral-mode Operation in Broad-area Lasers Having Built-in Lens-like Refractive Index Distributions

Shin'ichi NAKATSUKA and Kimio TATSUNO
Central Research Laboratory, Hitachi, Ltd.
1-280 Higashi-Koigakubo, Kokubunji-shi, Tokyo 185, Japan

ABSTRACT

High power fundamental lateral-mode operation up to 80 mW in CW condition is achieved in a broad-area laser diode. This diode has built-in lens-like effective refractive index distributions in the direction perpendicular to the laser beam. These distributions effectively suppress higher order lateral-mode generation.

INTRODUCTION

Recently, much effort has been made to develop high-power fundamental lateral-mode laser diodes operating at light output powers of several hundred mWs. One approach is the phase-locked array. However, light output powers achieved for continuous-wave (CW) fundamental lateral mode operation in such lasers has been limited to around 100 mW due to difficulty in suppressing the higher order super mode generation.

Another approach is single quantum well broad-area lasers. They are free from filamentary oscillation caused by self-focusing since the effective refractive index in the direction parallel to the junction plane has little dependence on the active layer's refractive index modulation. However, their fundamental mode output power under continuous operation has been limited to a few mW because they require a high nominal current density to obtain sufficient gain.

On the other hand, some authors have reported new methods to achieve fundamental lateral mode operation in broad-area lasers theoretically and experimentally. These methods utilize gain or refractive index distribution in the laser stripe resulting from laser heating, patterned electrodes, or curved facets.

This paper reports on the fundamental lateral-mode operation of a broad-area laser diode having built-in lens-like effective refractive index distributions in the direction perpendicular to the laser beam.

LASER STRUCTURE

The laser structure is shown in Fig. 1. The lens-like structures are in the p-Al Ga As cladding layer. The structures expand the laser beam in the direction parallel to the junction and suppress higher order mode oscillation.

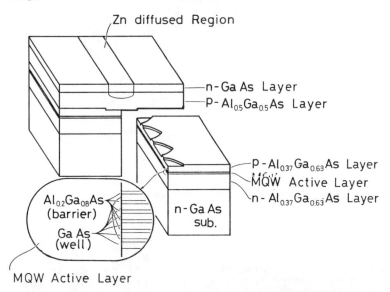

Fig. 1 Schematics of broad-area laser with built-i lens-like refractive index distributions.

The idea of beam expansion to suppress higher order lateral mode oscillation is similar to that of using an unstable resonator cavity in laser diodes. However, such diodes require a special technique such as reactive ion beam etching to fabricate the curved mirror facets. The present structure has no such requirement and is easy to fabricate.

The lasers were fabricated using a conventional two-step atmospheric pressure MOCVD technique. In the first growth step, an n-GaAs buffer layer, an n-$Al_{0.37}Ga_{0.63}As$ cladding layer (1.5 μm thick), a multiple quantum well active layer (six 10nm-thick GaAs well layers and six 4nm-thick $Al_{0.2}Ga_{0.8}As$ barrier layers), and a p-$Al_{0.37}Ga_{0.63}As$ cladding layer (0.4 μm thick) were fabricated on an n-GaAs substrate.

Convex lens patterns were made using conventional photo lithography. These patterns, each one of which consisted of two parabolic lines whose radius of curvatur was 40 μm, were placed every 20 μm in the stripe. The lens region of the p-$Al_{0.37}Ga_{0.63}As$ cladding layer was etched down. Lasers having lens etching depths of 0.15 μm and 0.3 μm were fabricated. Lasers without lens were also made for comparison.

Then, these structures were buried in a 1.5 um thick p-$Al_{0.5}Ga_{0.5}As$ layer and a 0.4 μm thick n-GaAs cap layer using the MOCVD technique. Next, Zn was diffused through the n-GaAs cap layer into the p-$Al_{0.5}Ga_{0.5}As$ layer in the stripe region to form a current path. The stripe width was about 40 μm. In the next step, p and n electrodes were evaporated on both sides of the wafer. After that, the wafer was cleaved into 400 um cavity length chips. Then, reflection and anti-reflection coatings were applied to the laser facets. The reflectivities of the front and rear facets were 8% and 90%, respectively.

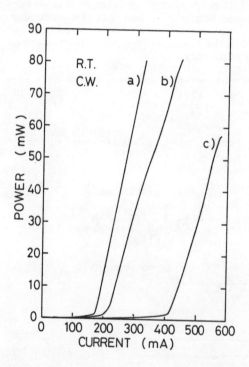

Fig. 2 Light output power versus current characteristics of broad-area lasers.

(a) without lens
(b) with 0.15 μm-deep lens
(c) 0.3 μm-deep lens

LASER CHARACTERISTICS

The light output power versus the current characteristics of the lasers (a) without lenses, (b) with a 0.15 μm-deep lens, and (c) with a 0.3 μm-deep lens, under room-temperature CW operation, are shown in Fig. 2. The refractive index step difference between the inside and outside of the lenses were about 1×10^{-3} and 5×10^{-3} for (b) and (c), respectively. The threshold current of lasers (a), (b) and (c) were 170, 210 and 420 mA, respectively. It can be seen in the figure that the laser threshold current increased with the lens depth. This may be caused by a cavity loss increase with beam expansion.

Despite the good linearity of the lensless laser's L-I characteristics as shown in Fig. 2 (a), the emitting beam consisted of many lateral modes. This was confirmed by measuring spectra-resolved far-field patterns. The far-field and near-field patterns of the laser with the 0.15 μm-deep lens are shown in Fig. 3. Narrow single-lobe far-field patterns up to 80 mW were obtained under CW operation, as shown in Fig. 3 (a). The full width at half maximum (FWHM) of the far-field pattern was about 3 degrees. This is almost double the diffraction limited angle of a 40-μm-wide broad-area laser.

The near-field pattern had a single lobe shape, as shown in Fig. 3 (b). The spectrum of this laser showed a single longitudinal mode at light output below 80 mW.

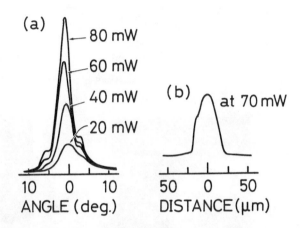

Fig. 3 Far-field and near-field patterns of broad-area laser with 0.15 μm-deep lens.

  (a) Far-field patterns at light output powers of 20, 40, 60, and 80 mW
  (b) Near-field pattern at light output power of 70 mW

For the laser with the 0.3 μm-deep lens, lateral mode deformation took place at an output power exceeding 20 mW, as can be seen in Fig. 4 (a). Corresponding to the far-field pattern change, the near-field pattern of the laser changed as shown in Figures 4 (b) and 4 (c).

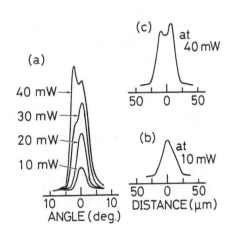

Fig. 4 Far-field and near-field patterns of broad-area laser with 0.3 μm-deep lens.

  (a) Far-field patterns at light output powers of 10, 20, 30, and 40 mW
  (b) Near-field pattern at light output power of 10 mW
  (c) Near-field pattern at light output power of 40 mW

PHASE FRONT OBSEBATION

To confirm the fundamental lateral mode operation of the lasers with the lens structures, wave front observations were carried out with a Mach-Zehnder interferometer (MZI). The interference pattern of the laser with the 0.15 µm-deep lens at an output power of 70 mW, just below the maximum output level, is shown in Fig. 5 (a). No phase shift in the wave-front was observed in this figure (The finer patterns in the photograph were caused by interfernce of the optical systems). This indicates the laser diode operated in the spatially coherent fundamental lateral mode. The astigmatism of the laser diode was measured by the MZI method as previously reported. For this laser, the astigmatic distance was about 90 µm.

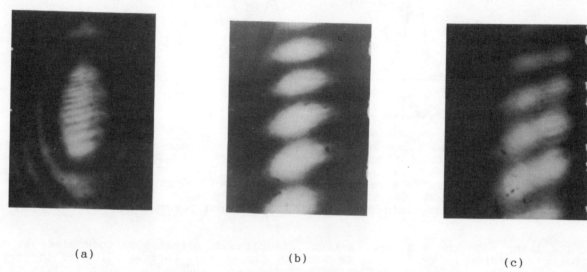

(a)   (b)   (c)

Fig. 5 Mach-Zehnder interference patterns of lasers

        (a) with 0.15 µm-deep lens at 70 mW
        (b) with 0.3 µm-deep lens at 10 mW
        (c) with 0.3 µm-deep lens at 40 mW

The interference patterns for the laser with the 0.3 µm-deep lens at light output powers of 10 and 40 mWs, respectively, are presented in Figures 5 (b) and (c). No phase shift is observed in Fig. 5 (b). This shows that the fundamental mode operation was also attained at a lower output range. However, beam shape distortion took place with an output power increase in this laser, as shown in Fig. 5 (c).

CONCLUSION

In conclusion, the fundamental lateral-mode oscillation in an broad-area laser having built-in lens-like refractive index distributions in the stripe has been attained for the first time. The lens-like refractive index distributions expand the laser beam to suppress the higher lateral mode. Moreover, fundamental lateral-mode oscillation at light output power of up to 80 mW has been achieved under room-temperature CW operation in the case of a laser with a 0.15 µm-deep lens. The fundamental lateral mode operation was confirmed with a Mach-Zehnder interferometer. The astigmatism of this laser was also investigated and found to be about 90 µm. The laser is simple in design and easy to fabricate. Therefore, it is a very promising one as a high power light source for various applications.

REFERANCE

1) S. Wang, J. Wilcox, M. Jansen, and J. Yang, Appl. Phys. Lett. 48, 1770 (1986)
2) S. Mukai, L. Katz, E. Kapon, Z. Rav-Noy, S. Marglit, and A. Yariv, Appl. Phys. Lett. 45, 834 (1984)

3) D. Welch, P. Cross, D. Scifres, W. Streifer, and R. Burnham, Appl. Phys. Lett. 49, 1632 (1986)
4) W. Tsang, Electro. Lett. 16, 939 (1980)
5) A. Larsson, J. Salzman, M. Mittelstein, and A. Yariv, Electro. Lett. 16, 79 (1986)
6) A. Chan, C. Lai, and H. Taylor, IEEE J. Quant. Electron. 24, 489 (1988)
7) J. Hohimer, G. Hadley, and A. Owyoung, Appl. Phys. Lett. 52, 260 (1988)
8) C. Lindsey, P. Derry, and A. Yariv, Electron. Lett. 21, 671 (1985)
9) A. Bogatov, P.Eliseev, M. Man'ko, G. Mikaelyan, and Y. Popov, Sov. Phys. Quant. Electro. 10, 620 (1980)
10) J. Salzman, A. Yariv, Appl. Phys. Lett. 49, 440 (1986)
11) K. Tatsuno, A. Arimoto, Appl. Optics 20 (20), 3520 (1981)
12) K. Tatsuno, et. al., Tech. digest CLEO'88 (Anaheim), 190 (1988)

Invited Paper

Two-Dimensional Surface-Emitting Arrays of GaAs/AlGaAs Diode Lasers

J. P. Donnelly, K. Rauschenbach, C. A. Wang, W. D. Goodhue and R. J. Bailey

Lincoln Laboratory, Massachusetts Institute of Technology
Lexington, MA 02173-0073

ABSTRACT

Three approaches to fabricating two-dimensional surface-emitting GaAs/AlGaAs diode laser arrays are discussed: a hybrid approach in which linear arrays of edge-emitting lasers with cleaved end facets are mounted on microchanneled Si heatsinks with integral 45° deflecting mirrors, a monolithic approach in which edge-emitting lasers are fabricated with deflecting mirrors adjacent to both end facets of each laser, and a monolithic approach in which horizontal-cavity lasers are fabricated with intracavity 45° deflecting mirrors. In both monolithic approaches, all the laser facets and deflecting mirrors are fabricated by ion-beam-assisted etching.

1. INTRODUCTION

Arrays of GaAs/AlGaAs diode lasers are currently of great interest, and several different approaches to developing such arrays are being investigated.[1-10] In this paper, a hybrid and two monolithic approaches to fabricating two-dimensional surface-emitting GaAs/AlGaAs laser diode arrays are discussed.

2. HYBRID SURFACE-EMITTING ARRAYS

A hybrid two-dimensional diode laser array[2,3] for high-power operation is illustrated in Fig. 1. The array consists of linear arrays of edge-emitting lasers with conventional cleaved end facets that are mounted in grooves with flat bottoms and 45° sidewalls etched in a Si substrate containing microchannels[11-15] for cooling fluid flow. The Cu bar on top of each linear array provides high electrical conductivity along the array.

The flat-bottom grooves with 45° sidewalls are etched in (100) Si by means of standard photolithography and an orientation-selective etch. A stripe pattern oriented in an (013) direction is first defined in a Si_3N_4 capping layer that serves as an etch mask. The Si is then etched in a KOH-isopropanol-H_2O solution at 80°C. The bottom (100) Si plane etches about 2.5 times faster than the (331) sidewalls. A sawed cross section of an etched groove is shown in Fig. 2(a). Since the etch ratio is only 2.5, the actual angles between the sidewalls and the top and bottom are closer to 45° than the theoretical angle of 46.5° between (331) and (100) planes. Fig. 2(b) shows a top view of a test GaAs/AlGaAs linear array mounted in a metallized groove. Reflections of the cleaved end facets of the GaAs/AlGaAs bar are clearly visible in the 45° deflecting mirrors.

Microchannels are cut into the bottom of the Si heatsink using a dicing saw. Figure 3 is a photomicrograph of the sawed cross section of a portion of a hybrid array showing a linear array mounted in an etched groove in a microchannel Si heatsink. The sawed microchannels are 100-µm wide on a 200-µm period. The top Cu conductor is tapered so it will not block any of the light emerging from the surface of the array.

The linear arrays used in the hybrid arrays are fabricated from GaAs/AlGaAs wafers that contain a single quantum-well symmetrically positioned in a large optical cavity. Following deposition of a top ohmic contact, 40-µm-wide stripe lasers on 250-µm centers are defined by a proton bombardment that penetrates to a depth approximately 0.2 µm above the top of the large optical cavity. A second proton bombardment at higher energies is performed to introduce sufficient optical loss in 10-µm stripes midway between the lasers to suppress lasing in the transverse direction. After the wafers are thinned to about 75 µm and ohmic contacts made to the n^+–GaAs substrates, linear arrays of the appropriate length are cleaved from the wafers.

Since separate-confinement quantum-well (SCH-QW) lasers have very low internal loss, it is advantageous from overall efficiency considerations to use linear arrays with longer cavities[16] than the 400 µm used in our initial demonstration (Ref. 2 and Figs. 2 and 3). Long cavities also increase the ratio of linear array area to total surface area of the hybrid array, an important advantage when heat removal capabilities are considered. Figure 4 is a photomicrograph of a hybrid array with eight 1-cm-long linear arrays with 720-μm laser cavities soldered in eight grooves on a microchanneled Si heatsink. The linear arrays have a top Pt layer that facilitates the soldering of the top Cu contacting bars. In this design, the 45° deflecting mirrors use only a small portion of the total active area, which is about 1 cm^2. The flat lip around the edge of the Si heatsink is used in mounting the array in a cooling fixture.

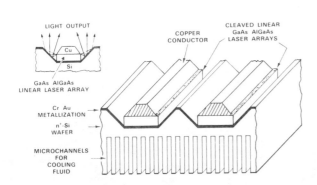

Fig. 1. Schematic diagram of hybrid two-dimensional surface-emitting diode laser array.

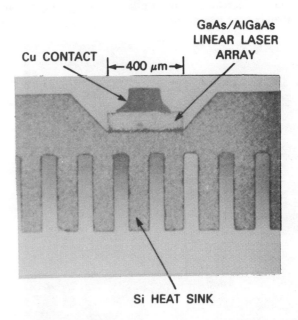

Fig. 3. Sawed cross section of a linear array with top Cu conductor mounted in an etched groove in a microchannel Si heatsink.

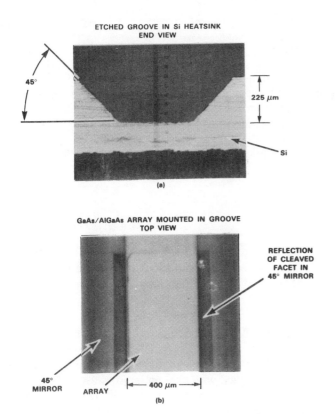

Fig. 2. (a) Sawed cross section of groove with flat bottom and 45° sidewalls etched in Si. (b) Top view of linear laser array mounted in metallized Si groove. Reflections of cleaved end facets of the linear array can be seen in the 45° deflecting mirrors.

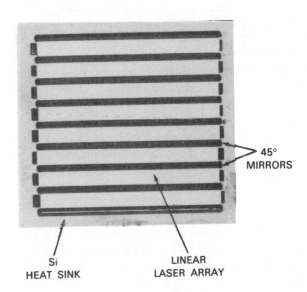

Fig. 4. Top view of eight 1-cm-long linear arrays with 720-μm cavities mounted on a microchannel Si heatsink. The metallized 45° deflecting mirrors (one on each side) are between the Pt-coated linear arrays and at each end. The flat outer lip is used for mounting purposes.

The near-field pattern of the laser emission from a completed 1-cm^2 hybrid array is shown in Fig. 5. The pulsed output power from several hybrid arrays was measured with all the linear arrays in parallel and also with each one driven separately. Because of limitations in current available from the pulser, higher output power per laser could be obtained by driving the linear arrays one at a time. Figure 6 shows output power vs pulsed current for the linear arrays with the highest and lowest overall differential quantum efficiencies. The average threshold current per laser for all the linear array bars was about 125 mA. Overall differential quantum efficiencies η_D ranged from 58 to 75%. Four of the eight linear arrays had η_D greater than 70% and all but one had η_D greater than 60%. Quasi-cw and cw measurements are underway.

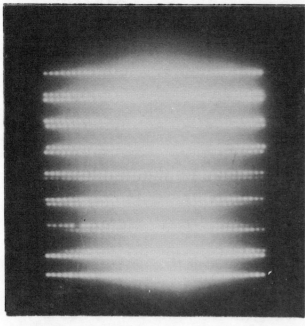

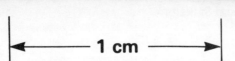

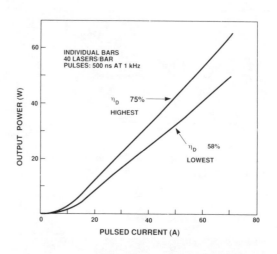

Fig. 6. Pulsed output power vs current for the linear arrays with the highest and lowest differential quantum efficiencies of a 1-cm^2 hybrid array composed of 8 linear arrays.

Fig. 5. Near-field pattern of a 1-cm^2 hybrid two-dimensional surface-emitting laser array with eight 1-cm-long GaAs/AlGaAs linear arrays.

Although all of the linear arrays are driven in parallel on the hybrid arrays presented here, it should be possible to drive them in series or series/parallel combination by using high-resistivity Si and/or selective implantation and metallization to electrically insulate the linear arrays from one another. It should also be possible to mount the lasers junction-side down by mounting the arrays on a pedestal and/or tapering the back of the arrays.

3. MONOLITHIC SURFACE-EMITTING DIODE LASER ARRAYS

Monolithic two-dimensional arrays of GaAs/AlGaAs diode lasers with light emission normal to the surface have been obtained by fabricating horizontal-cavity edge-emitting quantum-well lasers coupled with external mirrors that deflect the radiation from the laser facets by 90°.[9,10] In addition, several preliminary surface-emitting arrays with intracavity 45° deflecting mirrors[17-19] have been fabricated. In both types of arrays, all the laser facets and deflecting mirrors were formed by ion-beam-assisted etching (IBAE), a dry etching technique in which the chemically reactant species and the energetic ions can be independently controlled.[20-23]

The basic IBAE system has been described by Geis et al.[20]. Figure 7 is a schematic illustration of an IBAE system, with a load-lock, tiltable sample holder, cold trap and cryopump, that routinely reaches a background pressure of 10^{-7} Torr 15 min after sample loading. In this system, a chemically reactant species from a local jet and a separately controlled collimated ion beam from an ion source impinge simultaneously upon the sample. Both GaAs and AlGaAs can be etched at room temperature using Cl_2 as the reactant gas and argon as the source of ions. Since neither GaAs or AlGaAs is spontaneously etched by Cl_2 at room temperature, IBAE in this material system is highly directional and is determined essentially by the direction of the argon ion beam. Therefore almost any concave shape can be generated by using a computer-controlled sample stage that precisely varies the tilt angle between the sample and the ion beam.[22,23] Materials such as photoresist, phosphosilicate glass (PSG) and Ni, which have slow etch rates compared to GaAs, can be used as etch masks.

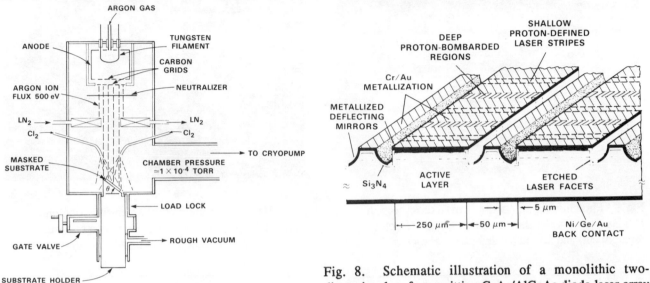

Fig. 7. Schematic of Cl_2-IBAE etching system.

Fig. 8. Schematic illustration of a monolithic two-dimensional surface-emitting GaAs/AlGaAs diode laser array with external cavity parabolic deflecting mirrors.

3.1 MONOLITHIC ARRAYS WITH EXTERNAL-CAVITY DEFLECTING MIRRORS

Monolithic two-dimensional surface-emitting GaAs diode laser arrays have been fabricated by using a combination of straight and angled IBAE to produce arrays of edge-emitting separate-confinement quantum-well lasers with deflecting mirrors adjacent to the laser facets, as shown schematically in Fig. 8. With photoresist as an etch mask, IBAE was used to etch pairs of straight-sided grooves 2 μm wide and 3-4 μm deep. The outer walls of each pair act as the facets for rows of laser cavities that are 250 μm long. Lines approximately 3 μm wide immediately adjacent to the inside edge of one of the grooves in each pair were then opened in a new layer of photoresist, and parabolic deflectors for one side of each row were formed by computer-controlled angled IBAE. The deflectors for the other side of each row were formed in a similar manner. Figure 9 is a photomicrograph of the cleaved cross section of an IBAE etched laser array wafer. The straight sidewall is the laser facet and the curved sidewall is the deflecting mirror.

The near-field pattern of a 100-element two-dimensional surface-emitting array is shown in Fig. 10. A shallow proton bombardment was used to confine the current to 40-μm-wide stripes on 180-μm centers, while a deep proton bombardment midway between the laser stripes was used to introduce sufficient optical loss to suppress transverse lasing. Futher details of the fabrication are given in Ref 9. The pulsed output power vs current for this array is plotted in Fig. 11. The power is limited to 15 W by the available pulsed current of 62 A. The output power vs current for an array consisting of only two rows, a total of 20 elements, fabricated from the same wafer is shown in Fig. 12. This smaller array has a pulsed power output of 16.5 W at 62 A, which corresponds to a power density of 1.5 kW/cm^2.

The external differential quantum efficiency of these arrays is about 20%. Several factors can limit the external quantum efficiency, including the quality of laser facets, the beam divergence of the laser emission and the effective F-number of the deflecting mirrors. The latter two affect the fraction of light emitted from the laser facets that is deflected by the deflecting mirrors. Although the quality of the laser facets can be a problem, this fraction is currently the major limitation on the external differential quantum efficiency. Several obvious changes can be made to increase the fraction of light collected and make this fraction less dependent on process variables. The first is to use laser material with a smaller output beam

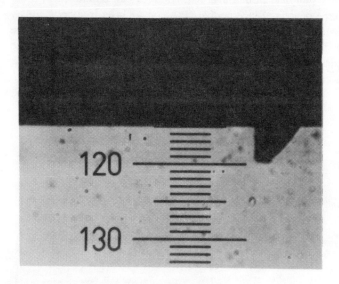

Fig. 9. Photomicrograph of the cleaved cross section of a laser array wafer showing an etched laser facet (straight cut) and the curved deflecting mirror.

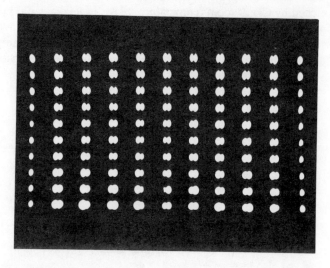

Fig. 10. Near-field pattern of 100-element monolithic surface-emitting GaAs/AlGaAs diode laser array with external-cavity deflecting mirrors.

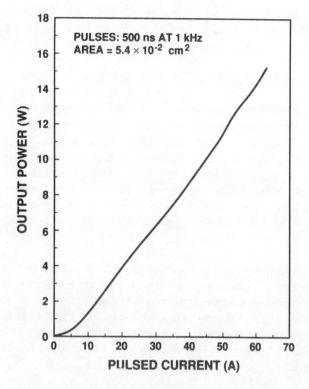

Fig. 11. Pulsed output power vs current for the 100-element array whose near-field pattern is shown in Fig. 10.

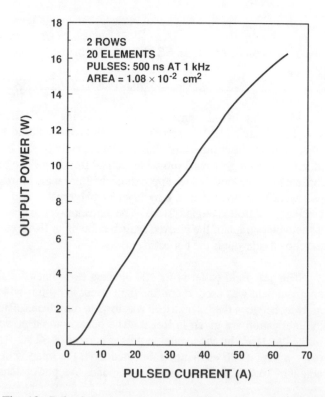

Fig. 12. Pulsed output power vs current for 20-element array.

divergence. Graded-index separate-confinement single-quantum-well laser material (GRIN-SCH-QW) is now being grown from which cleaved-facet lasers with less than a 35° beam divergence (full width at half maximum) have been fabricated. These lasers have differential quantum efficiencies greater than 75% which is higher than that of the lasers in the array whose near-field pattern is shown in Fig. 10. By making the junction slightly deeper (2.5 to 3 μm deep instead of 2 μm) and the facet etch narrower (1 to 1.5 μm wide instead of 2 μm), the collection efficiency of the deflecting mirrors should increase and become more tolerant of photolithograhic and etching inaccuracies. With these changes, it should be possible to fabricate parabolic deflecting mirrors with effective F- numbers less than one and arrays with external quantum efficiencies greater than 50%. A design of an integral parabolic deflecting mirror with an F- number less than 0.85 is shown in Fig. 13.

3.2 MONOLITHIC ARRAYS WITH INTRACAVITY DEFLECTING MIRRORS

Monolithic two-dimensional surface-emitting arrays with intracavity 45° mirrors, as illustrated in Fig. 14, have been fabricated using a combination of straight and 45° IBAE. The arrays were etched using one photolithography step. With photoresist as an etch mask, IBAE was used to etch straight-sided grooves 6 μm wide. Without removing the sample from the etch chamber, the sample was tilted at a 45° angle and the 45° intracavity mirrors etched.

The near-field pattern of a 100-element array is shown in Fig. 15. There is one bad element in the fourth row and some scattering in the fifth row. All the other lasers are operational. The pulsed output power vs current for the first row of the array (20 elements) is shown in Fig. 16. The average threshold current is high, about 1 A per laser, and the differential quantum efficiency is low, about 4%. One factor degrading the performance of this first array is the optical loss in the p^+-GaAs capping layer, which was not removed from the window region. Arrays are presently being fabricated with the capping layer removed.

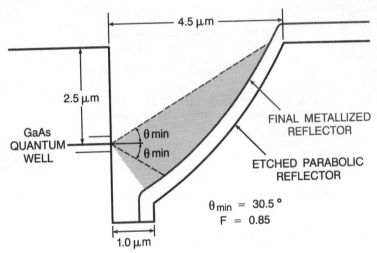

Fig. 13. Illustration of an external-cavity deflecting mirror with an effective F-number less than 0.85.

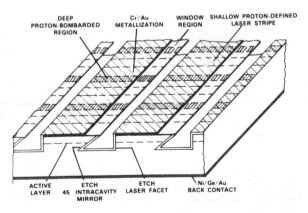

Fig. 14. Schematic illustration of a monolithic two-dimensional surface-emitting GaAs/AlGaAs diode laser array with intracavity 45° deflecting mirrors.

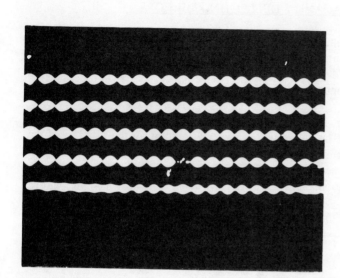

Fig. 15. Near-field pattern of 100-element monolithic surface-emitting GaAs/AlGaAs diode laser array with intracavity 45° deflecting mirrors.

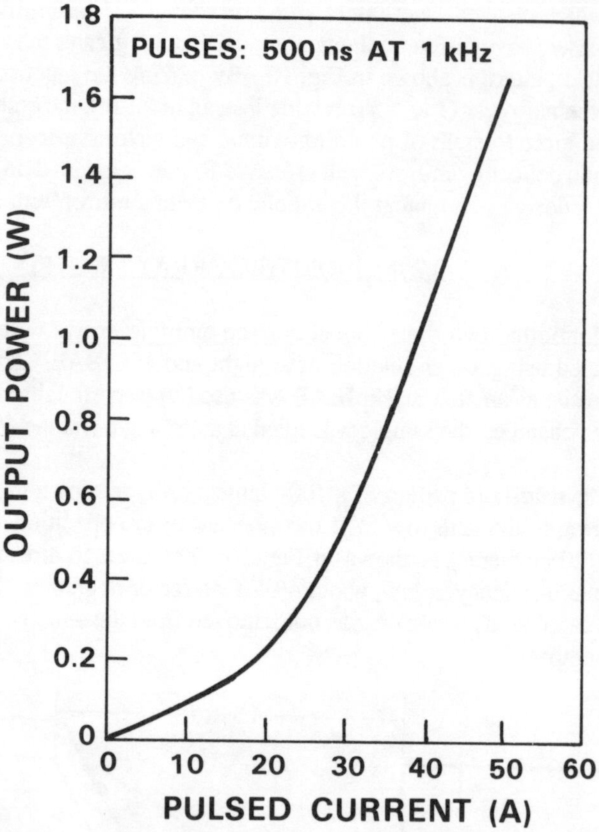

Fig. 16. Pulsed output power vs current for one row (20 elements) of the array whose near-field pattern is shown in Fig. 15.

4. SUMMARY

Three different approaches to fabricating two-dimensional surface-emitting GaAs/AlGaAs diode laser arrays have been discussed.

Large 1-cm^2 hybrid arrays have been fabricated. These arrays consist of linear laser arrays with conventional cleaved end facets mounted on Si microchannel heatsinks with integral 45° mirrors that deflect the laser radiation by 90°. Arrays of this type should be capable of 100-200 W/cm^2 cw and 500-1000 W/cm^2 pulsed.

Two monolithic approaches were presented. The first uses edge-emitting lasers with external-cavity deflecting mirrors adjacent to the laser facets. Both the laser facets and deflecting mirrors were etched by ion-beam-assisted etching. 100-element arrays capable of pulsed output powers greater than 1 kW/cm^2 have been fabricated.

Some preliminary results on monolithic arrays with intracavity 45° deflecting mirrors were also presented. Although the threshold currents and differential quantum efficiencies obtained on these initial intracavity deflecting mirror arrays were poor compared to those obtained on the external-cavity deflecting mirror arrays, they are somewhat easier to fabricate and are worth further investigation.

The authors wish to thank G. A. Simpson, G. A. Ferrante, G. D. Johnson, D. A. Seielstad, F. J. O'Donnell, C. D. Hoyt, D. B. Hoyt, L. J. Missaggia, J. N. Walpole, D. M. Tracy, J. D. Woodhouse and M. D. McAleese for technical assistance. This work was sponsored by the Departments of the Navy for SDIO and the Air Force.

5. REFERENCES

1. D. F. Welch, W. Streifer, R. L. Thornton and D. R. Scifres, Electron. Lett. 24, 113 (1988).
2. J. P. Donnelly, R. J. Bailey, C. A. Wang, G. A. Simpson and K. Rauschenbach, Appl. Phys. Lett. 53, 938 (1988).
3. J. P. Donnelly, R. J. Bailey, C. A. Wang, G. A. Simpson and K. Rauschenbach, Proc. 11th IEEE International Semiconductor Laser Conference, Aug. 29-Sept. 1, 1988 (IEEE, Piscataway, 1988), p. 170.
4. K. Iga, S. Kinoshita and F. Koyama, Electron. Lett. 23, 134 (1987).
5. G. A. Evans, N. W. Carlson, J. M. Hammer, M. Lurie, J. K. Butler, L. A. Carr, F. Z. Hawrylo, E. A. James, G. J. Kaiser, J. B. Kirk, W. F. Reichert, S. R. Chinn and P. S. Fory, Appl. Phys. Lett. 52, 1037 (1988).
6. A. J. SpringThorpe, Appl. Phys. Lett. 31, 524 (1979).
7. T. H. Windhorn and W. D. Goodhue, Appl. Phys. Lett. 48, 1675 (1986).
8. J. J. Yang, M. Sergant, M. Jansan, S. S. Ou, L. Eaton and W. W. Simmons, Appl. Phys. Lett. 49, 1138 (1986).
9. J. P. Donnelly, W. G. Goodhue, T. H. Windhorn, R. J. Bailey and S. A. Lambert, Appl. Phys. Lett. 51, 1138 (1987).
10. J. P. Donnelly, W. D. Goodhue, K. Rauschenbach, D. A. Seielstad, C. A. Wang and R. J. Bailey, presented at IEEE Laser and Electro-optic Society 1988 LEOS Annual Meeting, Nov. 2-4, 1988, Santa Clara, paper ThW. 4.
11. D. B. Tuckerman and R. F. W. Pease, IEEE Electron. Device Lett. EDL-2, 126 (1981).
12. R. J. Philips, The Lincoln Laboratory Journal 1, 31 (1988).
13. J. N. Walpole, Z. . Liau, V. Diadiuk and L. J. Missaggia, presented at IEEE Laser and Electro-optic Society 1988 LEOS Annual Meeting, Nov. 2-4, 1988, Santa Clara, paper ThW.4; see also, J. N. Walpole, Proc. SPIE. High Power Laser Diodes and Applications, vol. 893, 131 (1988).
14. L. J. Missaggia, J. N. Walpole and Z. L. Liau, to be published.
15. D. Mundinger, R. Beach, W. Benett, R. Solarz, W. Krupke, R. Staven and D. Tuckerman, Appl. Phys. Lett. 53, 1030 (1988).
16. J. Z. Wilcox, G. L. Peterson, S. Ou, J. J. Yang, M. Jansen and D. Schechter, Electron. Lett., 24, 1218 (1988).
17. J. J. Yang, L. Lee, M. Jansen, M. Sergant, S. J. Ou and J. Wilcox, Proc. SPIE - High Power Laser Diodes and Applications, vol. 893, 181 (1988).
18. T. Yuasa, H. Hamao, M. Sugimoto, N. Takadu, M. Vero, H. Iwatta, Y. Tashiro, K. Onobe and K. Asakawa, Tech. Summary of Conference on Laser and Electro-optics (CLEO'88), Apr. 25-29, 1988 (Optical Society of America, Washington, 1988), p. 258.
19. T. Takamori, L. A. Coldren and J. L. Merz, to be presented at Topical Meeting on Integrated and Guided Wave Optics (IGWO '89), Feb. 6-8, 1989, Houston, paper MCC 6.
20. M. W. Geis, G. A. Lincoln, N. Etremow and W. J. Pracentini, J. Vac. Sci. Technol. 19, 1390 (1981).
21. G. A. Lincoln, M. W. Geis, S. Pang and N. N. Efremow, J. Vac. Sci. Technol. B 1, 1043 (1983).
22. W. D. Goodhue, G. D. Johnson and T. H. Windhorn, in <u>Gallium Arsenide and Related Compounds 1986</u>, ed. by W. T. Lindley (Int. Phys. Conf. Ser. 83, Bristol, 1987), p. 349.
23. W. D. Goodhue, S. Pang, M. A. Hollis and J. P. Donnelly, Proc. IEEE/Cornell Conf. on Advanced Concepts in High Speed Semiconductor Devices and Circuits (IEEE, New York, 1987), p. 239.

Mode control of an array of AlGaAs lasers using a spatial filter in a Talbot cavity

F.X. D'Amato, E.T. Siebert, and C. Roychoudhuri

The Perkin-Elmer Corporation
100 Wooster Heights Road, Danbury, CT. 06810

1. INTRODUCTION

Coherence between elements of a laser diode array can be established either by coupling the individual oscillators together on-chip or by coupling the array as a whole to an external cavity. Several techniques for on-chip coupling have been demonstrated[1,2,3], however these approaches typically produce a output having low Strehl ratio due to the difficulty of maintaining adequate control of the phase and amplitude of the emitters across the length of the chip. Several authors have reported phase locking of small laser diode arrays by placing the diode array in an external cavity and making use of a spatial filter in a Fourier transform plane of the array to force mutual coherence between the diodes[4,5,6]. This technique works well for relatively small arrays, but becomes impractical for large scale arrays. Recently an external cavity technique has been demonstrated that takes advantage of the Talbot self-imaging effect[7] to phase lock an array of laser oscillators[8,9,10,11,12]. A significant advantage of the Talbot cavity as opposed to previous external cavity approaches is that the Talbot cavity can be scaled to accommodate arrays containing a large number of lasers if attention is paid to control of the oscillating modes of the array. In this paper we demonstrate how mode control of an array of diode lasers in a Talbot cavity can be achieved through the use of intracavity spatial filters or phase masks.

The Talbot (or "Self-Imaging") cavity makes use of the diffractive properties of the Fresnel (near-field) zone of a periodic array of coherent sources, which has a set of characteristic self-image planes associated with it. At distances $2nD^2/\lambda$ from the array an image of the array is formed (D is the separation between elements in the source array and n is an integer). In addition to these planes, there also exists a set of planes at distances $D^2/m\lambda$ (m=1,2,3,...) from the source array in which multiple images of the source are formed, we refer to these planes as "sub-image planes." In the "m-th" sub-image plane, "m" separate images of the source array are formed, the different images having relative phase shifts between them. Figure 1 shows the locations of the first few image planes and the relative phases of the images in the planes.

2. TALBOT CAVITY WITH SPATIAL FILTERS

The Talbot cavity as discussed by previous authors[8-10] consists of a flat mirror placed a distance D^2/λ from an array of lasers. Analysis of the normal modes of this cavity indicates that in general more than one array mode can oscillate within the cavity. Figure 1 shows the effective level of cavity feedback (as defined by the solutions of the eigenvalue equation in reference 9) for the normal modes of a 30 element array of laser diodes for which the ratio of diode separation to diode width parameter is 10:1. In this case the lowest order mode of the array (in which all the diodes oscillate in phase) and the highest order array mode (adjacent diodes oscillate 180° out of phase) have the same level of feedback from the external cavity, thus the external cavity is not able to discriminate between the two modes. Analysis shows that the fundamental mode is preferred over the highest order mode for arrays having relatively few diodes, however the degree of discrimination between the two modes decreases steadily as the number of diodes in the array is increased. Note that increasing the distance from the source to the mirror increases the number of low-loss modes in the cavity, for example placement of the output mirror at $2D^2/\lambda$ results in four low-loss cavity modes.

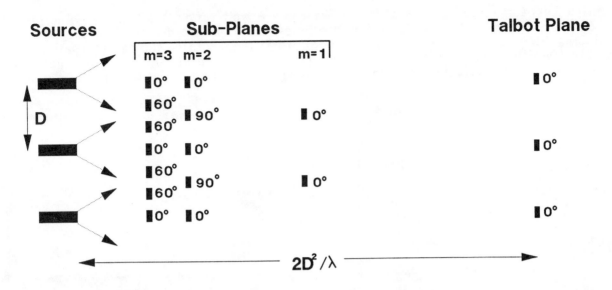

Figure 1. Positions and relative phases of the images of a coherent array of sources formed within the near-field zone of the array.

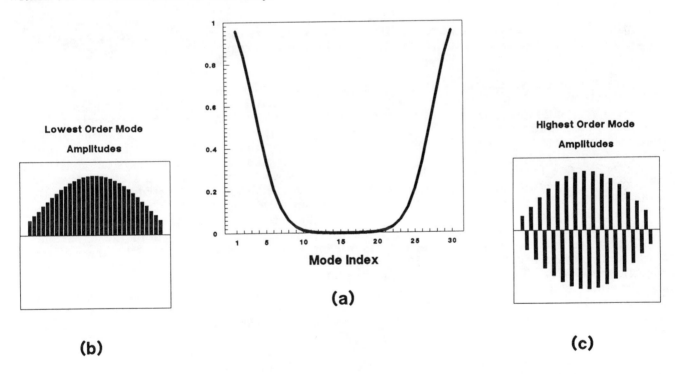

Figure 2. (a) Effective level of cavity feedback for the normal modes of a 30 element diode array in a Talbot cavity with no spatial filter. (b) Relative amplitudes for the array elements in the lowest order array mode. (c) Relative amplitudes for the array elements in the highest order mode.

To control the mode of a large array in a Talbot cavity a spatial filter must be placed in the cavity to suppress the highest order array mode. Figure 3 illustrates how the filter works. When the array is in either its lowest or highest order mode an image of the array is formed at the mirror of the Talbot cavity. In the highest order mode this image is aligned with respect to the source, in the lowest order mode the image is offset with respect to the source by one half of the separation between source elements. If the images are well resolved a spatial filter placed in front of the mirror as shown in figure 3 will suppress the highest order mode of the array, while introducing little loss to the lowest order mode. While this requires the cavity mode to have a relatively low fill factor at the cavity output plane (resulting in multiple lobes in the far-field) the fill factor can be increased through the use of aperture filling optics external to the cavity.

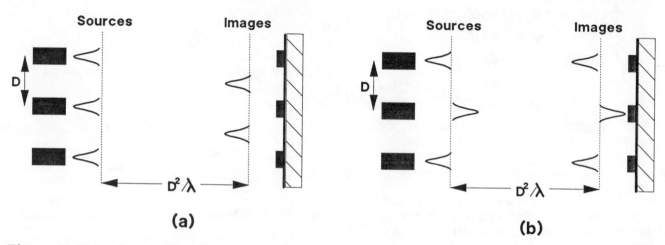

Figure 3. Use of a spatial filter placed in a Talbot cavity to suppress the highest order array mode. (a) The spatial filter introduces little loss to the lowest order mode of the array, (b) the spatial filter introduces significant losses to the highest order array mode.

Figure 4 shows a schematic of the apparatus used to demonstrate mode control in a Talbot cavity. The laser array used for this work was an AR coated 30 element array of index guided AlGaAs lasers that was manufactured by General Optronics. These diodes were not coupled together on-chip and were observed to oscillate incoherently without external feedback. The lasers were separated by 10 microns on the chip, which was too close together to permit simple construction of a Talbot cavity for the array. To overcome this problem a lens system consisting of a 0.6 N.A. wide field magnifying lens and a field lens was used to create a flat image of the array at a 38X magnification. The magnified image of the diode array acted as the effective source for the Talbot cavity, which consisted of a 40 mm focal length AR coated cylindrical lens (to control divergence of the beam perpendicular to the array junction plane) and a flat mirror 167 mm from the effective source array. Intracavity lenslets were not used in the experiment since they were not required to control the divergence of the effective sources (the array is long enough so that edge losses in the junction plane are low) and would have introduced unnecessary losses in the cavity. The spatial filter consisted of a chrome mask that had 180 micron wide clear apertures etched on 380 micron centers, the mask was supported on a flat AR coated fused silica substrate. The spatial filter plate was tilted slightly out of the array junction plane in order to prevent residual reflections from the chrome film from coupling back into the cavity mode.

Figure 5A shows the far-field pattern emitted by the diode array in the Talbot cavity with a spatial filter placed in the cavity. The positions and magnitudes of the lobes in the far-field pattern agree well with those predicted for the lowest order mode of the array. The structure beneath each of the lobes is an artifact of an aberration that was present in the magnification system at the time of the experiment. The measured full width at half maximum for the lobes (0.23 mrad.) was approximately 3 times the diffraction limit for the array, indicating either that not all of the diodes of the array were phase locked or that the phase front emitted by the diode array was somewhat aberrated. Several factors contributed to the observed width of the far-field lobes, the two most significant were the presence of aberrations in the cavity optics and large variations in the relative output intensities of the diodes in the array. The later of these factors was a direct by-product of material variations in the LPE grown wafer used for these diodes. Figure 5B shows the same far-field pattern when the spatial filter was removed. Here two separate sets of lobes were observed in the far-field, corresponding to the lowest and highest order modes of the diode array. In addition to the diffractive lobes, a broad background is observed in the far-field which corresponds to diodes that were not locked to the cavity mode and oscillated incoherently. The threshold current for the diode array with no feedback was 1.35 Amp., when the array was coupled to the external cavity with no spatial filter threshold dropped to 1.28 Amp. When the spatial filter was inserted into the cavity the threshold current remained at 1.28 Amp., indicating that the spatial filter did not introduce any significant loss into the lowest order array mode. As the bias current was increased the relative sizes and widths of the diffractive lobes did not change up to a bias current of 1.8 Amp. (thermal limit for the device), indicating that the array mode remained stable up to high levels of device gain.

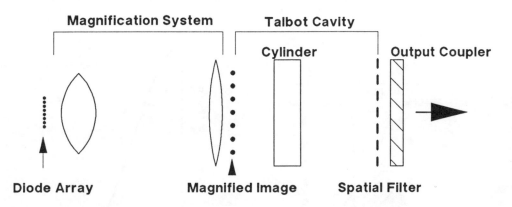

Figure 4. Schematic diagram of the apparatus used in these experiments.

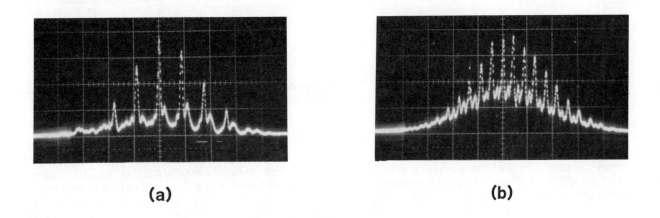

Figure 5. (a) Far-field pattern emitted by the laser diode array oscillating in its fundamental mode in a Talbot cavity with a spatial filter. (b) Far-field pattern emitted by the laser diode array in a Talbot cavity with no spatial filter. The two sets of lobes in the far-field pattern correspond to the lowest and highest order modes of the array.

3. SUB-IMAGE PLANE CAVITY WITH PHASE CORRECTOR

It is also possible to construct a cavity to phase lock a laser diode array by placing a mirror in the first sub-image plane of the source array (a distance $D^2/2\lambda$ from the array), using a binary phase mask to correct for the 90° phase shift between the two sets of images of the source array formed in this plane (figure 6a). This sub-image plane cavity has several potential advantages over the conventional Talbot cavity. It is shorter than the corresponding Talbot cavity, and is correspondingly less sensitive to misalignment of the cavity end mirror. This cavity has lower edge losses than the corresponding Talbot cavity. Since the spatial period of the cavity mode at the output plane of the cavity is 1/2 that of the source array itself, the far-field pattern from this cavity has only half the number of lobes as the far-field from the corresponding Talbot cavity.

Figure 6b shows the effective level of cavity feedback for the modes of a 30 element diode array in a sub-image plane cavity with a phase corrector. Note that in this cavity configuration the fundamental array mode is the only low-loss mode, additional filters are not required to suppress higher order modes of the array. When the phase mask is removed from the cavity the highest order array mode becomes the only low-loss cavity mode, the fundamental array mode is suppressed.

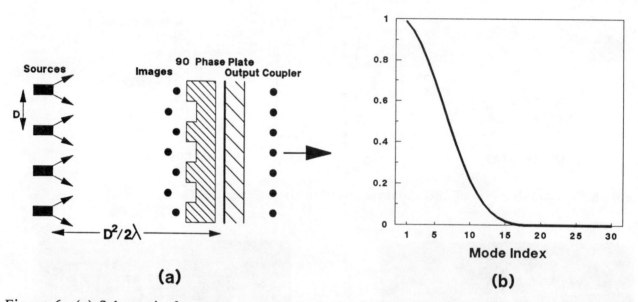

Figure 6. (a) Schematic for the Sub-Image Plane cavity. (b) Effective level of cavity feedback for the modes of a 30 element diode array in a Sub-Image Plane cavity with a phase corrector.

The apparatus that was previously described (figure 4) was modified to test the behavior of a diode array in a sub-image plane cavity. The same diode array and magnification system that were used to test the Talbot cavity were used to create an effective source having 30 elements separated by 380 microns. The output mirror was placed 84 mm from the effective source array and the spatial filter used in the previous experiment was replaced with a phase mask. This mask consisted of a flat fused silica plate that was ion milled to create a binary zone pattern having 90° phase shifts between adjacent zones, and a zone separation of 380 microns.

Figure 7 shows the far-field pattern emitted by the array in this cavity. The angular separation between lobes in the far-field corresponds to $2\lambda/D$ (4.6 mrad.) which agrees with the prediction of the theory. The observed width of the far-field lobes in this experiment was comparable to that observed in the Talbot cavity experiment using the same diode array. The far-field pattern was observed to be stable up to the maximum bias current for the device (1.8 Amp.).

Figure 8 shows a spectrally resolved near-field photograph of the array when phase locked in the sub-image plane cavity. Those diodes that couple to the external cavity mode oscillated on two common longitudinal modes separated by 3 Angstroms, those that are not coupled to the cavity typically oscillate independently on up to 12 longitudinal modes simultaneously. From the photograph it is apparent that roughly 15 of the 30 diodes in the array couple to the cavity mode. Measurements are currently in progress to establish the coherence between individual pairs of diodes in the array and will be reported at a later date.

This work was supported by the Department of the Air Force.

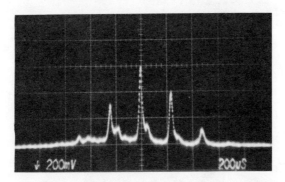

Figure 7. Far-field of the laser diode array in a sub-image plane cavity with phase corrector. The separation between the lobes corresponds to $2\lambda/D$.

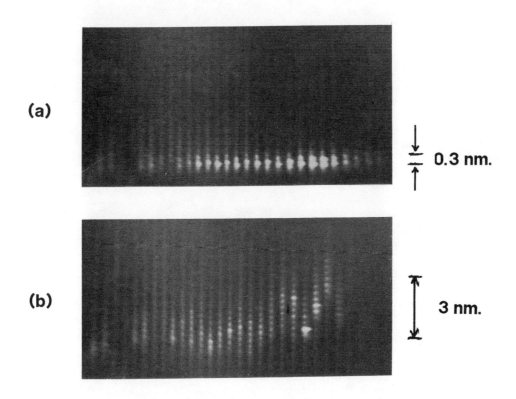

Figure 8. Spectrally resolved near-field of the diode array in a sub-image plane cavity: (a) with cavity feedback, (b) without cavity feedback.

References

1. N.W. Carlson, et. al., Appl. Phys. Lett. **52**(12), 939 (1988).
2. D. Botez, et. al., Appl. Phys. Lett. **53**(6), 464 (1988).
3. D.F. Welch, et. al., Electron. Lett. **22**, 293 (1986).
4. E.M. Philipp-Rutz, Jour. Appl. Phys. **46**(10) 4552 (1975).
5. R.H. Rediker, R.P. Scholss, and L.J. Van Ruyven, Appl. Phys. Lett. **46**(2), 133 (1985).
6. J. Yaeli, et. al., Appl. Phys. Lett. **47**(2), 89 (1985).
7. J.T. Winthrop and C.R. Worthington, Jour. Opt. Soc. Am. **55**(4), 373 (1965).
8. V.V. Antyukhov, et. al., JETP Lett. **44**, 78 (1986).
9. A.A. Golubentsev, V.V. Likhanskii, and A.P. Napartovich, Sov. Phys. JETP **66**(4), 676 (1987).
10. J.R. Leger, M.L. Scott, and W.B. Veldkamp, Appl. Phys. Lett. **52**(21), 1771 (1988).
11. C. Roychoudhuri, et. al., Meeting of the Optical Society of America, October 1988, Santa Clara, CA.
12. C. Roychoudhuri, et. al., International Conference on Lasers '88, December 4-9, Lake Tahoe, NV.

High Power AlGaAs Broad Area Laser Diodes
for Light Triggered Thyristor Valve System

Shin'ichi NAKATSUKA
Central Research Laboratory, HITACHI, LTD. Kokubunnji, Tokyo 185, Japan
Ryuuji IYOTANI
Hitachi Laboratory, HITACHI, LTD. Hitachi, Ibaragi 319-12, Japan
Chikara TANAKA
Hitachi Works, HITACHI, LTD. Hitach, Ibaragi 317, Japan

ABSTRACT

Application of a broad area laser for a light triggered thyristor valve system was investigated. The maximum light output powers of 1.8 W and 2.7 W were obtained in 80 um wide and 160 um wide laser, respectively. Lasers operated for more than 1000 hours in 100 times accerelated aging condition except for rapidly degraded ones. The rapidly degradation rate consistent with substrate defect dencity.

INTRODUCTION

Recently, a broad area lasers have attracted much attention as high power light sources for applications such as diode laser pumped solid state lasers. However, little has been reported on their reliability under actual work conditions. This paper reports on reliable AlGaAs broad area laser diodes and their application to light triggered thyristor valve systems.

THE LIGHT TRIGGERED THYRISTOR SYSTEM

Figure 1 shows a schematic of a light triggered thyristor valve system. This system consists of approximately 100 thyristors and potential divider circuit in series. A light pulse turn-on signal is output by a laser diode through an optical fibers (1 mm φ single core fiber with 200 μm core and bundle fiber with 21 cores) of more than twenty meters. This system can swich 1500 A at 125 kV.

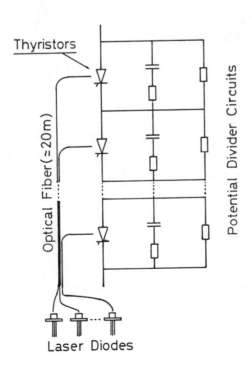

Fig. 1 Schematic of light triggered thyristor valve systems.

These systems have attractive features such as high noise immunity and few components and are suitable for a high-voltage direct current transmission systems. In conventional systems, light emitting diodes (LED) are used. However, when the emitted beam from the diodes is coupled with a thyristor through an optical fiber, the coupling efficiency is only about 15 %. Therefore, approximately 1 W of light power is required.

However, because LED energy conversion efficiency is low, junction temperatures rise during high power operation. In addition, the resistivity of LEDs is high because they require a large light emitting area without an electrode. Therefore LEDs can emit high power only in pulse mode, but even in this mode it is difficult to get reliable operation.

Because the broad area laser diodes have high energy conversion efficiency and narrow emission beam, this paper investigates thier application to a light triggered thyristor valve system.

LASER DIODES FOR LIGHT TRIGGERED THYRISTOR VALVE SYSTEM

Figure 2 shows a schematic of a broad area laser diode. The broad area lasers were fabricated by an atmospheric pressure metal organic chemical vapor deposition technique. An n-GaAs buffer layer (n= 2×10^{18} cm^{-3}, 0.5 μm thick), an n-AlGaAs cladding layer (n= 1×10^{18} cm^{-3}, 1.5 μm thick), an undoped multi-quantum well active layer (five 10-nm-thick GaAs well layers alternating with five 3-nm-thick AlGaAs barrier layers), a p-AlGaAs cladding layer (p= 7×10^{17} cm^{-3}, 1.5 μm thick), and an n-GaAs cap layer (n= 2×10^{18} cm^{-3}, 0.5 μm thick) were grown on an n-GaAs substrate. Then selective zinc diffusion was performed to fabricate a laser stripe using a conventional photo lithographic technique. The cavity length of the laser diode was 400 μm, and the stripe widths were 80 μm and 160 μm. A high reflection coating was deposited on the rear facet of the laser diode, giving a reflectivity of 90%, and an anti-reflection was deposited on the front facet, giving a reflectivity of 9%.

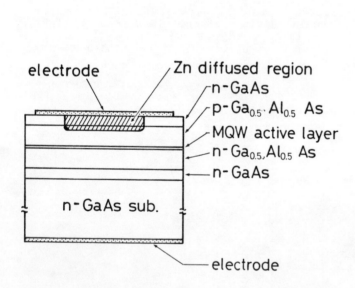

Fig. 2 Schematic of broad area laser diodes

diodes

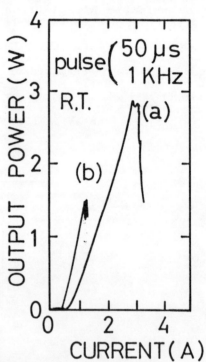

Fig. 3 L-I characteristics of the broad area laser in pulse mode

The laser diodes were operated at wavelengths of around 830 nm at room temperature. The light output power versus electric current characteristics in pulse mode (1 KHz, 50 usec) are shown in Fig. 3. The threshold currents of these lasers were about 400 mA and 700 mA for 80-um and 160-μm wide stripe lasers, respectively.

In pulse mode, the maximum light output powers were limited by catastrophic optical damage to 1.4 W for 80-μm wide stripes and 2.7 W for 160-μm wide stripes. On the other hand, with DC operation, output powers were limited by thermal saturation, and a maximum output power of about 0.8 W was obtained in the 80-um wide stripe laser as shown in Fig. 4(a). The far-field patterns of the laser diode are shown in Fig. 4(b). The emission angle parallel to the junction was 15° and perpencicular to the junction was 35 degrees. The far-field pattern parallel to the junction is a single lobed pattern. However, this beam consists of many modes in the lateral direction.

The laser beam's power coupling efficiency with an optical fiber was investigated. The optical fiber is a silica fiber (NA=0.55, 200 μm core diameter). An 80-μm wide laser diode with an output power of 600 mW was used in the experiment.

Figure 5 shows power coupling efficiency versus position of the fiber. Since the emission angles of the laser diode were small, a coupling efficiency of more than 60% was obtained. The tolerances of the fiber positions, where coupling efficiencies of more than 60% could be obtained, were +400 um in the direction parallel to the junction (X direction) and +600 μm in the direction perpencicular to the junction (Y direction).

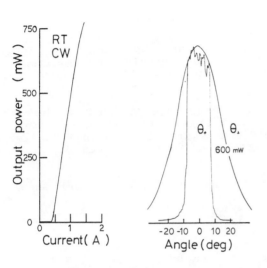
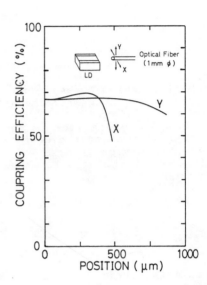

Fig. 4 L-I characteristic and far-field patterns of the broad area laser in DC condition

Fig. 5 Coupling efficiency versus fiber position characteristics in light triggered thyristor system

Considering the transmission loss of the optical fiber and coupling loss to the thyristor, the total coupling efficiency was about 40%, which is more than twice of the coupling efficiency of light emitting diodes.

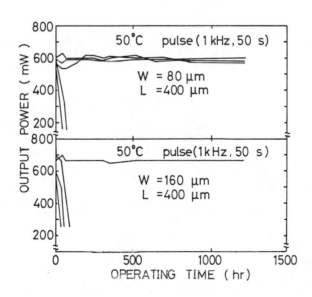

Fig. 6 History of 80 μm and 160 μm width laser under 600 mW, 50 C, pulse (1 KHz, 50 us pulse width) operation

RELIABILITY OF LASER DIODES

Because the light triggered thyristor system consists of handred of units, the reliability of each unit is very important. All thyristors should work stably for more than ten years under a wide range of conditions. Therefore, the reliability of the broad area lasers was investigated.

An accelerated aging test under a conditions similar to actual working conditions of a light trigger thyristor were performed. Figure 6 shows light output power versus operating time at 50 °C under constant pulsed current (1 kHz, 50 μs pulse). The aging rate could be accelarated by 100 times. The operating currents were about 800 mA for 80-um width lasers and 1100 mA for 160-μm lasers. The initial output power of these laser diodes was about 600 mW.

Two of five of the 80-um width lasers failed in the initial stage of the aging test, while four of six 160-um width lasers failed in the same stage. However, the remainding laser diodes have operated for more than 1000 hours without appreciabe degradation. This reliability, which coresponds to stable operation for more than 100000 hours under actual conditions, is enough for the actual system.

In spite of smaller optical power density and smaller injected current density in the wider stripe laser diodes, the probability of rapid degradation was larger than that of narrower stripe lasers. This suggests that rapid degradation depends on the existance of defects in the stripe. Therefore, the probability of defect existence in the laser stripe was calculated.

The probability P that there is no defects in the laser stripe can be written as

$$P = \left(\frac{A-S}{A}\right)^N$$

where, A is a unit area, N is the number of defects in the unit area, and S is area of the laser stripe. When N and A are sufficiently large, and the defect density $\sigma = N/A$ is constant, then ln(P) is

$$\ln(P) = N \cdot \ln\left(\frac{A-S}{A}\right) = -\frac{S}{\sigma}$$

and

$$P = \mathrm{EXP}\left(-\frac{S}{\sigma}\right)$$

The etch pit density of the GaAs substrate used in these experiments was about 2000 cm, and the probability of a defect-free stripe for 80-um stripe lasers is 52.7% and that for 160-nm stripe lasers is 27.8%. These probabilities were consistent with actual failure rates.

CONCLUSION

In conclusion, a new application of a broad area laser diode as a light source for a light triggered thyristor valve system was investigated. These laser diodes operated at light powers of up to 0.8 W under room temperature and DC conditions, and up to 1.4 W and 2.7 W in pulse mode for 80-μm and-160 μm width stripes, respectively. The coupling efficiency of the laser beam with a light guide was more than 60% in the 80-μm wide area. Lasers that did not fail in the initial stages of the accelerated test operated for more than 1000 hours. The probability of laser diodes degrading rapidly was consistent with the calculated probability of crystal defect exsistance in the laser stripe.

REFERANCES

1) W. Streifer et al., IEEE J. of Quant. Elec. 24 (1988) 883P
2) T. Fan et al., IEEE J. of Quant. Elec. 24 (1988) 924P
3) N. Konishi et al., Int. Power Elec. Conf. Tokyo (1983)

Invited Paper

OPTICAL CAVITY DESIGN FOR WAVELENGTH-RESONANT SURFACE-EMITTING SEMICONDUCTOR LASERS

S. R. J. Brueck, M. Y. A. Raja, M. Osinski, C. F. Schaus, M. Mahbobzadeh,
J. G. McInerney, and K. J. Dahlhauser

Center for High Technology Materials
University of New Mexico
Albuquerque, NM 87131

ABSTRACT

Recently, we have demonstrated a novel surface-emitting semiconductor laser with a wavelength-resonant periodic gain medium, which has performed significantly better than conventional double-heterostructure and multiple-quantum-well vertical-cavity devices. The gain medium consists of a series of half-wave-spaced quantum wells which provides enhanced longitudinal gain at a selected wavelength in the vertical direction, reducing transverse amplified spontaneous emission, lowering the threshold and raising the quantum efficiency. However, because the antinodes of the standing-wave optical field must coincide with the quantum wells, considerable attention must be devoted to designing the vertical cavity. Here we examine various cavity configurations in which the wavelength-resonant periodic gain medium has been incorporated. Multilayer epitaxial reflectors are particularly attractive for fabricating monolithic vertical-cavity surface-emitting lasers.

1. INTRODUCTION

Semiconductor lasers which emit from the top (epitaxial) surface [1-8] rather than from the end facets are of considerable interest for a variety of applications such as monolithic optoelectronic integrated circuits [9], optical chip-to-chip interconnects, optical logic devices [10] and high-power, large-area, two-dimensional arrays [11]. Because of their short cavity lengths, these lasers have large Fabry-Pérot mode spacings which favor single longitudinal mode operation. However, development of these systems has been impeded by the limitations of existing surface-emitting laser designs, particularly the high thresholds and low efficiencies of devices with vertical resonators, which are well suited for forming two-dimensional arrays. These problems are mostly due to short active-region lengths (a few micrometers), very large Fresnel numbers, lack of carrier and optical confinement, and generation of competitive amplified spontaneous emission (ASE) in the transverse plane.

The vertical cavity surface-emitting lasers developed to date have performed poorly compared with conventional edge-emitters, and considerable attention has been paid to alternative geometries whose active regions are configured in the same way as in edge-emitting lasers, but in which radiation is directed towards the surface either by 45° mirrors [12,13] or by second-order distributed Bragg reflectors [14-16]. While some of these designs have performed well, vertical-cavity surface-emitters offer potentially higher packing density, larger emitting areas, better beam quality, unconstrained arrangement of emitters, and planar integration with easier batch processing and on-wafer probe testing.

In this paper, we describe the novel concept of a vertical-cavity, resonant periodic gain surface-emitting semiconductor laser, with particular emphasis on how the gain medium is combined with an optical cavity. In Section 2, the concept of resonant periodic gain (RPG) is described briefly. Section 3 contains calculations of the reflectivity, phase and gain resonances which occur when the RPG medium is placed within an optical cavity, first for the structures used in the initial demonstrations of the RPG principle, then for projected cavity designs utilizing multilayer epitaxial high-reflectors which can be deposited in the same growth process as the gain medium.

2. RESONANT PERIODIC GAIN SEMICONDUCTOR LASERS

The gain experienced by a mode in a semiconductor laser resonator is determined by the interaction of the standing-wave optical field with the material gain distribution in the active region. This interaction is not spatially uniform, but is strongest at the antinodes of the standing-wave optical field and vanishes at the nulls. Hence the material gain in a homogeneous medium is not utilized efficiently by the resonant mode, *i.e.* the effective gain length is shorter than the overall physical length of the gain medium. To overcome this problem, we have developed a new multilayer structure: a resonant periodic gain (RPG) medium which maximizes the modal gain in a semiconductor laser by confining injected carriers, and hence the gain, to the antinode regions [17-21]. This will reduce spontaneous emission due to carriers normally present near the nodes. In addition, competition from amplified spontaneous emission (ASE) in the transverse directions is suppressed due to the poor modal overlap integral. This new design is particularly attractive for vertical-cavity surface-emitting lasers: it has already led to lower thresholds for optical pumping

[17-20], and may well be an important step towards room-temperature cw operation of electrically-pumped devices.

Details of the physics and fabrication of RPG vertical-cavity surface-emitting lasers have already been described elsewhere [17-20]. For completeness, we provide here a brief outline of the basic properties of RPG media, before proceeding to analyze how they are combined with various optical cavity configurations. The most straightforward RPG structure is formed by a series of localized gain regions consisting of single quantum-wells (QWs) or closely spaced groups of QWs, periodically arranged to coincide with the antinodes of the optical standing wave in the vertical cavity at the lasing wavelength. Fig. 1 illustrates the RPG structure schematically: the localized gain regions (GaAs quantum wells) are separated by passive AlGaAs spacers whose thickness determines the resonant wavelength λ_r, at which the interaction of the optical field with the periodic multiple quantum-well gain medium is maximized. This occurs when the gain medium has an optical periodicity of $\lambda_r/2$. For a properly designed structure, the resonant wavelength λ_r should be chosen to correspond to a particular transition in the quantum wells. In addition, it is essential that the RPG medium be placed within the cavity so that the antinodes of the optical standing-wave field coincide with the gain regions, i.e. that the optical thicknesses of the end layers be chosen carefully. In the worst possible case, misplacement of the RPG medium by a quarter-wavelength would result in a total absence of modal gain.

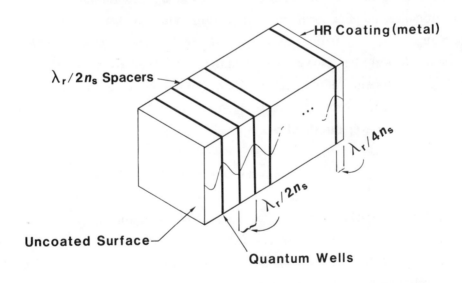

Fig. 1. Schematic diagram of resonant periodic gain (RPG) medium designed to enhance the effective gain length of a vertical-cavity surface-emitting laser. The thick lines represent the quantum wells, λ_r is the resonant wavelength and n_s is the refractive index of the spacer material.

To illustrate the effect of the RPG structure in a vertical-cavity surface-emitting laser, we calculate the effective gain of a single longitudinal mode propagating along the cavity (z) axis of the laser, for which the integrated gain coefficient $G(\lambda)$ (the product of active medium length and gain per unit length) is given by

$$G(\lambda) = \int_0^L g(z) \sin^2\left(\frac{2\pi n(z)z}{\lambda}\right) dz, \tag{1}$$

where λ is the free-space wavelength of the standing-wave optical field, L the cavity length, $g(z)$ and $n(z)$ the material gain and refractive index, respectively. If the medium were uniform, the integral (1) would give $G(\lambda) = gL/2$, i.e. only half of the available material gain would be utilized. For the RPG medium illustrated in Fig. 1, with N quantum wells of thickness L_z and separated by $D = \lambda_r/2n_s$, where n_s is the refractive index of the spacer material, we evaluate this integral assuming that each QW has the same constant gain coefficient g_w, to obtain the modal gain spectrum [18-20]

$$G(\lambda) = (Ng_w L_z/2)\{1 + \text{sinc}(2\pi L_z n_s/\lambda_r)\}, \tag{2}$$

where $\text{sinc}(x) = \sin(x)/x$, and we have ignored the wavelength dependence of the material gain for simplicity. The gain resonance becomes sharper as the number of quantum wells increases, much as the resolution of a diffraction grating is improved by illumination of more grating periods. Away from resonance, the sinc term averages to zero, and $G(\lambda)$ becomes $Ng_w L_z/2$, equal to the integrated gain in a uniform medium of length NL_z and material gain g_w. Hence, the integrated gain coefficient $G(\lambda_r)$ at the resonant wavelength is enhanced by a factor of two over that of a conventional, non-resonant MQW gain medium having equal active length. Because the gain anisotropy reduces ASE in the transverse plane, the RPG laser should have increased power efficiency as well as a lower threshold pump level.

3. OPTICAL CAVITY DESIGN FOR RPG LASERS

The basis for the RPG principle is alignment of the antinodes of the optical standing wave in the laser cavity with a periodic array of localized gain regions (single or multiple quantum wells), so that the effective gain is enhanced as described above. To optimize this arrangement, two conditions must be met simultaneously:

(1) the resonant wavelength, i.e. the period of the RPG medium, must correspond to a strongly amplifying transition in the quantum wells;

(2) the position of the RPG medium within the optical cavity, as determined by the phase shifting layers at the ends, must be such that the antinodes of the standing wave coincide with the quantum wells.

Satisfying these conditions ensures that the resonances of the cavity and gain medium overlap at a design wavelength where there is available gain. In this section we are primarily concerned with the second condition, that is, configuring the cavity with respect to the RPG medium. If the phase shift layers are not properly matched to the cavity resonance closest to the gain peak, the effective gain will degrade rapidly. The worst possible case would have the quantum wells located at the nodes of the optical standing wave, thereby reducing the usable gain to zero. It is therefore not sufficient to optimize the cavity and RPG medium separately: they must also be aligned with respect to each other. Another important consideration is that, because of the short gain length of the structure, the optical cavity must have extremely low losses. Mirror reflectivities must therefore be as close to unity as possible, and this imposes additional constraints on the cavity design.

We start by presenting a simple technique for calculating reflectivity and gain resonances for cavities enclosing RPG media. These calculations are performed for the RPG laser with a deposited aluminum mirror which was first used to demonstrate the principle of resonant periodic gain [19]. For this structure, the importance of correct choice of the thicknesses of the phase shifting end is demonstrated. Next, we consider optimization of the RPG laser by incorporating a high-Q cavity consisting of multilayer epitaxial reflectors, which can be deposited in the same growth run as that used to fabricate the RPG medium itself. The growth tolerances for such an optimized cavity are discussed, and reflectivity and gain resonances for the finished structure are calculated.

A. Method for Calculating Cavity Reflectivity and Gain

Many textbooks on thin film optical filters present techniques for the calculation of complex reflectivities of multilayer dielectric structures [22-24]. The approach used in this work is simply to express the fields E_{j+1} at each layer $(j+1)$ in terms of the fields E_j at the previous layer (j) and the optical phase shift Φ_j in traversing the jth layer, using a transfer matrix of the form

$$\begin{pmatrix} E_{j+1}^+ \\ E_{j+1}^- \end{pmatrix} = \frac{1}{2} \begin{pmatrix} \left[1 + \frac{n_j}{n_{j+1}}\right] e^{i\Phi_j} & \left[1 - \frac{n_j}{n_{j+1}}\right] e^{-i\Phi_j} \\ \left[1 - \frac{n_j}{n_{j+1}}\right] e^{i\Phi_j} & \left[1 + \frac{n_j}{n_{j+1}}\right] e^{-i\Phi_j} \end{pmatrix} \begin{pmatrix} E_j^+ \\ E_j^- \end{pmatrix} \quad (3)$$

where n_{j+1}, n_j are the respective (complex) refractive indices, E_{j+1}^+ and E_j^+ are the complex electric field amplitudes for waves propagating in the positive z-direction (to the right for definiteness), and E_{j+1}^-, E_j^- are the field amplitudes for waves propagating in the opposite direction. The layers are numbered from right to left, with the fields defined at the rightmost edge of each layer. The total cavity reflectivity for waves incident from the left can then be evaluated by imposing the boundary condition that there is only an outgoing wave in the medium beyond the right end of the cavity, and carrying out a straightforward series of matrix multiplications to evaluate the incident and reflected fields in terms of this outgoing wave. The effective gain in the structure is calculated by integrating the product of the intensity and gain factor through the layered structure and dividing by the incident intensity. Because we are interested only in matching resonances of the cavity and the RPG medium, we did not include dispersion of the material gain or index in any of these calculations. The additional requirement of placing these resonances close to the gain peak is less critical, and will not be dealt with explicitly in this paper.

B. Prototype RPG Cavity with Al End Reflector

The first structure used to demonstrate the resonant periodic gain principle consisted of a series of 32 GaAs quantum wells (L_z = 10 nm) separated by half-wave $Ga_{0.75}Al_{0.25}As$ spacers (D = 109 nm), designed for operation at the n = 2 subband transitions near ~825 nm [17,20]. One end of the structure was uncoated, so that its reflectivity was ~32%, while a layer of Al was deposited onto the other end to obtain a reflectivity of ~75%. The overall reflectivity and effective gain for this device have been calculated as described above, assuming a quarter-wave end spacer on the Al-coated side, and different spacer layer thicknesses on the other end. Figure 2 illustrates the results for a half-wave thick layer on the free (uncoated) end, which is expected to be close to optimum. As anticipated, the effective gain is enhanced by a factor of two at the resonant wavelength of ~825 nm. For comparison, we have performed similar calculations for the same RPG medium with a quarter-wave spacer layer at each end. This structure does not exhibit any enhancement in its effective gain, as shown in Figure 3. The normalized peak gain is given in Figure 4 as a function of the thickness of the final spacer layer on the free (uncoated) end of the resonator. In obtaining Fig. 4, the resonant wavelength was allowed to vary with the total cavity length, hence the observed periodicity in the gain as a function of and spacer thickness differs slightly from the nominal λ_r. The refractive indices used were $(2.75 + 8.31i)$ for Al [25], 3.64 for GaAs and 3.45 for $Al_{0.25}Ga_{0.75}As$ [26,27]. Note that the calculated resonances are relatively broad due to the poor cavity Q-factor; the round trip reflectivity product is only ~0.24. The variations in depth and width of the resonances are a manifestation of small distributed feedback effects due to reflections at the quantum wells. To estimate the magnitude of these distributed Bragg reflection effects, we have modeled the behavior of a structure in which the end reflections have been artificially suppressed by (computationally) attaching thick GaAs films to the ends. The results of these calculations are given in Figure 5. The effects of periodic reflections at the

32 quantum wells lead to effective reflectivity changes of ≤ 20% near the resonant wavelength.

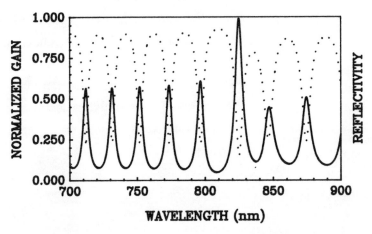

Fig. 2. Calculated normalized gain (solid line) and reflectivity (dotted line) spectra for RPG surface-emitting laser with a quarter-wave end spacer facing a metal reflector, and a half-wave spacer at the opposite end.

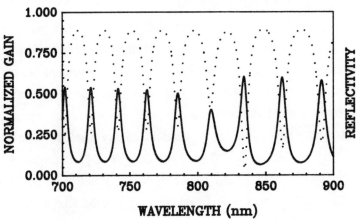

Fig. 3. Calculated normalized gain (solid line) and reflectivity (dotted line) spectra for RPG surface-emitting laser with a quarter-wave end spacer facing a metal reflector, and a quarter-wave spacer at the opposite end.

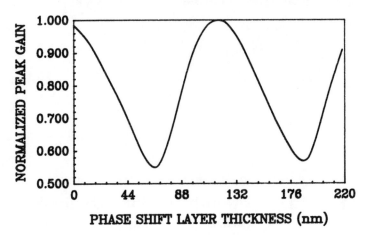

Fig. 4. Calculated variation in peak gain for a RPG surface-emitting laser with a quarter-wave end spacer facing a metal reflector, as a function of the thickness of the spacer at the opposite end.

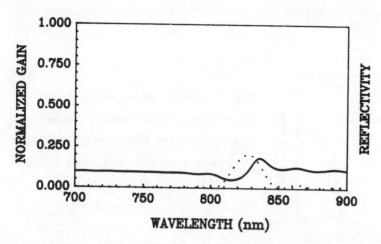

Fig. 5 Calculated normalized gain (solid line) and reflectivity (dotted line) spectra for RPG surface-emitting laser with semi-infinite GaAs layer at each end: this enables evaluation of the effects of distributed reflections at the quantum wells.

C. Improved Cavities Using Multilayer Epitaxial High-Reflectors

Because of its short cavity length, the vertical-cavity surface-emitting laser requires extremely high gain per unit length. The optimal way to configure a vertical-cavity surface-emitting laser is thus to provide a very high-Q cavity, which may be formed by bracketing the gain medium between a pair of epitaxial multilayer high-reflectors (MHRs) consisting of a stack of alternating high-and low-index quarter-wave layers [4,5,28]. The materials for these layers must obviously be chosen to have sufficiently wide bandgaps that excessive absorption losses in the reflectors are avoided. Simple calculations show that for a vertical cavity surface-emitting laser containing a series of ~30 quantum wells of thickness ~10 nm, the threshold gain required is of the order of 4 μm^{-1} when uncoated, 2.5 μm^{-1} when an Al reflector is deposited on one side, but drops to 0.03 μm^{-1} (300 cm^{-1}) when the active medium is bracketed by two MHRs with 99% reflectivity. The reflectivity spectrum for a typical MHR consisting of 20 pairs of alternating quarter-wave layers of indices n_L = 3.20 and n_H = 3.50, is shown in Figure 6.

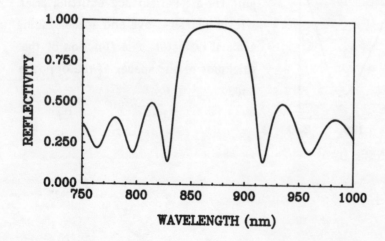

Fig. 6. Calculated reflectivity spectrum of an epitaxial multilayer high-reflector (MHR) consisting of 20 periods of alternating high- and low-index quarter-wave layers with indices n_H = 3.50 and n_L = 3.20, respectively.

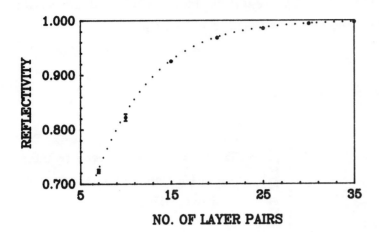

Fig. 7. Spread in reflectivity of a MHR at its design wavelength (825 nm) due to random ± 5% variation in optical thickness of the grown layers.

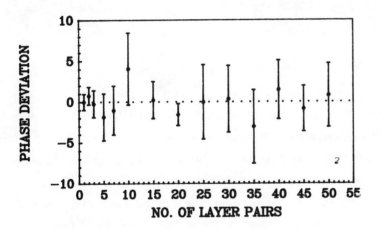

Fig. 8. Fluctuation in the phase shift (in degrees) of a MHR at its design wavelength (825 nm) due to a random ±5% variation in the optical thickness of the grown layers.

Since the inclusion of MHRs in the device dramatically increases the number of layers to be grown, the effects of uncertainties in layer thicknesses and compositions must be considered. In Figure 7 and 8 we plot the spread in the reflectivities (the dotted line is the ideal curve), and variations in the cavity phase shift at the peak, for AlGaAs/AlAs MHRs with different numbers of layer pairs, assuming a random variation of ± 5% in the optical thickness (combined uncertainties in physical thickness and refractive index). The solid curve is the theoretical result for a perfect stack of alternating quarter-wave layers of high-index (61.4 nm of $Al_{0.40}Ga_{0.60}As$, n_H = 3.36) and low-index (68.8 nm of AlAs, n_L = 3.00) materials, while the bars represent the spread in the quantity calculated. These data suggest that, while the spread in reflectivity is minimal when more than ten periods are used, the phase variations are of much greater concern for the RPG laser (refer also to Figure 5). Critical control of the cavity resonance is clearly required if the RPG structure is to be used to its best advantage.

Finally, we have calculated the reflectivity and effective gain for an improved RPG surface-emitting laser using a pair of MHRs. The results of these calculations are shown in Figure 9, and the threshold gain for the structure is estimated to be ~ 0.3 μm^{-1}.

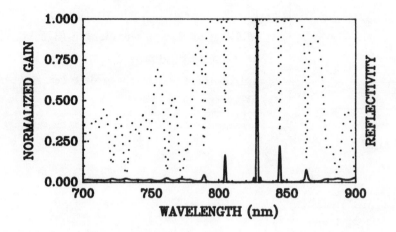

Fig. 9 Calculated reflectivity and gain spectra for improved laser structure using two MHRs.

4. Conclusions

In summary, we have described a novel resonant-periodic-gain (RPG) medium which optimizes the available gain in a vertical-cavity surface-emitting semiconductor laser. The basis for the gain enhancement is alignment of the antinodes of the standing wave optical field in a resonant cavity with periodic localized gain regions such as single or multiple quantum wells. Since the usual sine-square averaging in the overlap integral between the optical field and the spatial gain distribution is absent, the effective gain is increased by a factor of two. One critical condition which must be satisfied to optimize the gain in a RPG medium is that the gain medium must be positioned correctly within the optical cavity. If the RPG medium is misaligned within the cavity, the effective gain degrades rapidly and may actually become less than that of a conventional MQW structure.

Because of the need for very high Q cavities due to the short gain lengths in vertical-cavity surface-emitters, and due to the additional constraints on resonant periodic gain devices, cavity design is of the utmost importance. We have analyzed various cavity configurations for RPG lasers, including an optimized structure with epitaxial multilayer high-reflectors at either end. The tolerances in grown layer thicknesses and compositions required for successful fabrication of such devices are a few percent.

5. Acknowledgements

This work was partially supported by the U. S. Air Force Office of Scientific Research and by the National Science Foundation. Stimulating discussions with Dr. William Streifer of Spectra Diode Laboratories are also acknowledged.

6. REFERENCES

[1] H. Soda, K. Iga, C. Kitahara, and Y. Suematsu, "GaInAsP/InP surface emitting injection lasers", Japan. J. Appl. Phys., vol. 18, pp. 2329-2330, Dec. 1979.

[2] M. Ogura, T. Hata, and T. Yao, "Distributed feedback surface emitting laser diode with multilayered heterostructure", Japan. J. Appl. Phys., vol. 23, pp. L512-L514, 1984.

[3] S. Kinoshita and K. Iga, "Circular buried heterostructure (CBH) GaAlAs/GaAs surface emitting lasers", IEEE J. Quantum Electron., vol. QE-23, pp. 882-888, June 1987.

[4] P. L. Gourley and T. J. Drummond, "Visible, room-temperature, surface-emitting laser using an epitaxial Fabry-Perot resonator with AlGaAs/AlAs quarter-wave high reflectors and AlGaAs/GaAs multiple quantum wells", Appl. Phys. Lett., vol. 50, pp. 1225-1227, May 1987.

[5] M. Ogura, W. Hsin, M.-C. Wu, S. Wang, J. R. Whinnery, S. C. Wang, and J. J. Yang, "Surface-emitting laser diode with vertical GaAs/GaAlAs quarter-wavelength multilayers and lateral buried heterostructure", Appl. Phys. Lett., vol. 51, pp. 1655-1657, Nov. 1987.

[6] J. Faist, F. Morier-Genoud, D. Martin, J. D. Ganiere, and F.-K. Reinhart, "Optically pumped GaAs surface-emitting laser with integrated Bragg reflectors", Electron. Lett., vol. 24, pp. 629-630, May 1988.

[7] D. Botez, L. M. Zinkiewicz, L. J. Mawst, and T. J. Roth, "120 mW vertical-cavity surface-emitting diode laser", 11th IEEE International Semiconductor Laser Conf., Boston, MA, Aug. 29 - Sept. 1, 1988, Post-deadline paper PD3.

[8] K. Iga, F. Koyama, and S. Kinoshita, "Surface emitting semiconductor lasers", IEEE J. Quantum Electron., vol. QE-24, pp. 1845-1855, Sept. 1988.

[9] H. Matsueda, "AlGaAs OEIC transmitters", J. Lightwave Technol., vol. LT-5, pp. 1382-1390, Oct. 1987.

[10] J. Nitta, Y. Koizumi, and K. Iga, "GaAs/AlGaAs surface-emitting-laser-type optical logic and gate device", Digest of Technical Papers, CLEO'86 Conference on Lasers and Electro-Optics, San Francisco, 9-13 June 1986, paper FO4, pp. 382-383.

[11] S. Uchiyama and K. Iga, "Two-dimensional array of GaInAsP/InP surface-emitting lasers", Electron. Lett., vol. 21, pp. 162-164, Feb. 1985.

[12] Z. L. Liau and J. N. Walpole, "Surface-emitting GaInAsP/InP laser with low threshold current and high efficiency", Appl. Phys. Lett., vol. 46, pp. 115-117, Jan. 1985.

[13] Z. L. Liau and J. N. Walpole, "Large monolithic two-dimensional arrays of GaInAsP/InP surface-emitting lasers", Appl. Phys. Lett., vol. 50, pp. 528-530, March 1987.

[14] K. Kojima, S. Noda, K. Mitsunaga, K. Kyuma, and K. Hamanaka, "Continuous wave operation of a surface-emitting AlGaAs/GaAs multiquantum well distributed Bragg reflector laser", Appl. Phys. Lett., vol. 50, pp. 1705-1707, June 1987.

[15] N. W. Carlson, G. A. Evans, J. M. Hammer, M. Lurie, L. A. Carr, F. Z. Hawrylo, E. A. James, C. J. Kaiser, J. B. Kirk, W. F. Reichert, D. A. Truxal, J. R. Shealy, S. R. Chinn, and P. S. Zory, "High-power seven-element grating surface emitting diode laser array with 0.012° far-field angle", Appl. Phys. Lett., vol. 52, pp. 939-941, March 1988.

[16] G. A. Evans, N. W. Carlson, J. M. Hammer, M. Lurie, J. K. Butler, L. A. Carr, F. Z. Hawrylo, E. A. James, C. J. Kaiser, J. B. Kirk, W. F. Reichert, S. R. Chinn, J. R. Shealy, and P. S. Zory, "Efficient, high-power (>150 mW) grating surface emitting lasers", Appl. Phys. Lett., vol. 52, pp. 1037-1039, March 1988.

[17] M. Y. A. Raja, S. R. J. Brueck, M. Osinski, C. F. Schaus, J. G. McInerney, T. M. Brennan, and B. E. Hammons, "Wavelength-resonant enhanced gain/absorption structure for optoelectronic devices", in Post-Deadline Papers, XVI International Conference on Quantum Electronics IQEC'88, Tokyo, Japan, July 18-21, 1988, Paper PD-23, pp. 52-53.

[18] M. Y. A. Raja, S. R. J. Brueck, M. Osinski, C. F. Schaus, J. G. McInerney, T. M. Brennan, and B. E. Hammons, "Novel wavelength-resonant optoelectronic structure and its application to surface-emitting semiconductor lasers", Electron. Lett., vol. 24, pp. 1140-1142, Sept. 1988.

[19] M. Y. A. Raja, S. R. J. Brueck, M. Osinski, C. F. Schaus, J. G. McInerney, T. M. Brennan, and B. E. Hammons, "Surface-emitting, multiple quantum well GaAs/AlGaAs laser with wavelength-resonant periodic gain medium", Appl. Phys. Lett., Vol. 53, pp. 1678-1680, October 1988.

[20] M. Y. A. Raja, S. R. J. Brueck, M. Osinski, C. F. Schaus, J. G. McInerney, T. M. Brennan, and B. E. Hammons, "Wavelength-Resonant, Surface-Emitting Semiconductor Laser: A Novel Quantum Optical Structure," 1988 IEEE-LEOS Annual Meeting, Nov. 2-4, 1988, Santa Clara, CA.

[21] R. Geels, R. H. Yan, J. W. Scott, S. W. Corzine, R. J. Simes and L. A. Coldren, "Analysis and design of a novel parallel-driven MQW-DBR surface-emitting diode laser", in Conf. on Lasers and Electro-Optics, Tech. Digest Ser. 1988, Vol. 7 (Optical Society of America, Washington DC, 1988), paper WM1, p. 206.

[22] H. A. Macleod, "Thin-Film Optical Filters", 2nd Ed., pp. 50-52, New York: Macmillan 1986.

[23] Z. Knittl, "Optics of Thin Films", pp. 35-51, London: Wiley 1976.

[24] M. V. Klein and T. E. Furtak, "Optics", 2nd Ed., pp. 295-300, New York: Wiley 1986.

[25] "Handbook of Chemistry and Physics", 67th Ed., p. E-378, Boca Raton, FA: CRC Press 1986.

[26] D. E. Aspnes and A. A. Studna, "Dielectric functions and optical parameters of Si, Ge, GaP, GaAs, GaSb, InP, InAs, and InSb from 1.5 to 6.0 eV", Phys. Rev. B, vol. 27, pp. 985-1009, Jan. 1983.

[27] H. C. Casey, D. D. Sell, and K. W. Wecht, "Concentration dependence of the absorption coefficient for n- and p-type GaAs between 1.3 and 1.6 eV", J. Appl. Phys., vol. 46, pp. 250-257, January 1975.

[28] M. Ogura, T. Hata, N. J. Kawai, and T. Yao, "GaAs/Al$_x$Ga$_{1-x}$As multilayer reflector for surface emitting laser diode", Japan. J. Appl. Phys., vol. 22, pp. L112-L114, Feb. 1983.

Scanning Single-Slit and Double-Slit Phase Measurements of Grating Surface Emitter Diode Laser Arrays

Stanley L. Reinhold, J. Michael Finlan,
John G. Lehman, Jr. and Scott M. Hamilton

GE Astro-Space Division
P.O. Box 8555, Philadelphia, PA 19101

ABSTRACT

We report measurements of the near-field phase of a two-dimensional array of grating surface emitter diode lasers. The measurements were performed by scanning single and double slits. We use the individually measured phases over 300 μm x 50 μm emitting regions to predict the beam quality, and we compare the predictions with measured data.

1. INTRODUCTION

Measuring the phase of an optical source is generally a difficult task. It requires knowledge of the propagation distance between the source and the point of measurement as well as the calibration of aberrations introduced by optical elements in the measurement system. Dente et al. used a scanning double-slit technique to measure the near-field phase of a diode laser array.[1] In this paper, we utilize both single-slit and double-slit techniques to determine one-dimensional phase profiles without the use of any optics. These methods have particular appeal for our application, which is the measurement of the phase of Grating Surface Emitter (GSE) lasers.[2]

Conventional phase measurement systems such as radial shear interferometers or Mach-Zehnder interferometers have the advantage of providing two-dimensional phase profiles. However, these systems have entrance aperture requirements which are prohibitive for the sources we are testing. For example, the Zygo Wavefront Analyzer (radial shear) requires the beam cross section to be greater than 4 mm, but no larger than 15 mm. For an edge-emitting diode laser with a typical divergence of 10^0 by 30^0, a single collimating lens can produce a 4-mm by 12-mm collimated beam. However, for small sources with large aspect ratios, it may be necessary to use several cylindrical and spherical lenses to fill the entrance aperture of the interferometer. The introduction of lenses into the measurement path adds uncertainties to the measurement because of possible lens aberrations and misalignment. The scanning-slit approach to phase measurement removes the necessity of calibrating the system for lens aberrations and simplifies the alignment of the system.

2. THE SCANNING-SLIT PHASE MEASUREMENT TECHNIQUE

The scanning-slit conceptual diagram is shown in Figure 1 for the double-slit and single-slit approaches. The slit mask is placed in the path of the unknown wavefront. For a single-slit measurement, the centroid position of the single-slit diffraction is determined solely by the phase tilt across the slit. The plot of centroid location versus slit location yields the phase slope as a function of distance, and this can be integrated to determine the actual phase of the wavefront.

For the double-slit case, we expect to see an interference pattern in the far field of the two slits as shown in Figure 1. The location of the fringes depends upon the phase difference between the slits. The phase difference versus slit separation yields the phase derivative, and we can integrate to get the desired result.

The wavefront in Figure 1 is drawn as coming from an arbitrary source at an arbitrary distance. Indeed, the scanning-slit phase measurement is valid for the placement of the slit(s) anywhere on the optical axis. In addition to phase profile data, a by-product of the scanning-slit measurement is a record of the wavefront intensity profile. It is conceivable that the far field of an arbitrary source can be scanned with the single or double slit and that, from both the intensity and phase data, the source can be uniquely determined by simple inversion techniques such as Sommerfeld diffraction or Fast Fourier Transforms.

There are six major assumptions that have been made to simplify the explanation of the scanning-slit algorithms:

1. The centroid or fringe locator measurement device is in the far field of the slit(s).

2. The phase across a slit is locally flat to first order (constant phase plus a tilt).

3. For the double-slit case, the phase slopes for each slit are equal.

4. The phase profile is continuous.

5. The amplitude across a slit is uniform, and the two slits have equal amplitude.

6. The electric field is separable into longitudinal and lateral components.

For the most part, these assumptions are satisfied when the slits are smaller than the highest spatial frequencies (both phase and intensity) present in the wavefront.

3. PHASE OF THE GRATING SURFACE EMITTERS

The scanning-slit phase measurement technique is quite practical for sources that have large aspect ratios. Consider Figure 2, which depicts the conventional way to measure the phase of a long slender diode laser array. The introduction of aberrations from lenses as well as the alignment problem associated with the use of cylindrical lenses is more cumbersome than the scanning-slit approach, which utilizes no optics and is relatively trivial to align. The other disadvantage of radial shear interferometers is that they use the center 10% of the wavefront as the reference. Any phase perturbations present in the reference beam will corrupt the measurement.

The devices which were of interest to us were the Grating Surface Emitters fabricated at David Sarnoff Research Laboratories (DSRC).[2] The device consists of 10 groups of 10 diode lasers, monolithically grown in AlGaAs for operation in the near infrared. Figure 3 shows the geometry of the device, which uses a novel grating to serve three purposes: 1) to couple light longitudinally to the next group of ten lasers, 2) to reflect light to the preceding group of ten, and 3) to couple light out of the surface and subsequently provide a relatively large light emitting region (typically 300 μm by 50 μm). Each gain region in Figure 3 comprises 10 evanescently coupled stripes. The stripes are 3 μm wide on 5-μm centers. These stripes, which are in the lateral direction of the device, are not shown for simplicity of the diagram. In addition to the individual stripes in the gain region, there is also weak index guiding in the longitudinal direction of the grating. The near-field phase that was of interest to us was along the longitudinal direction, and we assumed that the electric fields in the evanescent and longitudinal directions were separable. The device tested was pumped uniformly at 600 mA for each gain region; it lased at 810 nm with a peak output of 100 to 200 mW for a 1% duty cycle and 100-ns pulses.

The setup for measurement of the near-field phase of the GSE is shown in Figure 4 where the subject grating was an end grating. Therefore, only one of the gain regions in Figure 4 was pumped. A translation stage with 1-μm precision was used to translate the slits. The slits utilized in the experiment were 25 μm for the single slit and 10 μm on 50-μm centers for the double slit. The slits were etched in chrome and gold on 15-mil quartz. The detector head was a 1024-element linear array with elements on 25-μm spacings. The slits were scanned in the near field of the GSE less than 5 mm from the array. The slits were preceded by a single light blocking mask to block all but one end grating. The scanning slits were aligned to traverse the 300-μm (longitudinal) direction of the grating region.

The phase derivative of the 300-μm source was determined where the ordinate was the location of the maximum intensity for the single-slit method or the fringe location for the double-slit method. The abscissa was the slit(s) position. The near-field phase was determined by integrating this result. The near-field phase of the single 300-μm grating is shown in Figure 5, where each division is $\lambda/10$. Over the majority of the 300-μm emitting region, the phase was flat to better than $\lambda/10$. The results for the single-slit and double-slit approaches agree within $\lambda/30$ inside the 300-μm aperture. In the limiting case of very small slits and separation of slits, the two approaches should yield identical results. The single-slit phase curve in Figure 5 was measured several times and was repeatable to better than $\lambda/50$.

4. CALCULATION VERSUS MEASUREMENT OF GSE FAR FIELD

The relative near-field intensity distribution for the grating region is plotted in Figure 6. The near-field intensity was measured by recording the peak irradiance from the slit(s) diffraction versus the slit(s) location. The far field of the grating region was calculated numerically from the measured near-field intensity and phase profiles. Scalar diffraction theory with the Fresnel-Kirchoff approximation was utilized. Partial coherence of the source was also modeled. The calculated far fields for the single-slit and double-slit data are plotted in Figure 7, where a 100% coherent source was assumed. Figure 8 compares the measured far field of the grating region with the calculated far field from single-slit phase and intensity data. Here, the spatial coherence of the source was measured and incorporated into the scalar diffraction model. We chose to model it as a geometric decrease of the form:

$$coh_{spatial} = .5^{\frac{x[\mu m]}{300}}.$$

5. LIMITATIONS OF SCANNING-SLIT PHASE MEASUREMENT

The resolution of the scanning-slit phase measurement techniques depends on :
1. Slit size, separation, and the quality of lithography used in the fabrication of the slits.
2. The difference in intensity between the slits as they scan across the wavefront.
3. The difference in slope between the phase of the two slits.
4. The resolution of the detector.
5. The degree of curvature of the phase of the wavefront.

These issues are presently being quantified and will be reported in a future paper.

6. APPLICATIONS OF PHASE MEASUREMENT TECHNIQUE

Because of the ability of the phase measurement setup to work for very small beams, it is useful for measuring small phase features in optical elements. For example, the features of a computer-generated optical lenses could be analyzed without the use of image or magnification lenses. This would give results similar to a profilometer. The design of low f-number lenses to collimate highly divergent sources, as well as correct for aberrations, could be achieved by characterizing the phasefront of the divergent source and calculating the appropriate computer-generated lens to correct for the phase curvature. Liquid crystal pixels could be analyzed for phase uniformity or to determine the presence of small, localized phase perturbations.

7. CONCLUSIONS

The use of a scanning single-slit or double-slit phase measurement technique has been demonstrated for the near-field phase characterization of a surface emitting diode laser. The phase of a 300-μm region was measured to an accuracy exceeding $\lambda/10$. The scanning-slit technique is well suited for situations in which beam sizes are smaller than the aperture requirements of conventional interferometric phase measurement schemes and when it is not desirable to use lenses. The radial shear measurement technique requires a flat phase reference, which is sheared from the center portion of the tested wavefront. This can result in degraded phase accuracy for wavefronts that exhibit localized phase perturbations.

The major limitations of the scanning-slit approach are the accuracy with which the slits can be fabricated and the resolution of the detector. The use of a scanning double-slit system, in which an optical matched filter can be utilized to reduce the detector to a single element (power meter), will be the topic of a future paper.

Finally, potential applications of this approach have been outlined in the fields of holography and liquid crystal characterization.

8. ACKNOWLEDGEMENTS

The authors extend thanks to Bill Cassarly and Kevin Flood for their insightful comments and to the David Sarnoff Research Center for the use of their devices. This work was funded in part by the Air Force.

9. REFERENCES

1. G. C. Dente, K. A. Wilson, T. C. Salvi, and D. Depatie, "Phase and spatial coherence measurements on diode arrays: Comparison to supermode theory," Appl. Phys. Lett. **51**, 9 (1987).
2. N. W. Carlson, G. A. Evans, J. M. Hammer, M. Lurie, S. L. Palfrey, and A. Dholakia, "Phase-locked operation of a grating-surface-emitting diode laser array," Appl. Phys. Lett. **50**, 1301 (1987).

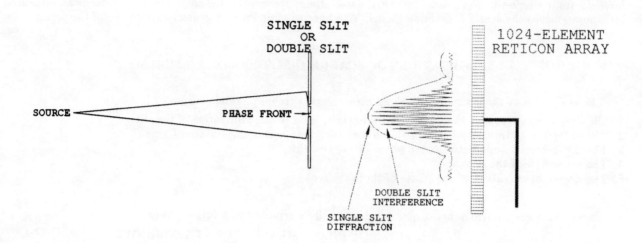

Figure 1: Scanning Slit Phase Measurement.

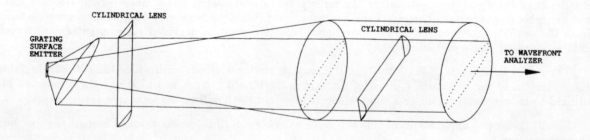

Figure 2: Phase Measurement of a Grating Surface Emitter Using a Shearing Interferometer Phase Measurement

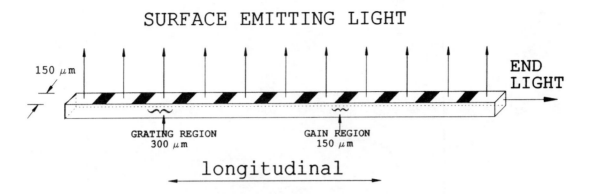

Figure 3: Grating Surface Emitter. Dark Regions Consist of Evanescently Coupled Stripes; White Regions Are Gratings.

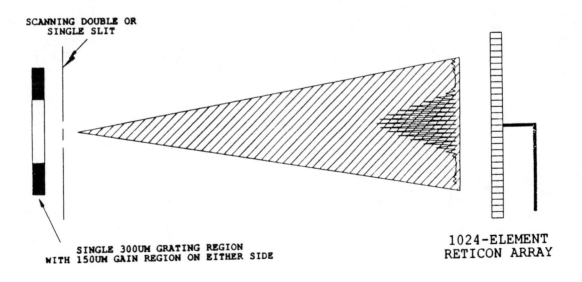

Figure 4: Near-Field Phase Measurement of a Grating Surface Emitter.

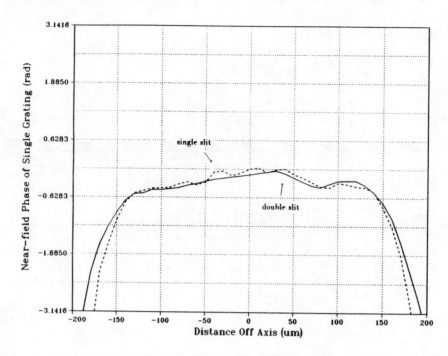

Figure 5: Phase of GSE Section Determined by Scanning Single and Double Slit.

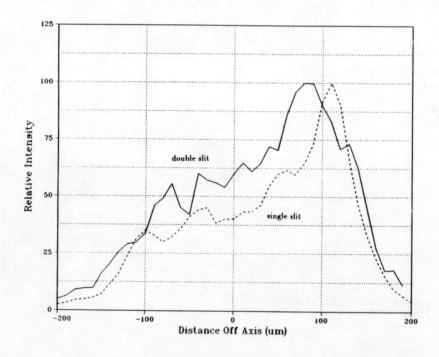

Figure 6: Near-Field Intensity of GSE Section Determined by Scanning Single and Double Slit.

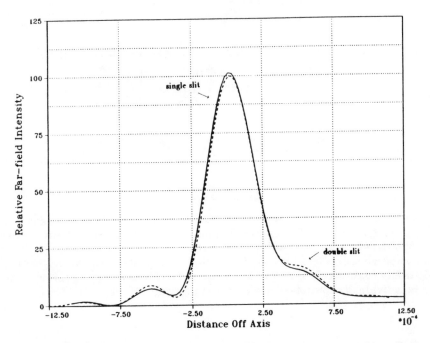

Figure 7: Calculated Far-Field Irradiance from a Single Grating (100% spatial coherence).

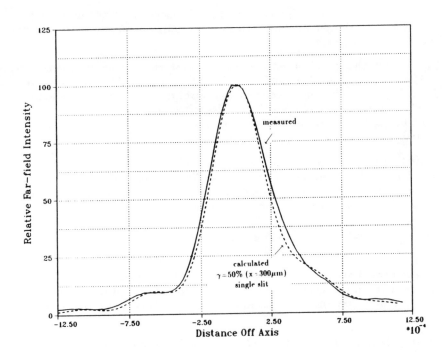

Figure 8: Calculated vs. Measured Far-Field Irradiance of a Single Grating (Geometric Falloff of Spatial Coherence to 70% at Grating Edges).

Phase Control of Coherent Diode Laser Arrays Using Liquid Crystals

Bill Cassarly and J. Michael Finlan
GE Astro-Space Division
P.O. Box 8555, Philadelphia, PA 19101

Michael DeJule and Charles Stein
GE Corporate Research and Development Center
Schenectady, NY 12345

ABSTRACT

The on-axis fields from separate elements of a coherent laser array can interfere either constructively or destructively, depending upon the relative phases. We describe thin film transistor (TFT) and direct-drive controlled arrays of liquid crystal phase shifters, which provide both phase matching and fine beamsteering. The transmissive liquid crystal devices contain homogeneously aligned layers of nematic liquid crystals sandwiched between two glass plates. The devices impart electrically controllable analog phase delays to laser beams passing through the cells. The devices are divided into arrays of individually controlled elements using separate transparent electrodes.

1. BACKGROUND

Coherent diode laser arrays are receiving increasing emphasis in many applications which require free space transmission over large distances and for applications requiring powers much greater than those possible from single-stripe lasers. To maximize the transmitted on-axis power, the individual elements of such an array must be both coherent and matched in phase. This paper addresses the phase-matching problem and assumes coherence.

To create a phase-matched array, the emitting surface of all the elements in the array must be coplanar. Guaranteeing fraction of a micrometer variations for large arrays is typically not practical. A transmissive liquid crystal phase plate provides the required phase correction.

In addition to the phase-matching problem, optical satellite-to-satellite communication systems require precise pointing angle control. At a wavelength of 0.8 μm, a 5-cm coherent array produces a beam for which the divergence of the central lobe is 10 μrad. It therefore becomes necessary to control the pointing to a few μrad. Microradian control of the beam is extremely difficult using conventional gimbals, but a phased array provides a method of obtaining such control. The spacing between elements and the fineness of control over the individual phases within the array determine the accuracy and resolution of the steering angle control.

This paper reviews how liquid crystals provide phase control, and it describes a 100 x 100 array controlled by thin film transistors (TFT) and a 1 x 25 element direct-drive array. Next, theory behind beamsteering with such arrays is included. This is followed by a discussion of the important insertion losses (reflections, uniformity, and absorption and scattering) and, finally, a description of our experimental results.

2. LIQUID CRYSTAL PHASE SHIFTER

To create an optical phased array, a method of introducing electrically controllable phase shifts is needed. The high birefringence of nematic liquid crystals and the ability to control this birefringence using small voltages makes them an excellent candidate material. The purpose of this section is to describe how this analog phase shift is produced.

A nematic liquid crystal phase cell is made by sandwiching a liquid material between two glass plates (Figure 1a). The molecules are aligned parallel to the glass surfaces. The application of an electric field causes the molecules to rotate (Figure 1b). When the molecules have rotated, the corresponding change in index of refraction produces a phase delay. The phase change is described by

$$\phi = \frac{2\pi}{\lambda} \int_0^d \Delta n(x) dx = \frac{2\pi d}{\lambda} \Delta n_{avg}, \tag{1}$$

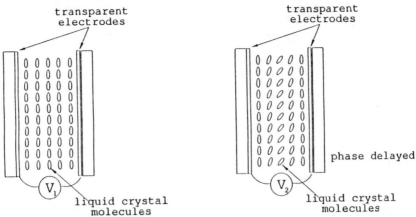

Figure 1: Liquid Crystal Phase Cell: a) Off State, b) Molecular Reorientation Induced Phase Change.

where d is the cell thickness, Δn is the voltage-controlled change in index of refraction, λ is the wavelength, and x denotes distance from the first glass/liquid crystal interface. The maximum birefringence of nematic liquid crystals can be greater than 0.25; this permits phase shifts greater than 2π (depending upon cell thickness). In our liquid crystal phase cell, the control voltages are applied via transparent ITO (indium tin oxide) electrodes. In the cell, the light polarization is oriented in the direction of the liquid crystal director (the local average orientation of the liquid crystal molecules) so that there is no polarization rotation, as is the case for twisted nematic devices.

The dependence of molecular orientation on voltage can be determined by minimizing the integral of the sum of the elastic and electrostatic energies. Once the molecular orientation is determined, the corresponding phase delay through the cell can be calculated using the index ellipsoid of a uniaxial crystal. A sample phase versus voltage curve, measured using Deuling's method[1], is shown in Figure 2. Notice the existence of a threshold voltage (V_{th}), a linear region, and a saturation region. Linearizing the elastic and electrostatic energy equations yields the slope of the phase-versus-voltage curve for voltages near threshold:

$$\frac{d\phi}{dV} = -\frac{2\pi d n_\|}{\lambda V_{th}} \left(\frac{n_\|^2}{n_\perp^2} - 1\right) \frac{1}{\kappa + \gamma + 1}, \qquad (2)$$

where $n_\|$ and $n_\perp$ are the indices of refraction parallel and perpendicular to the long axis of the liquid crystal molecule; the elastic constant anisotropy is $\kappa = (k_\| - k_\perp) / k_\|$, and the dielectric anisotropy is $\gamma = (\epsilon_\| - \epsilon_\perp) / \epsilon_\perp$. Experimental data and computer simulations show that the validity of this linear approximation depends upon the specific material parameters chosen, but it is typically correct to within 25% for voltages less than twice the threshold voltage.

3. DEVICE DESCRIPTIONS

The brute force approach for controlling 10000 elements is to run separate control electrodes to each element of the array. This direct control might be realizable for 10000 elements, but is somewhat impractical, especially for even larger arrays. One sophisticated method for reducing the number of control electrodes is to incorporate a nonlinear element, such as a transistor, into each element (Figure 3). In this way, row-column addressing can be used, thereby reducing the number of control lines from N^2 to $2N$. We are investigating control methods for applications which have a small number of elements and also for large arrays. Current devices for both types of applications are described in this section.

The compact size and low power requirements of TFTs make them an excellent choice for the nonlinear element. The approach we took was to utilize GE Corporate Research and Development's state-of-the-art amorphous silicon TFT technology. These TFT arrays are currently used in twisted nematic flat panel amplitude displays. However, instead of incorporating a twist in the molecular orientation (as is typical in current flat panel displays), the molecules are aligned parallel to each other, and parallel to the glass surfaces. A device with this homogeneous alignment is often referred to as a controlled birefringence device.

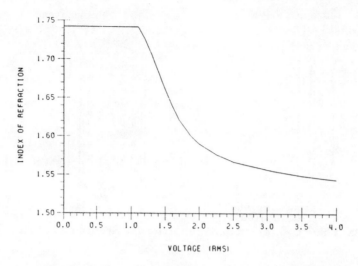

Figure 2: Index of Refraction versus Voltage Relationship.

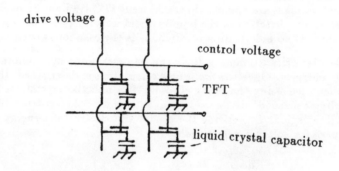

Figure 3: TFT Pixel Control.

The 100 x 100 element phase control array has pixels which are 220 μm x 220 μm, spaced on 250 μm centers. The pixels are 6 μm thick, yielding more than the required 2π phase variation at $\lambda = 0.8$ μm. Currently, twisted nematic liquid crystal TFT controlled arrays with 100-μm x 100-μm pixels are available, with some research focused on 50-μm x 50-μm pixels. Even smaller pixels are possible, but they may be limited by electric field fringing effects and elastic forces imposed by neighboring pixels.

In a TFT-controlled phase plate, the control (row) voltages are used to turn on/off the transistors, and the drive (column) voltages are applied across the transistor/capacitor pair. When the control voltage exceeds the transistor threshold, the transistor turns on, and the drive voltage is applied to the selected element. When the control voltage is below the transistor's threshold, the transistor turns off, and the applied information is retained by the selected element as a charge across a capacitor. In this device, the liquid crystal material is used as the capacitor (other designs have incorporated separate capacitors). By selecting a transistor/capacitor time constant much greater than the refresh time, the voltage stored on the capacitor is essentially constant.

For applications where the number of elements is small, the added complexity of TFT addressing is not warranted, and direct drive is appropriate. As an example of direct addressing, we built devices which correct the dissimilarities in the individual beams emitted from a AlGaAs Grating Surface Emitter (GSE) array. The GSE arrays are Distributed Bragg Reflectors with eleven grating regions (emitters) separated by ten gain regions. The GSE arrays were produced at the David Sarnoff Research Center[2], and each grating region consists of 10 individual 3-μm stripes on 6-μm centers. The length of each grating region is 300 μm, and the length of each gain region is 150 μm. Thus, the dimensions of one laser bar are 4.3 mm x 57 μm, and the bar contains 100 lasers.

The direct-drive liquid crystal array is designed with 25 pixels, where each pixel is 300 μm x 1000 μm. The rectangular shape was chosen to reduce the difficulty of aligning the liquid crystal array. There is a separate electrical contact to each of the pixels so that the phase from each pixel is controlled separately.

4. PHASED ARRAY BEAMSTEERING

Consider a linear array of identical elements with center-to-center spacing b. Assume the electric field amplitude of each element is $a_n(x)$, and let the elements have a linearly related phase term, $e^{j\phi n}$, where n is an integer which corresponds to the nth element, and ϕ is the element-to-element phase difference. If $a_n(x)$ is the same for all N elements, the aperture field, $a(x)$, is simply the convolution of the element field with a series of delta functions:

$$a(x) = [a_n(x)] * [\sum_{n=0}^{N-1} \delta(x - bn) e^{j\phi n}], \tag{3}$$

where $\delta(x)$ is the Dirac delta function, and the $*$ denotes convolution. Using the Fraunhofer approximation (the propagation distance $\gg \frac{(Nb)^2}{\lambda}$), and letting $a_n(x)$ be a circular aperture of diameter w, we find that the far field distribution resulting from the laser facet field described in Equation 3 is proportional to

$$A(u) \propto \frac{\sin[(\frac{N}{2})(\frac{2\pi}{\lambda}bu - \phi)]}{\sin[(\frac{1}{2})(\frac{2\pi}{\lambda}bu - \phi)]} \left(\frac{w}{2}\right)^2 \frac{J_1(\pi w u)}{\frac{wu}{2}}. \tag{4}$$

The $\frac{\sin(Nu)}{\sin(u)}$ term is called the array factor, and the second term, which is the transform of the element field distribution and includes the first-order Bessel function J_1, is called the element factor.

A normalized plot of $|A(u)|^2$ is shown in Figure 4 with $N = 21$, $w = 150$ μm, $b = 250$ μm, $\lambda = 0.6328$ μm, and $\phi = 0, \frac{\pi}{2}$, and π. Because of the array factor's periodicity, the unique range of ϕ's is $-\pi < \phi < \pi$, and the maximum deflection angle is

$$\theta_{max} = \sin^{-1} u = \sin^{-1}(\frac{\lambda}{2b}). \tag{5}$$

Notice in Figure 4 that the intensity decreases as the main lobe is steered off axis. This amplitude decrease is due to the element factor falloff. A phase gradient (tilt) across each element is needed to control this falloff. We are currently investigating a device which provides tilt across each element, and we will report on it at a later date.

5. INSERTION LOSSES: REFLECTIONS

Analogous to impedance mismatches in electrical circuits, mismatches in dielectric constants will create reflections. If both the exact thickness and the surface variations of the two sheets of glass are controlled to a fraction of a wavelength, the reflections can be reduced to a few percent. Such control is difficult in practice, but necessary. Without it, the index of refraction mismatches of typical liquid crystal phase cells can yield reflections as high as 30%. In addition, the percent reflection will vary as the liquid crystal index of refraction is varied, thereby producing an undesired amplitude variation in addition to the phase modulation (see Figure 5). To reduce these undesired amplitude effects, a wavelength-tuned antireflection coating is required for the phase cell. In addition, to reduce ITO layer reflections, silicon nitride layers are incorporated into the cell.

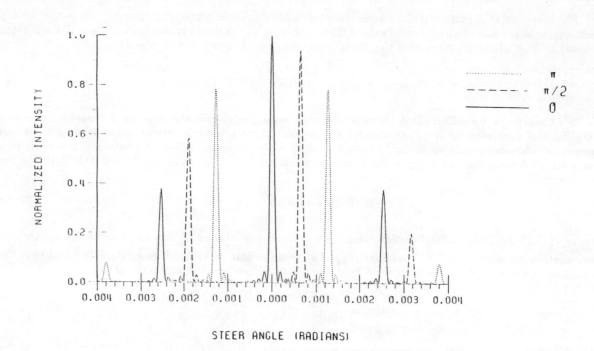

Figure 4: Calculated Beam Deflection Curves for a Phased Array Antenna: Element-to-Element Phase Difference of (a) 0, (b) $\frac{\pi}{2}$, and (c) π

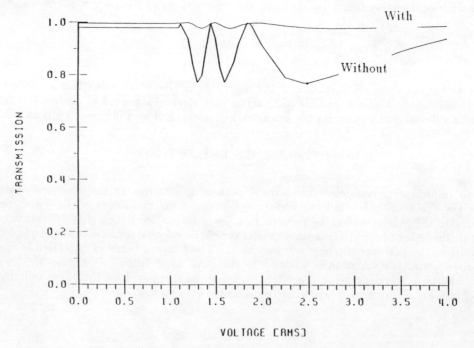

Figure 5: Amplitude Variation Due To Dielectric Mismatches: With and Without an Antireflection Coating

6. INSERTION LOSSES: NONUNIFORMITIES

Even with an antireflection coating, the glass surface flatness will affect the phase cell's performance in three ways: 1) Each pixel will have a different off-state phase delay, 2) The phase-versus-voltage relationship (shown in Figure 2) will vary from pixel to pixel, and 3) Each pixel will introduce a phase tilt. Each of these ideas is discussed below.

1) The off-state phase delay (the delay when the control voltages are zero) does not pose any significant problems because these delays affect the system performance in the same way as the laser diode surface flatness. The process of correcting the laser diode element-to-element phase mismatches will also correct the phase cell off-state thickness variations.

2) The pixel-to-pixel liquid crystal layer thickness differences in a phase cell can easily be controlled to within 0.2 μm. In the 100 x 100 element array, this thickness control is accomplished via polyimide spacers, which are incorporated into the area between pixels. Because the shape of the index-of-refraction-versus-voltage profile scales linearly with thickness, the thickness variations create an error which is directly proportional to the thickness error. The maximum error then occurs when the largest birefringence change is attempted. This phase error is

$$\phi_{error} = \frac{2\pi}{\lambda}(\Delta n_{max})(d_{error}), \tag{6}$$

where d_{error} is the liquid crystal layer variation. For $\lambda = 0.8$ μm and $\Delta n_{max} = 0.25$, the peak error is less than 0.4 radians.

The effect of element-to-element phase errors upon the on-axis normalized intensity is described by

$$I_{norm} = 1 - \frac{1-N}{N}(2\pi\sigma_\phi)^2, \tag{7}$$

where N is the number of elements, and σ_ϕ is the standard deviation of ϕ_{error}. If the phase errors from an array of emitters are uniformly distributed between plus and minus 0.2 radians, the on-axis intensity will be reduced by less than 1.3 percent. This small on-axis degradation creates a slight broadening of the far-field beamwidth and a corresponding increase in the sidelobe intensity.

3) Once the random element-to-element "piston" phase variations are removed, the residual phase error is dominated by the phase tilt error. To understand how dependent the on-axis irradiance is upon the residual tilt errors, consider an array of slits. If the tilt errors are uncorrelated and small, then the element tilt error creates a change in the normalized on-axis intensity, described by

$$I_{norm} = 1 - \frac{\sigma_\theta^2}{\lambda^2}\frac{A''(0)}{A(0)} \tag{8}$$

where σ_θ^2 is the variance of the tilt error (in rad^2), $A(0)$ is the on-axis far-field aperture function, and $A''(0)$ is the spatial second derivative of A across a plane in the far field. For a slit of width w, the decrease in on-axis intensity described by Equation 8 is

$$\frac{\sigma_\theta^2}{\lambda^2}\frac{(2\pi w)^2}{3}. \tag{9}$$

This error is less than 1% for $\sigma_\theta = \frac{0.01\lambda}{w}$ when the aperture is uniformly illuminated, and the error is even smaller if the aperture illumination is nonuniform (e. g., Gaussian).

7. INSERTION LOSSES: ABSORPTION AND SCATTERING

Indium tin oxide is an alloy of indium oxide (In_2O_3) and tin oxide (SnO_2). Both indium oxide and tin oxide are more transparent than indium tin oxide at 0.8 μm. Their absorption coefficients are less than 10,000 m^{-1}, whereas the coefficient for the alloy is between 10,000 and 1,000,000 m^{-1}. However, indium tin oxide is a better conductor, which is desirable. Fortunately, the two ITO thicknesses are very thin, so that the ITO losses can be less than 0.2%.

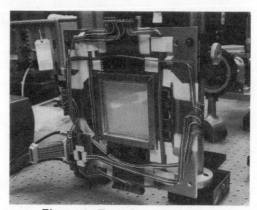

Figure 6: Experimental Setup

Three loss mechanisms exist in liquid crystal materials: 1) scattering due to thermally induced time and space fluctuations of the liquid crystal director, 2) absorption due to the tails of the ultraviolet absorption, and 3) scattering due to disclinations and other nonuniformities. For temperatures much less than the liquid crystal clearing point (the transition from nematic to isotropic), the thermally induced scattering will be the most significant loss mechanism for a carefully aligned cell. The scattering coefficient is approximately 700 m^{-1} for the liquid crystal mixture E7.[3] For a 6-μm thick cell, the loss is less than 0.5%.

For optical communication applications, frequency variations caused by the beam control optics must be considered. Because of the liquid crystal time fluctuation, a frequency shift on the order of a kHz can arise, and this shift varies with angle.[4] Since the optical spectrum of current laser diodes is significantly larger than 1 kHz, this frequency shift can be neglected for most systems.

8. EXPERIMENTAL RESULTS

To demonstrate beam steering, we passed the output of a collimated HeNe laser through an array of 150-μm circular apertures, which were aligned in front of the liquid crystal phase plate. A photograph of the phase plate is shown in Figure 6. The far-field intensity when all phases are matched is shown in 7. A plot of the far-field profile when the beam is steered to $\frac{\lambda}{4b}$ radians is also shown along with a plot of the profile when the central lobe is steered to $\frac{\lambda}{2b}$ radians. The plots show excellent agreement with the theoretical curves.

The curves in Figure 7 show horizontal steering; we also demonstrated vertical steering with similar results. In addition, a collimated 0.8-μm diode laser was also steered in both directions with excellent agreement to theory. The control voltages for the diode laser experiments were significantly different from the HeNe experiments. This difference is due to the longer wavelength and the lower birefringence of the liquid crystal at 0.8μm.

The direct-drive array produced similar results with both a HeNe source and an array of surface emitting diode lasers.

9. CONCLUSIONS

We have described how liquid crystals can provide phase matching and beam steering for a coherent array of laser sources. A large scale TFT-driven liquid crystal phase plate was demonstrated experimentally, and we described possible insertion losses for such a device. These results show that liquid crystals can be used for beam control of diode laser arrays.

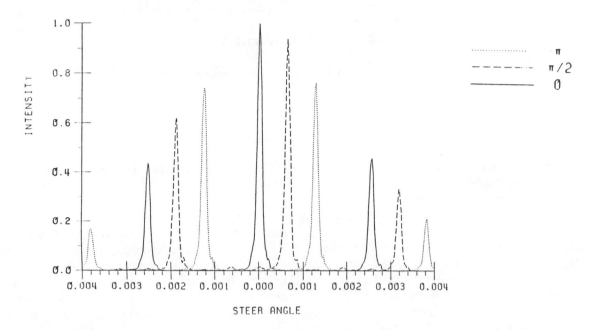

Figure 7: Experimental Results: Element-to-Element Phase Difference of (a) 0, (b) $\frac{\pi}{2}$, and (c) π

10. REFERENCES

1. H. J. Deuling, "Deformation of Nematic Liquid Crystals in an Electric Field", Mol. Crys. Liq. Crys., **19**, 123-131, 1972
2. N. W. Carlson, G. A. Evans, J. M. Hammer, M. Lurie, S. L. Palfrey, and A. Dholakia, "Phase-locked operation of a grating-surface-emitting diode laser array," Appl. Phys. Lett. **50**, 1301 (1987).
3. S. T. Wu and K. C. Lim, "Absorption and scattering measurements of nematic liquid crystals", Appl Opt., **26**, 1722-1727, 1987
4. L. Leger-Quercy, *Etude experimentale des fluctuations thermiques d'orientation dans un cristal liquide nematique par diffusion inelastique de la lumiere*, thesis, University of Paris, France, 1970

ACKNOWLEDGEMENTS

The authors thank the invaluable contributions made by the individuals at Astro-Space Division and the GE Corporate Research and Development Center. Funding was provided by GE IR&D.

Coupling of index-guided lateral modes in
three-stripe gain-guided laser diode arrays

Donald G. Heflinger and Wayne R. Fenner

The Aerospace Corporation, Electronics Research Laboratory
P.O. Box 92957, MS M2-246, Los Angeles, CA 90009

ABSTRACT

Experimental results are presented which indicate the existence of index-guided lateral modes between stripes in multistripe laser diode arrays fabricated from planar double heterostructure material. Through a comparison to measurements made on twin-stripe arrays, each adjacent pair of stripes in a three-stripe array is observed to support index-guided modes. A comparison of the measured far-field intensity pattern with the calculated far-field diffraction pattern from the three-stripe array suggests that out-of-phase coupling between the two index-guided modes has been observed just above threshold, while at higher currents the two modes run independently. The presence of higher-order index-guided modes has also been observed as the current is increased. Measurements made on a commercially available ten-stripe laser also suggest the presence of index-guided lateral modes.

1. INTRODUCTION

Laser diode arrays, fabricated from planar double heterostructure (DH) material, have been at the forefront of the revolution in high-power semiconductor lasers. As single-stripe lasers, they operate on the gain-guided regime; as closely spaced stripes, they have been characterized as coupled arrays of gain-guided lasers. They are relatively easy to fabricate compared with index-guided devices which are typically nonplanar. Unfortunately, the range of applications for these devices has been limited because they typically produce a double-lobed, rather than the desired single-lobed, far-field intensity pattern.

This paper presents experimental evidence that lateral array modes of a laser array fabricated from planar DH material may also arise from coupling between index-guided modes positioned between the stripes. These index-guided modes differ from the gain-guided modes positioned under the stripes in that they are better confined and have a lower lasing threshold[1]. Since the index-guided modes form between the stripes while the gain peaks lie under the stripes, it seemed possible that the in-phase array modes might have a lower threshold current than the out-of-phase modes.

We review here the data which clearly identifies the index-guided modes of the twin-stripe laser. We then present experimental evidence which shows that two index-guided modes exist in three-stripe devices, that these modes couple together in an out-of-phase array mode (instead of the hoped for in-phase array mode), and that at conditions of high drive current, the individual modes do not coherently combine (i.e., lock) even though they exhibit nearly identical spectra.

2. THE FORMATION OF INDEX-GUIDED LATERAL MODES

Recent studies made on twin-stripe laser diodes fabricated from planar DH material have shown that the changes in the refractive index due to the injected current can form a waveguide between the stripes which supports index-guided modes[1]. Experiments were carried out with devices fabricated using both Si_3N_4 defined and Schottky barrier defined stripes on an MOCVD (metal-organic chemical vapor deposition) grown wafer of GaAlAs/GaAs. The width of the stripes was set by a 4 μm wide mask with a center-to-center spacing of 8 μm. The Schottky barrier stripes were defined by etching away the heavily p⁺-doped GaAs cap layer everywhere except for the stripe. A uniformly evaporated metal contact formed a Schottky barrier to the lighter p-doped isolation layer and allowed the two stripes to be driven together. The width of each Schottky barrier defined stripe was reduced to 3 μm by the etch.

The characteristics of both the Si_3N_4 and Schottky barrier defined devices were the same as long as care was taken to avoid etching the Schottky barrier deep enough to induce ridge waveguiding. The Schottky barrier defined devices were also convenient for determining the exact position of the lasing mode relative to the stripe since the location of the stripes could be determined by viewing the output facet.

The lasing mode of the twin-stripe laser just above threshold was tightly confined between the stripes and occurred at a lower threshold than that for a single-stripe laser. Figure 1 compares the near-field facet images of the single and twin-stripe lasers. The etched ridges of the Schottky barrier allow the stripe location to be

      (a) Single-stripe   (b) Twin-stripe

Figure 1. Facet images of the near-field intensity for single and twin-stripe lasers.

determined in the output facet photographs. Figure 2 displays the intensity profiles of these two lasers. In the twin-stripe laser, the lateral mode is confined between the two stripes in an index-guide formed between the stripes[2]. The injected current

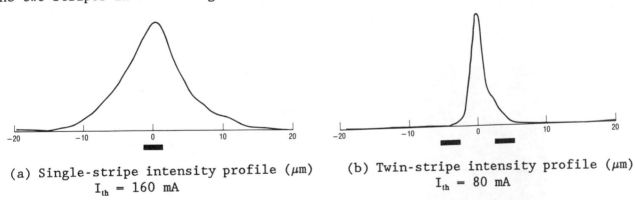

(a) Single-stripe intensity profile (μm)   (b) Twin-stripe intensity profile (μm)
I_{th} = 160 mA I_{th} = 80 mA

Figure 2. Near-field intensity profiles for single and twin-stripe laser diodes.

lowers the refractive index under the stripes leaving the region between the stripes at a slightly higher index to form a waveguide. The improvement in optical confinement provided by this waveguide overcomes the lower gain produced by current spreading and reduces the lasing threshold current below that of a gain-guided single-stripe laser.

Figure 3 displays the contrasting far-field patterns from these two laser diodes. The injected current in the single-stripe laser lowers the refractive index under

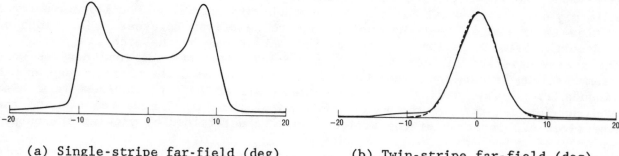

(a) Single-stripe far-field (deg) (b) Twin-stripe far-field (deg)

Figure 3. Far-field intensity profiles in single and twin-stripe lasers. The dashed curve is the calculated Fraunhofer diffraction assuming a best fit Gaussian near-field profile to the near-field profile in Fig. 2(b).

the stripe forming an anti-waveguide[3]. The light propagating in this anti-waveguide has a curved wavefront which interferes to form a "rabbit-eared" far-field pattern. In contrast, the propagating light in the waveguide formed in the twin-stripe laser has a flatter wavefront and diffracts into a single-lobed far-field pattern. If one assumes that the twin-stripe near-field intensity profile in Fig. 2(b) represents the waist of a Gaussian beam, Fraunhofer diffraction predicts a far-field intensity profile depicted by the dashed curve in Fig. 3.

3. HIGHER-ORDER INDEX-GUIDED MODE DEPENDENCIES

The twin-stripe element can also support higher-order index-guided modes. The size of the index-step defining the waveguide between the stripes increases as the current to the laser is increased which allows higher-order modes to propagate and lase simultaneously with the fundamental mode.

Figure 4 depicts the spectrally resolved near-field pattern from a twin-stripe laser operating at a current large enough to support three index-guided modes. The

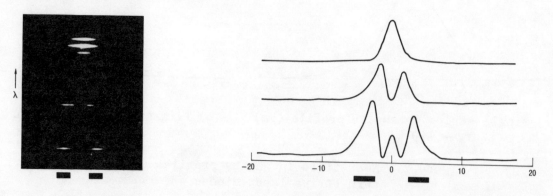

(a) Spectrally resolved near-field (b) Intensity profiles of each mode (μm)

Figure 4. Spectrally resolved near-field images and mode profiles of three index-guided modes in a twin-stripe laser.

higher-order modes were always separated by roughly 2 nm enabling an intensity profile of each mode to be taken. As the current was increased, the first mode to lase was the single-lobed fundamental. Increasing the current increased the index-step of the waveguide allowing the first order transverse electric mode (TE_{01}) to be supported simultaneously with the fundamental. Increasing the current further allowed the next higher-order mode (TE_{02}) to lase.

The lateral extent of these index-guided modes can be seen to be limited to the region between and under the stripes. This limited extent of the near-field intensity is a consequence of the mode confinement provided by the index-guide. Array modes from coupled gain-guided elements can also give rise to multi-lobed near-field intensities through interference of the curved wavefronts[4]. These would appear similar to the higher-order mode intensity profiles, but the intensity profile would extend beyond the outer edges of the stripes.

The effect of the center-to-center stripe separation was also studied. As the stripe separation was increased, the width of the index-guide increased and the order of the index-guided modes also increased. Figure 5 shows the higher-order modes observed at the output facet just above lasing threshold as the stripe separation, S, was increased from 12 μm to 18 μm.

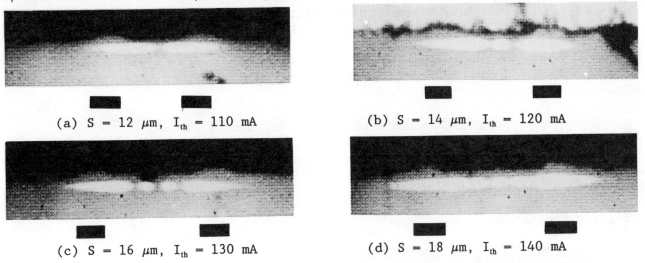

(a) S = 12 μm, I_{th} = 110 mA

(b) S = 14 μm, I_{th} = 120 mA

(c) S = 16 μm, I_{th} = 130 mA

(d) S = 18 μm, I_{th} = 140 mA

Figure 5. Facet images of twin-stripe lasers with increasing stripe separation showing the preference of higher order modes with increasing separation.

The highest-order mode that the index-guide could support was the one which lased first because the gain under the stripes has the best overlap with this mode. As the current was increased, additional higher-order modes were allowed by the increase in the index-step defining the waveguide. Each additional mode occurred roughly 2 nm shorter in wavelength than the initial lasing mode. The spectrally resolved near-field images obtained from twin-stripe lasers with increasing stripe separation are shown in Fig. 6.

The spectral separation of the higher-order index-guided modes may be due in part to band filling[5]. The current density increases in the region under the stripes placing the available states at a higher energy. The optical fields of the higher-order modes must draw from this region forcing them to have a shorter wavelength. The wavelength separations of the lateral modes of a waveguide also force the higher-order modes to be at shorter wavelengths; however, separations of roughly 2 nm for a waveguide several microns wide are some what surprising. In addition, the

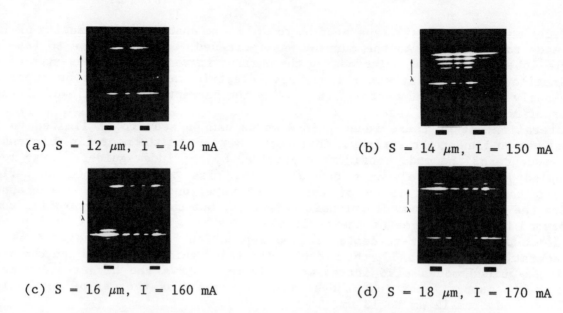

(a) S = 12 μm, I = 140 mA

(b) S = 14 μm, I = 150 mA

(c) S = 16 μm, I = 160 mA

(d) S = 18 μm, I = 170 mA

Figure 6. Spectrally resolved near-field images of twin-stripe lasers at several stripe separations.

presence of gain may be influencing the spectral separations in a way other than band filling. In any case, the spectral separation of the higher-order modes made it possible to identify and study them.

4. INDEX-GUIDED MODES IN THREE STRIPE ARRAYS

Three-stripe laser arrays were fabricated using Schottky barrier defined stripes on MOCVD grown DH material. All three stripes were driven together. Figure 7 is a photograph of the output facet showing the typical near-field intensity just above lasing threshold. Two index-guided modes confined between the three stripes are clearly discernible.

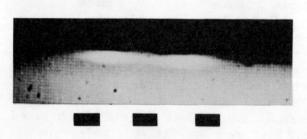

(a) Facet image

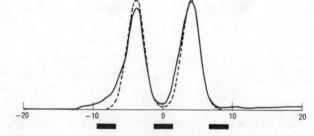

(b) Intensity profile (μm)

Figure 7. Facet image and experimentally measured intensity profile (solid curve) of the near-field from a three-stripe array superimposed over the calculated best fit double Gaussian intensity (dashed curve) from a three-stripe laser array.

The presence of just two intensity lobes positioned between the three stripes is best described by the fundamental index-guided modes of the two waveguides formed by the two twin-stripe elements, in which the center stripe is shared. The near-field intensity has been modeled using a best fit double Gaussian depicted by the dashed curve in Fig. 7(b).

5. EVIDENCE FOR OUT-OF-PHASE COUPLING OF THE FUNDAMENTAL INDEX-GUIDED MODES

The close proximity of the two fundamental index-guided modes suggests that they should phase lock together. The large gain present between each mode from the current injected under each stripe would suggest that the two modes should couple in-phase[6]. However, the double-lobed far-field intensity measurement depicted in Fig. 8(a)

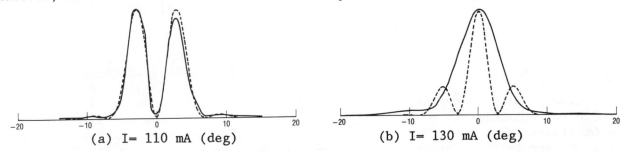

(a) I= 110 mA (deg)   (b) I= 130 mA (deg)

Figure 8. Far-field intensity profiles from a three-stripe gain-guided laser array (solid curves) and calculated far-field diffraction patterns (dashed curves) for (a) out-of-phase and (b) in-phase coupling of the double Gaussian depicted in Fig. 7(b).

indicates that just above threshold these two modes initially lock together out-of-phase. Increasing the current further resulted in a single-lobed far-field intensity profile as shown in Fig. 8(b). Fraunhofer diffraction intensity profiles from the double Gaussian near-field profile fitted in Fig. 7(b) are depicted for coupling both in-phase and out-of-phase by the dashed curves superimposed on Figs. 8(a) and 8(b) respectively. As illustrated in Fig. 8(b), the single-lobed far-field obtained at higher currents is not from in-phase locking of the two fundamental index-guided modes. The broad extent and lack of side lobes indicate that the light is not coherent over the width of the three-stripe array. The single-lobed far-field could be simply the incoherent sum of two Gaussians resulting in a Gaussian with the same extent as the single Gaussian obtained from the twin-stripe laser shown in Fig. 3(b).

6. HIGHER-ORDER MODES IN THREE-STRIPE ARRAYS

The incoherent superposition of two Gaussian modes is not the only contribution to the broad single-lobed far-field pattern of the three-stripe array at higher currents. Spectrally resolved near-field measurements indicate that as the current is increased,

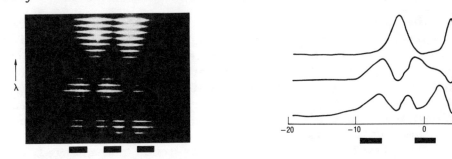

(a) Spectrally resolved near-field   (b) Intensity profiles of each mode (μm)

Figure 9. Spectrally resolved near-field image and intensity profiles of a three-stripe array.

the twin-stripe elements support higher-order index-guided modes. Figure 9 shows the spectrally resolved near-field of a three-stripe array.

The additional modes which begin to lase as the current is increased occur at shorter wavelengths, just as in the twin-stripe lasers. The spectra of the higher-order modes suggests that coupling may be taking place between them. However, the wavelength resolution was not sufficient to prove this conclusion. Two possible couplings of the adjacent first-order index-guided modes appear to be possible. The first, suggested by the middle profile, could have adjacent fields locked in phase, and the second, suggested by the bottom profile, could have adjacent fields locked out-of-phase.

7. INDEX-GUIDED MODES IN A GAIN-GUIDED TEN-STRIPE LASER DIODE ARRAY

The presence of higher-order index-guided modes in the three-stripe array prompted a preliminary examination of a gain-guided ten-stripe laser commercially available from Spectra Diode Labs[7]. This device, a SDL-2100-E1, differed from the previously studied lasers in that the stripes were defined by proton bombardment. Thus it was not possible to determine the exact location of the stripes relative to the near-field light intensity. However, spectrally resolved near-field measurements do suggest that index-guided modes are being formed between the stripes in these ten-stripe laser diode arrays. Figure 10 depicts the spectrally resolved near-field from the ten-stripe array.

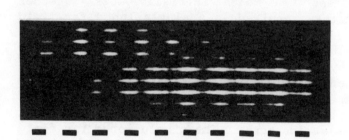
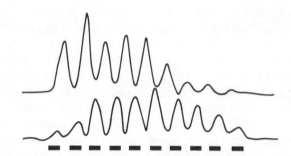

(a) Spectrally resolved near-field (b) Intensity profiles of each mode

Figure 10. Spectrally resolved near-field and intensity profiles of a Spectra Diode Labs ten-stripe array (SDL 2100-E1). The stripe positions are assumed based on the location of modes.

The pattern in Fig. 10 indicates that there are two distinct, spectrally resolved, lateral intensity profiles. The longer wavelength pattern appears to have intensity peaks centered between the peaks of the shorter wavelength pattern. A comparison to the three-stripe results suggests that the longer wavelength pattern (upper profile in Fig 10(b)) is comprised of the fundamental index-guided modes centered between each stripe while the shorter wavelength pattern (lower profile) is from the first-order lateral modes of each adjacent pair of elements. The location of the stripes shown in Fig. 10 has been assumed using this interpretation.

The far-field from this laser was basically double-lobed and changed some with increasing current. Spectrally resolved far-field measurements would be necessary to determine the phase coupling relations of the two lateral near-field patterns depicted in Fig. 10.

8. CONCLUSION

We have observed that a simple multistripe laser diode fabricated from planar DH material can support index-guided lateral modes. In a twin-stripe laser, an index-guide is formed between the stripes from the dip in the injected current density. The width of this index-guide, established by the stripe separation, determines the lateral mode on which the laser initially begins to lase. The size of the index-step, determined by the level of injected current, determines how many higher-order index-guided modes will be supported.

Three-stripe lasers have been observed to operate on the index-guided modes supported between the stripes. Just above threshold, the two fundamental index-guided modes appear to couple out-of-phase as evidenced by a double-lobed far-field pattern. At higher currents, the two lasing elements decouple to form a single-lobed far-field. The presence of higher-order index-guided modes in a three-stripe laser has also been observed.

From a comparison to our three-stripe results, spectrally resolved measurements on a commercially available gain-guided ten-stripe laser suggest that index-guided modes are also present.

9. ACKNOWLEDGMENTS

The authors wish to thank M. Van Loan and R. D. Real for their assistance in fabricating and testing and Prof. E. M. Garimre and Dr. M. B. Chang for helpful discussions.

10. REFERENCES

1. D. G. Heflinger and W. R. Fenner, "Simultaneous operation of gain- and index-guided lateral modes in twin-stripe laser diode arrays," J. Appl. Phys. 64, 3750-3751, (1988).

2. G. H. B. Thompson, Physics of Semiconductor Laser Devices, John Wiley and Sons, New York, 1980.

3. P. A. Kirkby, A. R. Goodwin, G. H. B. Thompson and P. R. Selway, "Observations of self-focusing in stripe geometry semiconductor lasers and the development of a comprehensive model of their operation," IEEE J. Quantum Elect. QE-13, 705-719 (1977).

4. E. Kapon, C. Lindsey, J. Katz, S. Margalit and A. Yariv, "Coupling mechanism of gain-guided integrated semiconductor laser arrays," Appl. Phys. Lett. 44, 389-391 (1984).

5. H. Kressel and J. K. Butler, "Semiconductor Lasers and Heterojunction LEDs, Academic Press, Inc., New York, 1977.

6. L. Figueroa, T. L. Holcomb, K. Burghard, D. Bullock, C. B. Morrison, L. M. Zinkiewicz, and G. A. Evans, "Modeling of the optical characteristics for twin-channel laser (TCL) structures," IEEE J. Quantum Elect. QE-22, 2141-2149 (1986).

7. Spectra Diode Labs, Inc., 80 Rose Orchard Way, San Jose, CA 95134-1356.

LASER DIODE TECHNOLOGY AND APPLICATIONS

Volume 1043

SESSION 3

Semiconductor Laser Modeling and Design

Chair
Gary A. Evans
David Sarnoff Research Center

Invited Paper

Analysis of Double-Heterostructure and Quantum-Well Lasers Using Effective Index Techniques

Jerome K. Butler
Southern Methodist University
Dallas, TX 75275

Gary A. Evans
David Sarnoff Research Center
Princeton, NJ 08543-5300

Abstract

The effects of geometrical and compositional properties of semiconductor lasers are analyzed using the effective index method. The effective index method of analysis is explained by separating the two-dimensional wave equation into transverse and lateral differential equations. The near- and far-field patterns show the effects of asymmetries when the optical fields have strong coupling to the lossy substrates. Emphasis is placed on channeled-substrate-planar lasers fabricated with aluminum gallium arsenide compounds.

1 Introduction

Channeled-substrate-planar (CSP) AlGaAs/GaAs semiconductor lasers are important, established, commercial products and have been extensively studied both experimentally and theoretically.[1]-[12] They have single spatial mode output powers as high as any single element semiconductor laser[4],[5] and have demonstrated long life at very high power.[6] They have been used as the elements in linear[13],[14] and Y-guide[15],[16] arrays. Originally grown by liquid phase epitaxy (LPE) on n-type[1] and later p-type[2] GaAs substrates, functionally equivalent structures are also grown by metalorganic chemical vapor deposition (MOCVD)[17],[18] and molecular beam epitaxy (MBE).[19]-[20] In this paper, we review the lateral guiding mechanism of CSP double-heterostructure quantum-well lasers. The main mechanism for the lateral guiding is the fact that the optical mode in the center of the laser is relatively lossless, whereas, it is high lossy in the lateral "wing" positions due to coupling of optical power from the active region to the lossy substrate.

2 The Effective Index Method

Early approaches of analyzing two-dimensional dielectric waveguides, other than those encountered in optical fibers, treated the two perpendicular waveguide modes independently[21]. More sophisticated approximate methods have been refined to what is generally now recognized as the effective index method [22,23]. The effective index method yields field solutions which accurately approximate the actual fields when the transverse dielectric variations are large compared to the lateral ones. In semiconductor lasers, the lateral dielectric dependencies are due to the structure geometry, lateral gain variation, and temperature gradients. The lateral gain variations affect the imaginary part of the dielectric constant while temperature and carrier injection [24] affect the real part of the dielectric constant.

The relative dielectric constant κ in each layer of a semiconductor laser is generally assumed to be uniform, except in the active layer (Region 2 of Fig. 1), which must account for the gain distribution. The active layer dielectric constant can be written as

$$\kappa_2(y) = n_2^2 + 2n_2 \delta n_2 + i n_2 g(y)/k_0 \quad (1)$$
$$\equiv \kappa_{20} + \kappa_{2v} \quad (2)$$

where n_2 is the bulk refractive index of the active layer, $g(y)$ is the lateral gain distribution, k_0 is the free-space propagation constant ($k_0 = 2\pi/\lambda$), and $\kappa_{02} = n_2^2$. The variable κ_{2v} is the difference between the dielectric in the active layer with current injected ("hot cavity") and with no current injected ("cold cavity"). Index changes due to temperature could be included in κ_{2v} as a real part. However, to make our analysis more general in nature, the dielectric constant of the ith layer is written as

$$\kappa_i(y) = \kappa_{oi} + \kappa_{vi}(y), \qquad i = 1, 2, 3, 4 \quad (3)$$

where κ_{vi} contains only "lateral" variations.

Solutions to Maxwell's equations will be restricted to fields polarized along the junction plane and will be assumed to have the form

$$E(x,y) = \psi(x,y)\exp(i\omega t - \gamma z) \quad (4)$$

where $\gamma(y) = \alpha(y) + i\beta(y)$ is the complex propagation constant. The wave equation is

$$\nabla_t^2 \psi + [k_0^2 \kappa(x,y) + \gamma^2]\psi = 0 \quad (5)$$

where $\kappa(x,y)$ defines the complex dielectric constant of all space and ∇_t^2 is the two-dimensional Laplacian operator. In the spirit of the effective index method, we write

$$\psi(x,y) = u(x,y)\,v(y) \quad (6)$$

where $u(x,y)$ describes the transverse fields and its y dependence occurs because of the layer thickness variations. The functional dependence of $u(x,y)$ is determined by the layer thickness $d_i(y)$ and the dielectric constant of each layer $\kappa_i(y)$. Substituting (5) into (4) gives

$$v\frac{\partial^2 u}{\partial x^2} + u\frac{\partial^2 v}{\partial y^2} + [k_0^2 \kappa(x,y) + \gamma^2]uv = 0 \quad (7)$$

where we have neglected derivatives of $u(x,y)$ with respect to y (the change in propagation constant due to layer thickness variations is very small compared to changes in the propagation constant due to dielectric variations in the x direction). Equation (6) can be rearranged in the following form:

$$v\left[\frac{\partial^2 u}{\partial x^2} + [\gamma_0^2 + k_0^2 \kappa_0(x,y)]u\right]$$
$$+ u\left[\frac{\partial^2 v}{\partial y^2} + [\gamma^2 - \gamma_0^2 + k_0^2 \kappa_v(x,y)]v\right] = 0 \quad (8)$$

which is satisfied when

$$\frac{\partial^2 u}{\partial x^2} + [\gamma_0^2 + k_0^2 \kappa_0(x,y)]u = 0 \quad (9)$$

$$\frac{\partial^2 v}{\partial y^2} + [\gamma^2 - \gamma_0^2 + k_0^2 \kappa_v(x,y)]v = 0 \quad (10)$$

Equations (9) and (10) define the effective index concept and they have a simple physical interpretation. The first is the wave equation for a planar dielectric waveguide at each point y. The effective index along the lateral direction is defined as $n_{eo}(y)$. It is obtained by repeated solutions of the differential equation for all values of y, yielding a lateral effective index profile which is now contained in the second equation. The x dependence of the second equation can be eliminated by weighting with $|u(x,y)|^2$ and integrating over the interval $(-\infty,\infty)$. In each layer we assume that κ_v has only y dependence. Therefore, upon integration, the second equation becomes

$$\frac{\partial^2 v}{\partial y^2} + [\gamma^2 - \gamma_0^2 + k_0^2 \sum_i \Gamma_i(y)\kappa_{vi}(y)]v = 0 \quad (11)$$

which is equivalent to the result derived by a more rigorous method [45]. The overlap parameter $\Gamma_i(y)$ satisfies

$$\Gamma_i(y) = \int_{i^{th}\,layer} |u(x,y)|^2\,dx \quad (12)$$

The transverse function $u(x,y)$ has been normalized so that $\sum_i \Gamma_i = 1$. This above procedure characterizes the effective index method and reduces a two dimensional dielectric waveguide problem into two one dimensional problems. For layered waveguides with no ohmic losses, the effective propagation constant $\gamma_0 = i\beta_0$ is imaginary for all proper modes.

For typical laser structures, we can neglect temperature effects and consider that $\kappa_{vi} = 0$ except for layer 2 (active layer), and then (9) assumes a form

$$\frac{\partial^2 v}{\partial y^2} + [\gamma^2 - \gamma_0^2 + k_0^2 \Gamma_2(y)\kappa_{v2}(y)]v = 0 \quad (13)$$

where $\Gamma_2(y)$ is the active layer confinement factor (ratio of the mode power in the active layer to the total mode power). Defining $n_{e0} = -i\gamma_0/k_0$ as the complex effective index in the absence of injected current, the net lateral effective index is

$$n_{eff}^2(y) = (i\gamma_0/k_0)^2 + \Gamma_2(y)\kappa_{v2}(y) \quad (14)$$

3 The Four Layer Slab Model

The four-layer model can be applied to many contemporary laser structures. The four layers are associated with the epitaxial grown layers, the: n-type GaAs substrate, n-type AlGaAs cladding layer, and undoped AlGaAs active layer, and a p-type AlGaAs cladding layer, as shown in Fig. 2. Although actual devices have a GaAs p-type "capping" layer for electrical contact, this final layer has negligible influence on the optical fields, assuming the top p-clad layer is greater than $1\,\mu m$ in thickness.

The transverse field function $u(x,y)$ defined above is a solution of the wave equation (9) and the secular equation for the modes in the four-layer waveguide is

$$[(r^2 - q^2)\tan rd_2 - 2qr](p+q)\exp(qd_2) +$$
$$[(r^2 + q^2)\tan rd_2](p-q)\exp(-qd2) = 0 \quad (15)$$

where

$$r^2 = \gamma_0^2 + k_0^2 \kappa_2 \quad (16)$$
$$q^2 = -[\gamma_0^2 + k_0^2 \kappa_i]; \quad i = 1, 3 \quad (17)$$
$$p^2 = -[\gamma_0^2 + k_0^2 \kappa_4] \quad (18)$$

We have assumed for proper modes, i.e., modes that decay exponentially as $|x| \to \infty$, that the real parts of p and q are positive. Generally the solutions are complex with complex eigenvalues[25] and the fields in the substrate are damped sinusoidal functions. The solutions for the transverse field functions $u(x, y)$ are obtained in both the channel region ($|y| < W/2$) and the wing region ($|y| > W/2$) by matching the fields and their derivatives at the three interfaces located at $x = 0$, d_2, and d_3. The lateral field functions $v(y)$ are computed after the complex effective index profile is determined. In the analysis of the transverse mode functions, we assume the absorption losses in the p-cladding, active layer, and n-cladding layers have values $\alpha_1 = 10\,\text{cm}^{-1}$, $\alpha_2 = 200\,\text{cm}^{-1}$, and $\alpha_3 = 10\,\text{cm}^{-1}$. (The actual value of loss/gain in the active layer has an insignificant effect on the value of the complex effective index. However, the lateral distribution of the gain in the active layer above threshold is very important in determining the optoelectronic characteristics of the device.) The Al content of the active layer is approximately 7 percent in order to give a lasing wavelength $\lambda_0 = 0.83\,\mu\text{m}$. The Al content of the cladding layers is 33 percent while the Al content of the substrate (normally 0 percent for CSP lasers), is varied from 0 to 40 percent. This variation allows for a study of the coupling of light from the lasing region to the substrate. Because the mole fraction of AlAs in the substrate is variable, the value of the substrate absorption coefficient (at $\lambda_0 = 0.83\,\mu\text{m}$) ranges from about $10{,}000\,\text{cm}^{-1}$ (p-type GaAs substrate) or $5{,}000\,\text{cm}^{-1}$ (n-type GaAs substrate)[26] down to $10\,\text{cm}^{-1}$ as the mole fraction of AlAs in the substrate increases beyond 0.10. A material absorption value of $10\,\text{cm}^{-1}$ is nominally assigned to the cladding layers and the AlAs containing substrates to account for free-carrier losses.

4 Near and Far-Field Patterns

The above analysis provides a good approximation of the near-field distribution on the laser facet. The far-field intensity pattern is found from the two dimensional Fourier transform of the aperture field and the obliquity factor $g(\theta)$[27]. The two dimensional Fourier transform of the aperture field at the laser facet lying in the $z = 0$ plane is

$$F(k_x, k_y) = \iint_{-\infty}^{\infty} u(x, y)\, v(y)\, \exp(ik_x x + ik_y y)\, dx\, dy \quad (19)$$

where $k_x = k_0 \sin\theta' \cos\phi'$ and $k_y = k_0 \sin\theta' \sin\phi'$ and r, θ, and ϕ are the observation point coordinates in the far-field defined by $z = r\cos\theta$, $x = r\sin\theta\cos\phi$, and $y = r\sin\theta\sin\phi$. The transverse radiation pattern is obtained by placing $\phi = 0$ and varying θ. The lateral pattern is obtained by placing $\phi = \pi/2$ and varying θ.

If we focus our attention on the transverse patterns by placing $\phi = 0$, then

$$F(k_x, 0) = \iint_{-\infty}^{\infty} u(x, y)\, v(y)\, \exp(ik_x x)\, dx\, dy \quad (20)$$

represents an "average transform" of the transverse field function $u(x, y)$ where $v(y)$ is the weighting term. In the special case of a square channel CSP, the function $u(x, y)$ can be written as

$$u(x, y) = \begin{cases} u_{ch}(x), & |y| < W/2 \\ u_w(x), & |y| > W/2 \end{cases} \quad (21)$$

For this case, Eq. (20) reduces to:

$$F(k_x, 0) = F_{ch}(\theta)\, \zeta_{ch} + F_w(\theta)\, \zeta_w \quad (22)$$

where

$$F_i(\theta) = \int_{-\infty}^{\infty} u_i(x)\, \exp(ik_x x)\, dx, \quad i = ch, w \quad (23)$$

The quantities ζ_{ch} and ζ_w represent the fraction of the lateral fields concentrated in the channel and wing regions respectively. Thus the transverse far-field radiation pattern perpendicular to the junction $I_p(\theta) = |g(\theta)|\, F(k_x, 0)|^2$ for the square channel CSP laser can be written as

$$I_p(\theta) = I_{ch}(\theta)|\zeta_{ch}|^2 + I_w(\theta)\, |\zeta_w|^2 + 2|g(\theta)|^2 \text{Re}[F_{ch}(\theta) F_w(\theta) \zeta_{ch} \zeta_w] \quad (24)$$

where $I_{ch}(\theta) = |g(\theta) F_{ch}(\theta)|^2$ and $I_w(\theta) = |g(\theta) F_w(\theta)|^2$. For typical laser structures, ζ_{ch}, the fraction of the lateral field confined to the channel, is almost unity. For the conventional CSP lasers studied, $|\zeta_{ch}|^2$ ranges from 0.97 to 0.99 for channel widths of 4 to 6 microns. Therefore the transverse far-field pattern of the laser will be almost totally shaped by the Fourier transform of the transverse field in the channel region.

5 Lateral Optical Confinement

Waveguiding in CSP lasers appears paradoxical at first glance: Based on intuition for bound modes in dielectric waveguides, one expects that the CSP geometry has a larger effective index (real part) in the region outside the channel since a significant portion of the perpendicular field distribution there "averages in" the high index of the GaAs substrate. In addition, one expects that the large imaginary component of the effective index outside the channel region is due to high absorption (because $\alpha_4 = 5000 - 10000 \, \text{cm}^{-1}$ at a lasing wavelength of $0.83 \, \mu\text{m}$[26]) in the GaAs substrate. However, analysis of the CSP structure shows that 1) the effective index (real part) is higher inside the channel than outside (producing a positive index step and corresponding bound lateral modes), and 2) the mode loss outside the channel region increases as the substrate absorption is decreased.

The reason for these apparent contradictions is that the transverse field in the regions outside the channel is not a conventional bound mode, but a complex field which radiates some power into the substrate. The conventional bound mode of a passive dielectric waveguide has decaying exponential field solutions in the first and last (the outermost, semi-infinite) layers. A leaky mode[28] has sinusoidal solutions with exponential growth in one or both of the outermost layers. When the outermost layers of an otherwise leaky waveguide have sufficient loss, the field solution is proper (referred to here as a "bound leaky mode") because the fields exponentially decay, albeit the decay is due to the absorption. Conventional bound modes have normalized transverse propagation constants β_0/k_0 that are greater than the refractive indices of the outermost layers. The complex transverse fields ("bound leaky modes") outside the channel have normalized propagation constants less than the refractive index of one or both outermost layers.

In Fig. 3, the index of refraction profile of the layers outside the channel region is shown superimposed on a plot of the real (3a) and imaginary (3b) parts of the electric field for the fundamental mode. The magnitude (3.4163) of the normalized longitudinal propagation constant β_0/k_0 (at $y > W/2$) for the fundamental mode, also shown in Fig.3, corresponds to sinusoidal solutions in both the active layer and the substrate. The oscillatory behavior of the fields for $x > 0.36 \, \mu\text{m}$ is characteristic of a complex field which radiates some power into the substrate. Even in the channel region, the mode perpendicular to the junction is also, strictly speaking, a complex field, but the electric field is so isolated from the substrate by the thick n-clad region that the amplitude of the field oscillations in the substrate are negligible (see Fig. 3).

Figure 4 shows the near-field intensities for the fields perpendicular to the junction in both the regions inside and outside the channel for a CSP structure with $d_2 = 600 \, \text{Å}$ and $\alpha_4 = 10,000 \, \text{cm}^{-1}$. Plots of the near fields show that there is a wavefront tilt of about $1°$ for $-1.5 < x < 0$ microns and is tilted at about $20°$ for $x > 0.3 \, \mu\text{m}$ for the mode in the regions outside the channel. Since the direction of wave propagation is perpendicular to the wavefront, the wave outside the channel is therefore tilted away from the z-axis of the waveguide and is radiating some energy into the substrate. As the wavefront tilt increases, the guide wavelength λ_z increases (see Fig. 5). Correspondingly, the propagation constant and the effective index decrease.

As a further illustration of the guiding mechanism, three structures are considered. All three models have the same dimensions: a $600 \, \text{Å}$ active layer, $1.5 \, \mu\text{m}$ channel depth, and a $0.3 \, \mu\text{m}$ thick n-clad in the "wing" regions ($|y| > W/2$). The first model is that of a real CSP with losses of $10,000 \, \text{cm}^{-1}$ in the GaAs substrate. The second model (CSPNL) is the same as the first model, except that there are no losses in the GaAs substrate. The third model (CSPNIC) is the same as the first model except that the "substrate" has the same AlAs composition as the n-clad layer (no index change between the n-clad and the substrate). The last two models are not physical, but are pedagogically chosen to show the various effects of complex field distributions and substrate absorption on the complex effective index that provides lateral confinement in a CSP laser. The lateral optical confinement is due to the difference Δn and $\Delta \alpha$ in the real and imaginary parts of the complex effective index (γ_0/k_0) between the channel and wing region.

The near-field intensities, phases, and far-field intensities in the channel region are nearly identical for all three cases. However, the near-field intensities in the wing region, plotted in Fig.6a differ, primarily for $x > 0.36 \, \mu\text{m}$, where the bound mode (CSPNIC) is the strongest damped, the CSP leaky mode is moderately damped, and the CSPNL leaky mode is undamped. The near-field phases in the wing region are plotted in Fig. 6b. They are similar for the CSP and CSPNL cases, with the CSPNL case having slightly more tilt for $x > 0.36 \, \mu\text{m}$. The near-field phase of the CSPNIC has considerably less tilt than the other cases. The far-field intensities corresponding to the near-field in the wing region are shown in Fig. 6c. The far-field peaks are all shifted from 0° to about 4°. Because the far-field pattern in the transverse direction obtained from either Eq. (20) or (22) is due to the field in the channel and wing regions, the asymmetries in the far-fields produced by the wing regions will always add a slight asymmetry to the far-field produced by CSP lasers. Other causes of asymmetries in semiconductor far fields are thin cladding layers[29]-[31], material composition variations[11], and asymmetries in the device geometry[10],[12]. Although these far-field equations also hold for other laser geometries such as the ridge guide, the transverse fields inside and outside an ideal ridge structure both have symmetric transforms, and therefore ideal ridge (and most other) laser structures should have symmetric transverse far-field patterns.

Of the three models, the first two (CSP and CSPNL) give almost identical results, with the "no loss" model having a slightly larger complex effective index step. The third model does show that only high losses outside the channel region are sufficient to provide a lateral positive index, in agreement with an earlier qualitative calculation[9]. The index step of the third model is less than half the complex effective index step of the other two models for a substrate loss of $10,000\,cm^{-1}$. If the substrate absorption is $5000\,cm^{-1}$, the result is a positive index step of only 1.25×10^{-3} for the CSPNIC model, which is comparable to the amount of gain induced index depression[24] expected at threshold.

These results are reasonable since from Fig. 6a the CSPNL structure has a larger fraction of the mode intensity in the substrate, has slightly more tilt in the near-field phase, and has slightly more off- axis tilt in the far-field than the CSP case. As the substrate absorption is decreased, more energy is radiated into the substrate resulting in an increased average wavefront tilt, and therefore both the positive index step and the mode absorption (imaginary part of the effective index) in the region outside the channel increases. Another way to view the increasing mode loss with decreasing substrate absorption is that the "skin depth" of the "bound leaky mode" increases as the substrate becomes less like a perfect conductor. The mode loss and the lateral index step only increase by about 13 percent and 8 percent as the substrate absorption decreases from $10,000\,cm^{-1}$ to 0. This increase, although slight, is unexpected from an earlier explanation[9] of CSP waveguiding which predicts that the magnitude of the complex lateral effective index step approaches zero as the substrate absorption decreases towards zero.

6 CSP Design Curves

Figure 7(a) is a plot of the real part of the effective index for the mode perpendicular to the junction as a function of the n-clad thickness (d_3 in Fig. 2) for active layer thicknesses of 300, 400, 600, 800, and 1000 Å. For a CSP laser to have stable near- and far-field patterns with increasing drive current, the lateral index step should be large compared to index variations due to gain. The gain induced index depression will typically reduce the index of refraction of the active layer by 10^{-2}, which in turn reduces the "cold cavity" effective index by about 10^{-3}. For this reason, a "cold cavity" lateral index step greater than 3×10^{-3} is desired to provide lateral mode stability. From Fig. 7, this is obtained for n-clad thicknesses (outside of the channel) of $0.3\,\mu m$ or less for channel depths greater than $1.0\,\mu m$.

Figure 7(b) is a plot of the imaginary part of the effective index, which increases with decreasing cladding thickness. The resulting magnitudes of the real and imaginary parts of the lateral effective index step for a CSP are always the same order of magnitude. Although a large imaginary component of the effective index is beneficial for stability of single laser diodes, it is detrimental to the operation of coherent CSP arrays in the fundamental array mode[33,34].

Figure 8 is a plot of the active layer confinement factor as a function of the n-clad thickness (d_3) for active layer thicknesses (d_2) of 300, 400, 600, 800, and 1000 Å.

References

[1] K. Aiki, M. Nakamura, T. Kuroda, J. Umeda, R. Ito, Naoki Chinone, and M. Maeda, "Transverse mode stabilized $Al_xGa_{1-x}As$ injection lasers with channeled-substrate-planar structure," *IEEE J. Quantum Electron.* QE-14, 89-94,(1978).

[2] S. Yamamoto, H. Hayashi, S. Yano, T. Sakurai, and T. Hijikata, "Visible *GaAlAs* V-channeled substrate inner stripe laser with stabilized mode using p-GaAs substrate," *Appl. Phys. Let.* 40, 372-374(1982).

[3] S. Yamamoto, N. Miyauchi, S. Maei, T. Morimoto, O. Yamamoto, S. Yano, and T. Hijikata, "High output power characteristics in broad-channeled substrate inner stripe lasers," *Appl. Phys. Let.* 46, 319-321 (1985).

[4] K. Hamada, M. Wada, H. Shimizu, M. Kume, F. Susa, T. Shibutani, N. Yoshikawa, K. Itoh, G. Kano, and I. Teramoto, "A 0.2 W cw laser with buried twin-ridge substrate structure," *IEEE J. Quantum Electron.* QE-21, 623-628 (1985).

[5] B. Goldstein, M. Ettenberg, N.A. Dinkel, and J.K. Butler, "A high- power channeled-substrate-planar AlGaAs laser," *Appl. Phys. Let.* 47, 655-657 (1985).

[6] T. Shibutani, M. Kume, K. Hamada, H. Shimizu, K. Itoh, G. Kano, and I. Teramoto, "A novel high-power laser structure with current-block regions near cavity facets," *IEEE J. Quantum Electron.* QE-23, 760-764 (1987).

[7] T.Kuroda, M. Nakamura, K. Aiki, and J. Umeda, "Channeled-substrate- planar structure $Al_xGa_{1-x}As$ lasers: an analytical waveguide study," *Applied Optics* 17, 3264-3267 (1978).

[8] K. A. Shore, "Above-threshold analysis of channelled-substrate-planar (CSP) laser," *IEE Proc.* Part I, 9-15 (1981).

[9] S. Wang, C. Chen, A.S. Liao, and L. Figueroa, "Control of mode behavior in semiconductor lasers," *IEEE J. Quantum Electron.* QE-17, 453-468 (1981).

[10] J. K. Butler, G. A. Evans, and B. Goldstein, "Analysis and performance of channeled-substrate-planar double-heterojunction lasers with geometrical asymmetries," *IEEE J. Quantum Electron.* QE-23 1890-1899 (1987).

[11] G. A. Evans, B. Goldstein, and J. K. Butler, "Observations and consequences of non-uniform aluminum concentrations in the channel regions of AlGaAs channeled-substrate-planar lasers," *IEEE J. Quantum Electron.* QE-23, 1900-1908 (1987).

[12] T. Ohtoshi, K. Yamaguchi, C. Nagaoka, T. Uda, Y. Murayama, and N. Chinone, "A two dimensional device simulator of semiconductor lasers," *Solid-State Electron.* 30, 627-638 (1987).

[13] T. Kadowaki, T. Aoyagi, S. Hinata, N. Kaneno, Y. Seiwa, K. Ikeda, and W. Susaki, "Long-lived phase-locked laser arrays mounted on a Si-submount with Au-Si solder with a junction-down configuration," IEEE International Semiconductor Laser Conference, Kanazawa, Japan, Conference Program and Abstract of Papers, 84-85 (1986).

[14] B. Goldstein, N. Dinkel, N. W. Carlson, G. A. Evans, and V. J. Masin, "Performance of a channeled-substrate-planar-high-power phase-locked array operating in the diffraction limit," Conference on Lasers and Electro-Optics, Baltimore, Technical Digest, 330-331 (1987).

[15] M. Taneya, M. Matsumoto, S. Matsui, S. Yano, and T. Hijikata, "0° phase mode operation in phased-array laser diode with symmetrically branching waveguide," *Appl. Phys. Let.* 47, 341-343 (1985).

[16] D. F. Welch, P. Cross, D. Scifres, W. Streifer, and R. D. Burnham, "In-phase emission from index-guided laser array up to 400 mW," *Electron Lett.* 22, 293-294 (1986).

[17] K. Uomi, S. Nakatsuka, T. Ohtoshi, Y. Ono. N. Chinone, and T. Kajimura, "High-power operation of index-guided visible GaAs/GaAlAs multiquantum well lasers," *Appl. Phys. Let.* 45,818-821 (1984).

[18] J. J. Yang, C. S. Hong, J. Niesen, and L. Figueroa, "High-power single longitudinal mode operation of inverted channel substrate planar lasers," *J.Appl. Phys.* 58, 4480-4482 (1985).

[19] H. Tanaka, M. Mushiage, Y. Ishida, "Single-longitudinal-mode selfaligned (AlGa)As double-heterostructure lasers fabricated by molecular beam epitaxy," *Japanese J. of Appl. Phys.* 24, L89-L90 (1985).

[20] K. Yagi, H. Yamauchi, and T. Niina, "High external differential quantum efficiency (80%) SCH lasers grown by MBE," IEEE International Semiconductor Laser Conference, Kanazawa, Japan, Conference Program and Abstract of Papers, 158-159 (1986).

[21] E. A. J. Marcatili, "Dielectric rectangular waveguide and directional coupler for integrated optics," *Bell Syst. Tech. J.* 48, 2071-2102, (1969).

[22] G. B. Hocker and W. K. Burns, "Mode dispersion in diffused channel waveguides by the effective index method," *Appl.Opt.* 16, 113-118, (1977).

[23] W. Streifer and E. Kapon, "Applications of the equivalent-index method to DH diode lasers," *Appl. Opt.* 18, 3724-3725, (1979).

[24] J. Manning and R. Olshansky, "The carrier-induced index change in AlGaAs and 1.3 μm InGaAs diode Lasers," *IEEE J. Quantum Electron.* QE-19, 1525-1530, (1983).

[25] A. Sommerfeld, *Partial Differential Equations in Physics*, New York:Academic Press, New York, 1949.

[26] H. C. Casey, Jr., D. D. Sell, and K. W. Wecht, "Concentration dependence of the absorption coefficient for n- and p-type GaAs between 1.3 and 1.6 eV," *J. Appl. Phys.* 46, 250-257, (1975).

[27] L. Lewin, "Obliquity-factor correction to solid-state radiation patterns," *J. Appl. Phys.* 46, 2323-2324, (1975).

[28] T. Tamir, "Leaky waves in planar optical waveguides," *Nouv. Rev. Optique* 6, 273-284, (1975).

[29] J. K. Butler, H. Kressel, and I. Ladany, "Internal optical losses in very thin cw heterojunction laser diodes," *IEEE J. Quantum Electron.* QE-11, 402-408, (1975).

[30] W. Streifer, R. D. Burnham, and D. R. Scifres, "Substrate radiation losses in GaAs heterostructure lasers," *IEEE J. Quantum Electron.* QE-12, 177-182, (1976).

[31] D. R. Scifres, W. Streifer, and R. D. Burnham, " Leaky wave room-temperature double heterostructure GaAs:GaAlAs diode laser," *Appl. Phys. Let.* 29, 23-25, (1976).

[32] W. Streifer, D. R. Scifres, and R. D. Burnham, "Channelled substrate non planar laser analysis," *IEEE J. Quantum Electron.* QE-17, 1521-1530 (1981).

[33] W. Streifer, D. R. Scifres, and R. D. Burnham, "Channeled substrate non-planar laser analysis, Part I: for modulation," *IEEE J. Quantum Electron.* QE-17, 736-744, (1981).

[34] C. B. Su, "An analytical solution of kinks and nonlinearities driven by near field displacement instabilities in stripe geometry diode lasers," *J. Appl. Phys.* 52, 2265-2673.

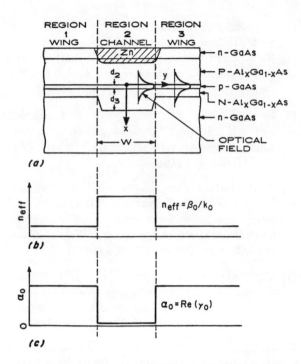

Fig. 1 (a) Geometrical cross section of a CSP laser, (b) real part of the lateral effective index profile, and (c) imaginary part of the lateral effective index profile.

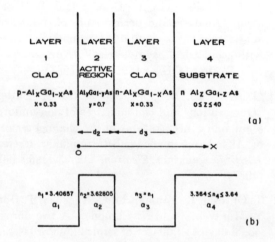

Fig. 2 The four-layer waveguide structure with (a) the layer geometry and (b) the refractive index profile.

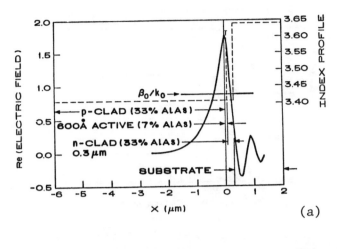

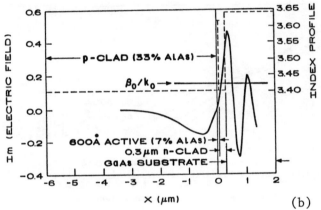

Fig. 3 The (a) real and (b) imaginary part of the electric field distribution for the transverse profile shown in Fig. 2 with $d_2 = 600\,\text{Å}$ and $\alpha_s = 5000\,\text{cm}^{-1}$.

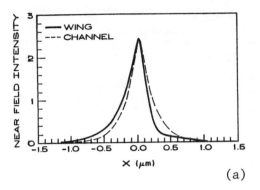

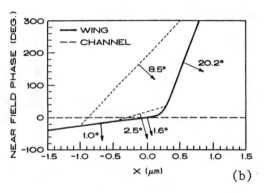

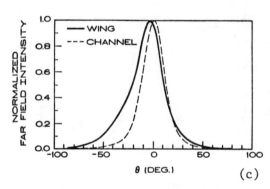

Fig. 4 The transverse (a) near field intensity, (b) near-field phase, and (c) far-field intensity $I_{ch}(\theta)$ and $I_w(\theta)$ for a conventional CSP laser with an active layer thickness of 600 Å in the region inside (—) and outside (---) the channel.

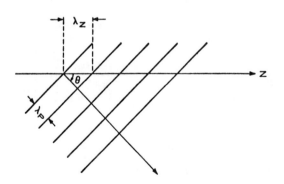

Fig. 5 Relationship of the guide wavelength λ_z to the wavelength in the direction of propagation λ_p for a wave propagating at an angle θ with respect to the guide axis.

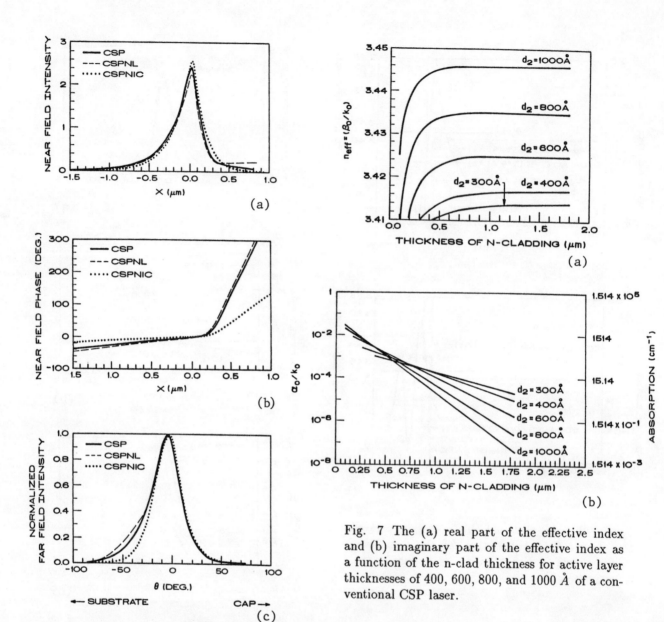

Fig. 6 The transverse (a) near-field intensity, (b) near-field phase, and (c) far-field intensity in the region outside the channel region for a conventional CSP laser (—), a CSP laser with no absorption in the GaAs substrate (---) and a structure with the same index in the substrate as the channel region, but with high losses (10,000 cm^{-1}) in the substrate (···). All structures have an active layer thickness of 600 Å.

Fig. 7 The (a) real part of the effective index and (b) imaginary part of the effective index as a function of the n-clad thickness for active layer thicknesses of 400, 600, 800, and 1000 Å of a conventional CSP laser.

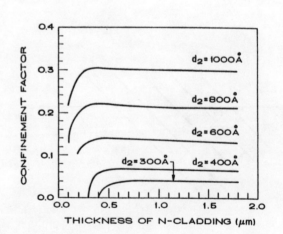

Fig. 8 The active layer confinement factor as a function of the n-clad thickness for active layer thicknesses of 400, 600, 800, and 1000 Å of a conventional CSP laser.

Computer modeling of GRIN-SCH-SQW Diode Lasers

S. R. Chinn, P. S. Zory*, and A. R. Reisinger

General Electric Company, Electronics Laboratory
Syracuse, NY 13221

*University of Florida, Dept. of Electrical Engineering
Gainesville, FL 32611

ABSTRACT

A computer model for the optical gain of graded-index, separate-confinement-heterostructure, single-quantum-well (GRIN-SCH-SQW) $Al_xGa_{1-x}As$ diode lasers is presented, and compared with experimental data. The model combines many individual features not heretofore included together, and gives good agreement with gain vs current density data for two different structure variations. In addition, the threshold temperature dependence agrees well with data for typical laser conditions, the observed high-gain discontinuity in T_o vs temperature is explained, and new predictions are made concerning T_o discontinuities at gain cross-overs.

1. INTRODUCTION

Quantum-well (QW) semiconductor lasers offer the advantages of low threshold current density and high power capability with good efficiency. In this paper, we describe a new model for one particular type, the graded-index separate-confinement-heterostructure single-quantum-well (GRIN-SCH-SQW) laser. Rather than summarize the properties of QW lasers, we refer the reader to a recent review paper (ref. 1).

A principal feature of the QW laser is the extremely high optical gain that can be obtained in the QW for very low current densities. This arises partly from greater population inversion at a given carrier density because of the lower quantized density of states, but mostly from the high carrier density in the QW because of its small width. Equally important, however, in determining laser properties are modal gain, determined by the optical confinement factor, and the ability to collect injected carriers efficiently. In this paper we will discuss the case in which a single quantum well active layer is embedded in a linear-graded-index waveguide layer, which is in turn sandwiched between outer cladding layers. All calculations are done for the $GaAs/Al_xGa_{1-x}$ materials system, although the general model should apply equally well to many other III-V lasers such as $InP/In_xGa_{1-x}As_yP_{1-y}$. We have attempted to start from a point of view as fundamental as possible, yet consistent with practical computational effort and time. The primary goal was to obtain a model for the laser gain as a function of excitation current density, which could describe the laser threshold current data measured for different variations of the GRIN-SCH-SQW structure and for different temperatures. In Section 2 we describe the features of the model, and its approximations and assumptions. In Section 3 we present the computational results and compare them with experimental data. Finally, in Section 4 we discuss the results, their implication for laser design, and a comparison with other calculations. In this paper we will emphasize new results concerning the gain vs current density relation and the characteristic temperature. Additional details of other aspects of the model can be found in reference 2, along with more extensive references.

2. FEATURES OF GRIN-SCH-SQW MODEL

In the GRIN-SCH-SQW structure a narrow (50-400Å) quantum well parallel to a crystallographic (100) plane is located in the center of a considerably wider symmetric graded-band-gap (GRIN) layer. We assume a symmetric potential appropriate for high injection and lightly doped cladding layers. Excitonic effects are not considered in this gain model because laser operation at the high carrier densities and temperatures examined here should lead to almost complete ionization of the two-dimensional excitons into single-particle band states.

The energy levels of the complete GRIN-SCH-SQW structure are found using the most accurate single-band approximation that avoids a more complete but more complicated band-mixing type of analysis[3]. Our present method follows that of ref. 4, and uses a type of "effective mass" Schrödinger equation:

$$[\varepsilon(-i\nabla) + V(x)] \psi = E \psi. \qquad (1)$$

In equation (1) the kinetic energy term, ε, is written as a function of the momentum operator; $\varepsilon(k)$ describes the non-parabolic energy dispersion for Bloch states in the unperturbed, bulk lattice, V represents the band potential energy from the GRIN-SCH-SQW structure, E is the energy eigenvalue, and ψ is the envelope wave function. The lowest quantized energies are found by taking the lateral wave vector (parallel to the QW plane) to be zero. We assume that the envelope wave functions are sinusoidal in the QW, Airy functions in the graded layers, and decaying exponentials is the cladding layers. We neglect the non-parabolicity in the linearly graded regions outside the QW and in the cladding. The eigenvalue equation is obtained by imposing the proper boundary conditions on the wave functions in their respective regions, namely the continuity of ψ and the probability current $(1/m) \partial\psi/\partial x$ across each heterojunction. A similar procedure is followed for the quantized light and heavy hole states. We have taken a value of 0.65/0.35 for the ratio of conduction to valence band offsets, consistent with more recent data[5] (0.66/0.34) and close to the ~0.60/0.40 ratio recommended in ref. 6. The low lying levels in the QW are widely separated, whereas the levels in the GRIN region are more closely spaced as the layer becomes wider.

For each quantized level, there is a continuum of energies arising from the lateral kinetic energy of the carriers in the plane of the QW. Associated with each discrete level, the resulting sheet density of states for energies above that minimum level is[7]

where
$$\rho_n = m_n / (\pi \hbar^2), \qquad (2)$$

m_n = effective carrier mass,   n = quantized state label
$\hbar$ = $(1/2\pi) \times$ Planck's constant .

This sheet density gives the number of states per unit energy interval (for both spin directions) per unit area. It is more appropriate to work with sheet densities than volume densities because different quantized states (particularly in the GRIN layer) have different spatial extents in the direction perpendicular to the QW plane. When considering only the states localized in the QW, it is a good approximation to divide their sheet density by L, to find the volumetric density of states.

From a perturbation analysis, we take the lateral effective carrier mass to be an average of that of the QW and graded material, with local inverse masses weighted by the corresponding wavefunction confinement factor. Once the energy levels and densities of states are known for each band minimum, the sheet carrier density in that minimum can be related to the quasi-Fermi level:

$$n_i = \sum_j kT \rho_j \ln[1 + \exp(F - \Delta_i - E_j/kT)], \qquad (3)$$

kT = Boltzmann constant × temperature.

In eq. (3), n_i refers to either Γ or 'L' electrons, or light or heavy holes. F is the quasi-Fermi energy for the conduction or valence band, measured positive into the band from the k=0 band edge. The quantum levels E_j are also measured positive into their respective bands with respect to the edge of the band minima, and Δ_i gives the displacement of the 'i'th minimum with respect to k=0 for the conduction band states. The different case of the 'X'-minimum is discussed below. We assume undoped QW layers with high injection, and charge neutrality of all carriers in the GRIN-SCH-SQW structure. From charge neutrality and equation (3) the quasi-Fermi levels for the conduction and valence bands can be related to the total carrier excitation.

The indirect 'L' and 'X' conduction band minima play an important role in determining non-equilibrium quasi-Fermi levels, non-radiative recombination rates, and carrier leakage. We find the quantized levels of the 'L' minimum as described above. The 'X' valley presents a more complicated problem however, because use of our present band parameters predicts that for many of our typical high-aluminum GRIN and cladding compositions, there is no confinement in the X-valley quantum well; i.e. the QW potential is higher than that of the cladding layer. If this were the case, carriers which thermalized into the 'X' minimum in the QW would transfer out into the AlGaAs cladding layers. Our assumption is that this process is limited by the charge imbalance that must be created when such transfer occurs. A self-consistent relation is then found between the population of this triangular-potential Coulombic 'X' minimum and the conduction band quasi-Fermi level. We have found values for n_x of about 10% of the total conduction band population under typical injection conditions for 71% Al cladding composition (structure II, described below) and less than 1% of the population for 40% cladding (structure I, described below). By comparison, the 'L'-valley populations in both cases increase to nearly 20% at current densities near 1 kA/cm^2. The rest of the computation is simplified by starting with an assumed value for the conduction band quasi-Fermi level. The conduction band sheet densities in each band minimum are then found using equation (3). This gives the total hole sheet density, and the procedure is reversed to find the valence band quasi-Fermi level in terms of 'p'.

The present model calculates laser gain on the basis of band-to-band transitions. Transitions between the quantized band states are assumed to obey lateral wave-vector conservation. Because the lattice periodicity is removed in the perpendicular direction by the presence of the GRIN-SCH-SQW structure, the perpendicular wave vector components for the bound states describe the envelope function parameters. The electric dipole transitions occur between the unit cell wavefunctions having opposite parity (between conduction band 's' functions and valence band 'p' functions), so the envelope functions must have the same parity[8]. This allows coupling between quantum well states having the same symmetry, but does **not** require that the states have the same quantum number. If bound states in the QW are well confined, the overlap between their sinusoidal envelopes does give an approximate Δn=0 selection rule. However, in the present case we also wish to consider the possibility of radiative transitions between states in the GRIN region. For the same quantum number, such electron and hole states will have very different spatial extents, and an overlap factor for the transition must be included. Conversely, non-zero overlap exists between electron and hole states of differing quantum number. Factors such as weak confinement, high excitation, and high temperature all contribute to significant thermal population of the GRIN states. For each laser structure we calculate the matrix of overlap integrals for the normalized electron and hole envelope functions at Γ, described by eq. (1) for each spatial region. Typically, there may be only one or two states confined to the QW, and from 50 to 200 states in the different GRIN band minima.

Another significant issue in calculating QW laser gain is anisotropy. We follow the derivations of Asada et al[8] and Yamada et al[9,10] in calculating the anisotropy of the dipole matrix element for both the light hole and heavy hole transitions, using Kane's wave functions[11].

The optical gain is calculated using standard perturbation theory (Fermi's golden rule). Since the gain anisotropy favors lasing in TE modes, we calculate the gain only for this polarization. The spectrally dependent gain coefficient for the quantum well region is:

$$g(E) = \frac{q^2 |M|^2}{E \varepsilon_o m^2 c_o \hbar N L} \sum_{i,j} m_{r,ij} C_{ij} A_{ij} [f_c - (1-f_v)] H(E-E_{ij}) \quad , \tag{4}$$

where
- $|M|^2$ = bulk momentum transition matrix element,
- ε_o = free space permittivity,
- m = free electron mass,
- c_o = vacuum speed of light,
- N = effective refractive index,
- i,j = conduction, valence quantum numbers (Γ),
- $m_{r,ij}$ = spatially weighted reduced mass for transition i,j.
- C_{ij} = overlap factor between states i and j
- A_{ij} = anisotropy factor for transition i,j
- f_c = Fermi factor for conduction electrons
- f_v = Fermi factor for valence holes
- H = Heaviside step function
- E_{ij} = transition energy between states i and j

Note that the i=j selection rule is no longer imposed, and all symmetry-allowed transitions are considered. The reduced mass parameter is given by

$$m_{r,ij}^{-1} = m_i^{-1} + m_j^{-1} \quad , \tag{5}$$

where m_i is the weighted effective electron mass for quantized conduction level 'i' and m_j is the weighted effective hole mass for quantized valence level 'j'. The angular anisotropy factor is normalized so that its angular average (bulk limit) is unity. For TE transitions, with the electric field vector in the plane of the QW, its values are:

$$A_{ij} = (3/4)(1 + \cos^2\Theta_{ij}) \quad \text{(heavy hole)}$$
$$= (1/4)(5 - 3\cdot\cos^2\Theta_{ij}) \quad \text{(light hole)}. \tag{6}$$

The angular factor is $\cos^2\Theta_{ij} = E_{ij}/E$, and shows decreasing anisotropy between nearby heavy and light hole transitions as the photon energy increases deeper into the band. The Fermi conduction band factor gives the occupancy probability for electrons at an energy $(m_{r,ij}/m_i)(E-E_{ij})$ into the i-th quantized conduction band; similarly, the valence band Fermi factor gives the **hole** occupancy probability at an energy $(m_{r,ij}/m_j)(E-E_{ij})$ into the j-th quantized valence band. $|M|^2$ is a momentum matrix element between conduction $<s|$ and valence $|x>$ states, averaged over spatial orientation and summed over spin. Equation (4) gives the spectral dependence of the gain on energy as a function of the excitation level, as related to the quasi-Fermi levels.

Up to this point we have neglected the effects of carrier intra-band scattering on broadening the transition spectra. A common assumption is that each individual transition contributing to the gain continuum is itself broadened by scattering, and has a Lorentzian line shape. The net effect of this broadening can then be found by convolving the Lorentzian function with the previously calculated gain distribution[8,10]. As has recently been pointed out, however, this assumption is a simplification of the true situation in which the broadening of each state, rather than the transition pair, should be considered[12]. Consequences of the simplification include a shift in the energy crossover from gain to absorption away from the true quasi-Fermi separation. From a mathematical point of view this occurs because the wide Lorentzian tails sample too large a loss from the absorptive part of the gain spectrum during the convolution process. On the other hand, use of the exact theory would require another level of spectral integration, making computation prohibitively long. The solution proposed in ref. 12 and which we adopt is to keep the convolution procedure, but to use the appropriate lineshape found by a more exact calculation of the induced dipole phase damping. This lineshape, found by Fourier transforming the appropriate phase diffusion function, is intermediate between a Gaussian and Lorentzian. The final spectral convolution calculation is most conveniently done using multiplication of fast Fourier transforms of the spectrum and lineshape, followed by inverse transformation.

For most cases of practical interest, the above equations give the material gain of the quantum well, since most of the carriers are confined to the QW layer. In the present situation, we evaluate the **modal** gain, $G(E)=\Gamma\cdot g(E)$, of the GRIN-SCH-SQW laser by finding the optical overlap factor, Γ, between the gain in the QW and the wider TE waveguide mode. The waveguide modes are found from an Airy function analysis quite similar to the above solution for the electronic eigenstates. In addition we have applied a minor correction factor, N_{QW}/N_g (N_{QW} = refractive index of QW, N_g = effective mode index) to the geometrical overlap factor to account for the tilt of the plane wave component in the QW with respect to its longitudinal axis. This factor can be rigorously derived for conventional double-heterostructure lasers by perturbation analysis of the modal waveguide equation. To save computation time, in most of the calculations of mode gain vs photon energy we have applied the confinement factor found at the energy of the material gain peak and neglected the variation of Γ with photon energy.

The above elements of the model give results in terms of carrier density, which is not directly measurable. Since we wish to calculate properties of semiconductor injection lasers, a relation between carrier density and current must be obtained. This is done by the equilibrium requirement that current must balance the total carrier recombination rate, which consists of radiative and non-radiative components.

The radiative component of carrier recombination is found from the spectrally dependent spontaneous emission rate:

$$R(E) = \frac{16\pi^2 N q^2 E |M|^2}{\varepsilon_o m^2 c_o^3 h^4 L} \sum_{i,j} m_{r,ij} C_{ij}[f_c\cdot f_v] H(E-E_{ij}) \quad, \tag{7}$$

Equation (7) is an expression for the total spontaneous emission density into all angles and at all polarizations, and therefore does not contain the polarization anisotropy, which has been removed by angular integration. The total spontaneous emission rate is found by integrating eq. (7) over the photon energy, E. Note that it is not necessary to convolve eq. (7) with the intraband scattering lineshape, since the integrals over the unconvolved and convolved spectra are the same. This spontaneous emission rate includes only the summation over bound states at the Γ minimum (including those in the GRIN layer). In fact, the inclusion of all the GRIN transitions was motivated more by the requirement to include them in the emission rate, than for their negligible effect on gain near the QW transition energies. The effect of the thermal populations of the 'X' and 'L' indirect minima is included by assuming a non-radiative recombination time of 10 ns for all non-Γ electrons. In discussion of the results below, the 'radiative' case includes this small, generally negligible non-radiative part as well. The more important non-radiative contributions to the current come from thermal leakage of the carriers over the confining potential barriers, and from Auger recombination.

The calculation of leakage currents follows that of Casey and Panish[13] and Dutta[14] for double heterostructure lasers, modified for the GRIN-SCH-SQW structure. The procedure is to find the minority carrier densities in the cladding layer at the GRIN interfaces, and then find the minority drift and diffusion currents in the n- and p-cladding layers in the presence of the ohmic electric field. We include the non-negligible leakage contribution from the 'L' valley.

Auger processes in III-V semiconductors allow for non-radiative recombination of electron-hole states via three-particle interactions. Generally, such recombination has been considered to have an important effect on laser operation only for small-gap materials, where the Auger coefficients are much larger[15]. However, since the Auger rates are proportional to the third-order product of various carrier concentrations (n or p), this process can be significant in a large-band-gap QW laser, since the carrier concentrations in the QW can be an order of magnitude larger than in a conventional double heterostructure. We find the Auger contribution to the non-radiative current as in ref. 16, with slight modification from the presence of the QW. We use for the relevant carrier densities the respective electron and heavy hole sheet densities in the confined QW levels, divided by the QW thickness. Note that these electron and hole densities are not equal, because we use only the heavy holes and because the GRIN levels and 'L' and 'X' minima may become significantly populated.

3. RESULTS

The calculation of the peak mode gain requires a calculation of the spectral dependence of the mode gain, followed by spectral convolution to include the intra-band relaxation. The radiative component of the excitation current density at the various drive levels is found from the integral over energy of the total spontaneous emission spectrum. Non-radiative components of the current density include contributions from indirect-gap non-radiative recombination, Auger recombination, and leakage of carriers over the confining energy barriers. The radiative and non-radiative recombination rates can all be calculated for each value of carrier density. Since the peak gain is a function of carrier density, each value of peak gain can be associated with a current density whose components can be added sequentially for modeling purposes, to examine their relative sizes. The carrier density, while a necessary variable for the model, does not appear in the final result for the peak mode gain G as a function of current density J.

Calculating the spectral gain curves over a closely spaced range of current densities leads to the resulting G versus J plots shown in figure 1. In figure 1 we have also indicated the different effects of intra-band scattering, current leakage, and Auger recombination on the gain-current relation. A structure with GaAs QW, 20% lower GRIN Al mole fraction, and 40% cladding Al mole fraction (structure I) was chosen for evaluation because it is highly sensitive to all of these effects, and has been characterized experimentally. The topmost dotted curves **do not** include intra-band scattering. In order of decreasing gain they represent currents calculated on the basis of radiative recombination (RR) alone (including a small contribution from indirect-gap non-radiative recombination) ; RR and Auger recombination (AR); and RR, AR, and carrier leakage. The lower solid curves follow the same sequence as above, but **do** include the intra-band scattering described above. The lowest solid curve represents the results of the full model, whose parameters are not adjustable except to the degree of uncertainty of the various AlGaAs material-related coefficients (band gaps, effective masses, diffusion coefficients, etc.). We have also plotted experimental data points obtained by other workers[17,18], on the basis of evaluating the threshold gain for wide-stripe GRIN-SCH-SQW lasers of different cavity lengths, using the mode reflectivity and measured mode loss coefficient. Specifically, the peak of the mode gain at threshold is given by the total cavity loss,

$$G_{th} = \Gamma g_{th} = \alpha_i + (1/L) \ln (1/R) , \qquad (8)$$

where α_i is the internal waveguide loss coefficient, L is the device length, and R is the mode reflectivity at the facet. In reducing the threshold current vs length data of references 17 and 18 to obtain the values of threshold mode gain and current density used in figure 1, we have used α_i ~4 cm^{-1}, a stripe width of 60 µm, and a mode reflectivity of 0.32. The agreement between theory and data is quite good, considering that no adjustable parameters were used.

If our convolution procedure were perfect, we would expect that each pair of convolved/unconvolved spectral gain curves would change from gain to loss at the same high energy (at the quasi-Fermi energy separation, ΔF). That is, with a correct model we would not expect the convolution procedure to change ΔF. Such an effect, when translated to figure 1, gives rise to the difference in transparency current density (value of J at zero gain) between convolved and unconvolved curves. This minor defect could be remedied by using a more exact theory involving another level of spectral integration.

Similar G(J) results for another GRIN-SCH-SQW structure with higher confinement are shown in figure 2. This structure (II) has a 75-Å quantum well, ~0.15µm GRIN half-thickness, and GRIN composition grading from $Al_{0.33}Ga_{0.67}As$ to $Al_{0.71}Ga_{0.29}As$. The data plotted in figure 2 were obtained as above, using lasers from one of our OMVPE-grown wafers. Our value for mode loss coefficient, α_i, derived from data for long lasers, is 10 cm^{-1}. This wafer differs from the generic GRIN-SCH-SQW structure described previously in that both the GRIN and cladding layers are actually composed of GaAs/AlAs superlattices[19]. The higher energy barriers of this structure (either the model II or actual epitaxy, when averaged over the superlattice) provide better electronic confinement properties than structure I, and both the calculated and experimental gains are about two times larger, for the same current density. The agreement with theory and data, while not as good as for structure I, is nevertheless quite reasonable, given the many parameters entering the theory and some uncertainty in the actual laser structure. An interesting difference between structures I and II is the significant decrease in leakage current in the latter, because of its better electronic confinement. Structure II also has a larger optical confinement factor, both from the wider QW and larger refractive index steps. We have used no changes in parameters in the calculations for the two structures, except those occurring within the model as compositions and thicknesses change.

In general, there is no single optimum quantum well thickness. Thinner wells generally have lower thresholds, but not necessarily higher gains well above threshold. In figure 3 we show the calculated dependence of G(J) on the quantum well thickness, keeping other parameters of the type-II laser structure constant. At small thicknesses, the threshold and low level gain is nearly independent of QW thickness, because of the trade-off between QW gain and optical confinement factor. At larger thicknesses, higher index QW transitions contribute more to the gain, and the curves become more nearly linear as a tendency toward bulk behavior takes place. Gain-crossovers occur when the peak of the gain spectral dependence shifts from a transition energy associated with one lateral continuum of quantized two-dimensional electron-hole states (e.g. n=1) to an energy in the next higher continuum (e.g. n=2). Note that the gain in the higher lateral energy continuum still has contributions from transitions in the lower continua. At each such gain cross-over, a kink, or change in slope of G vs J occurs, as seen in figure 3.

One of the primary applications of our model has been to find the characteristic temperature, T_o, the exponential coefficient of the threshold current density temperature dependence, according to

$$J(T) = J(T_r) \exp[(T-T_r)/T_o] , \qquad (9)$$

where T_r is an arbitrary reference temperature. One of the earliest works discussing such temperature dependence in QW lasers[20] (and even very recent work[21]) calculated that a semi-logarithmic plot of threshold current vs temperature had a decreasing slope, meaning that the characteristic temperature of a QW laser was not a constant, but an **increasing** function of temperature. Recent experimental work[19,22], however, indicates that T_o is actually a **decreasing** function of temperature. Also, it has been found that T_o for a GRIN-SCH-SQW increases with cavity length[22,23]. Both of these features are predicted by our model, simply by calculating G(J) at several temperatures, and finding the required threshold current density at those temperatures **for a specified threshold gain**.

A difficult test for the model is to predict the abrupt change in T_o which shows up at a critical temperature (T_c) in log J_{th} vs T plots for **high gain**, wide-stripe, **thin** quantum well AlGaAs GRIN-SCH devices[22]. For example, for devices with structure I having uncoated facets and cavity lengths about 150 μm, T_c is near 60°C and abrupt changes in T_o of about 25K are observed. This abrupt change in T_o at T_c is accompanied by a change in threshold wavelength of about 50 nm, which is attributed to a gain cross-over from an n=1 electron to light hole transition to an n=2 electron to heavy hole transition[22]. Consequently, there is little doubt that the change in T_o is associated with the temperature dependence of the lowest slope discontinuity of the G(J) curve.

In our previous paper[2] we demonstrated good agreement of our model's results for threshold current vs temperature, including the T_o discontinuity, with the data of ref. 22 for a structure-I laser. In figure 4, we show the predictions of our model for the more highly confining structure II. The characteristic temperature is plotted as a function of QW thickness at two values of threshold gain, 20 and 40 cm^{-1}. Here, the characteristic temperature is evaluated at 300K. There is a general tendency for T_o to decrease with thinner quantum wells. This trend is due primarily to the non-radiative currents which become more important at the higher carrier densities associated with thinner wells.

For the larger gain value, 40 cm^{-1}, there is a discontinuity in T_o associated with the gain crossover from n=1 to n=2 transitions at a QW thickness between 17.5 and 20 nm. At the lower gain value, 20 cm^{-1}, this jump occurs for a QW thickness between 25 and 27.5 nm. This behavior can be understood from the original G(J) curves, since the kinks, or slope changes, in gain vs current density associated with the n=1 to n=2 transition change occur at lower values of gain for thicker quantum wells.

4. SUMMARY AND CONCLUSIONS

We have presented a model for GRIN-SCH-SQW lasers which is in good agreement with experimental data from operating injection lasers. We find that an accurate gain model requires several factors which strongly affect the gain vs current relation: (1) carrier relaxation, and the resulting spectral smoothing, significantly lowers the peak gain; (2) gain anisotropy is very significant near the edges of the heavy hole transitions, where it is 50% larger than the corresponding bulk value; (3) non-radiative processes must be included, and may even dominate the current, for weakly confining structures at high gain or high temperature.

In GRIN-SCH-SQW lasers, the largest peak gain for a given current density occurs for structures with the largest energy barriers, both in the QW and GRIN regions, which give better optical and carrier confinement. The advantages of higher barriers can be seen from the G(J) curves for structures I and II. The mode gain is approximately twice as high for the 33%/71% confining structure as for the 20%/40% structure. Changes in the QW thickness between I and II **do not** contribute significantly to this improvement. Both Auger recombination and carrier leakage are significant, but the leakage contribution to injection current dominates at high gains and temperatures when thermal population of high energy levels becomes significant. In these circumstances, the GRIN levels may become important in determining the carrier population distribution.

In predicting which GRIN-SCH-SQW structure will give a minimum J_{th} for a given cavity loss, the thickness of the QW in the range we have examined is less significant than the confining structure. For mode gains less than ~60 cm^{-1} we have found relatively small mode gain differences using quantum wells from 50Å to 100Å. With a given confining structure, the optical confinement factor increases approximately proportional to the QW thickness. On the other hand, the current needed to supply the required carrier density also increases with QW thickness, so the two factors in a calculation of mode gain vs current density tend to balance each other. At larger QW thicknesses, the threshold current density increases but the average G(J) slope does as well. Ultimately, a quasi-linear relation develops as the active layer takes on three-dimensional (bulk) character.

Of course, one is usually interested in maximizing T_o as well as minimizing J_{th} and as our results show, this will generally occur at larger QW thickness. A discontinuity in T_o will occur near the n=1 to n=2 gain crossover, which will take place at lower gains for larger QW thickness. Consequently, an optimal design for a given threshold requirement is a complex undertaking and requires a full exercising of all aspects of the model.

In summary, we have presented a comprehensive model of unsaturated gain for GRIN-SCH-SQW lasers in good agreement with a wide range of experimental data. We conclude that a simple model using only sharp quantized gain spectra and radiative recombination cannot provide an accurate model for quantum well lasers. If carrier relaxation and non-radiative currents are included, a quantitative model in the low to medium gain regime can be obtained.

5. REFERENCES

1. H. Okamoto, "Semiconductor quantum-well structures for optoelectronics - recent advances and future prospects," Jap. J. Appl. Phys. **26**, 315-330 (1987).
2. S. R. Chinn, P. S. Zory, and A. R. Reisinger, "A model for GRIN-SCH-SQW diode lasers," IEEE J. Quantum Electron. **QE-24**, 2191-2214 (1988).
3. R. Eppenga, M. F. H. Schuurmans, and S. Colak, "New k·p theory for GaAs/$Ga_{1-x}Al_x$As-type quantum wells," Phys. Rev. **B36**, 1554-1564 (1987).
4. T. Hiroshima and R. Lang, "Effect of conduction-band nonparabolicity on quantized energy levels of a quantum well," Appl. Phys. Lett. **49**, 456-457 (1986).
5. P. Dawson, K. J. Moore, and C. T. Foxon, "Photoluminescence studies of type II GaAs/AlAs quantum wells grown by MBE," SPIE **792** Quantum Well and Superlattice Physics, 208-213 (1987).
6. For a recent review see G. Duggan, "A critical review of heterojunction band offsets," J. Vac. Sci. Technol. **B 3**, 1224-1230 (1985).
7. N. Holonyak, Jr., R. B. Kolbas, R. D. Dupuis, and P. D. Dapkus, "Quantum-Well Heterostructure Lasers," IEEE J. Quantum Electron. **QE-16**, 170-186 (1980).
8. M. Asada, A. Kameyama, and Y. Suematsu, "Gain and intervalence band absorption in quantum-well lasers," IEEE J. Quantum Electron. **QE-20**, 745-753 (1984).
9. M. Yamada, S. Ogita, M. Yamagishi, K. Tabata, N. Nakaya, M. Asada, and Y. Suematsu, "Polarization-dependent gain in GaAs/AlGaAs multi-quantum-well lasers: theory and experiment," Appl. Phys. Lett. **45**, 324-325 (1984).
10. M. Yamada, S. Ogita, M. Yamagishi, and K. Tabata, "Anisotropy and broadening of optical gain in a GaAs/AlGaAs multi-quantum well laser," IEEE J. Quantum Electron. **QE-21**, 640-645 (1985).
11. E. O. Kane, "Band structure of indium antimonide," J. Phys. Chem. Solids **1**, 249-261 (1957).
12. M. Yamanishi and Y. Lee, "Phase dampings of optical dipole moments and gain spectra in semiconductor lasers," IEEE J. Quantum Electron. **QE-23**, 367-370 (1987).
13. H. C. Casey and M. B. Panish, Heterostructure Lasers, , Part A, pp. 248-253, Academic, New York (1978).
14. N. K. Dutta, "Calculated temperature dependence of threshold current of GaAs-Al_xGa_{1-x}As double heterostructure lasers," J. Appl. Phys. **52**, 70-73 (1981).
15. A. Sugimura, "Auger recombination effect on threshold current of InGaAsP quantum well lasers," IEEE J. Quantum Electron. **QE-19**, 932-941 (1982).
16. A. R. Reisinger, P. S. Zory, and R. G. Waters, "Cavity length dependence of the threshold behavior in thin quantum well semiconductor lasers," IEEE J. Quantum Electron. **QE-23**, 993-999 (1987).
17. D. K. Wagner, R. G. Waters, P. L. Tihanyi, D. S. Hill, A. J. Roza, Jr., H. J. Vollmer, and M. M. Leopold, "Operating characteristics of single-quantum-well AlGaAs/GaAs high-power lasers," IEEE J. Quantum Electron., **QE-24**, 1258-1265 (1988).
18. P. S. Zory, A. R. Reisinger, L. J. Mawst, G. Costrini, C. A. Zmudzinski, M. A. Emanuel, M. E. Givens, and J. J. Coleman, "Anomalous length dependence of threshold for thin quantum well AlGaAs diode lasers," Electron. Lett. **22**, 475-476 (1986).
19. J. R. Shealy, "Optimizing the performance of AlGaAs graded index separate confining heterostructure quantum well lasers," Appl. Phys. Lett. **50**, 1634-1636 (1987).
20. N. K. Dutta, "Temperature dependence of threshold current of GaAs quantum well lasers," Electron. Lett. **18**, 451-453 (1982).
21. P. Blood, S. Colak, and A. I. Kucharska, "Temperature dependence of threshold current in GaAs/AlGaAs quantum well lasers," Appl. Phys. Lett. **52**, 599-601 (1988).
22. P. S. Zory, A. R. Reisinger, R. G. Waters, L. J. Mawst, C. A. Zmudzinski, M. A. Emanuel, M. E. Givens, and J. J. Coleman, "Anomalous temperature dependence of threshold for thin quantum well AlGaAs diode lasers," Appl. Phys. Lett. **49**, 16-18 (1986).
23. M. M. Leopold, A. P. Specht, C. A. Zmudzinski, M. E. Givens, and J. J. Coleman, "Temperature-dependent factors contributing to T_o in graded-index separate-confinement-heterostructure single quantum well lasers," Appl. Phys. Lett. **50**, 1403-1405 (1987).

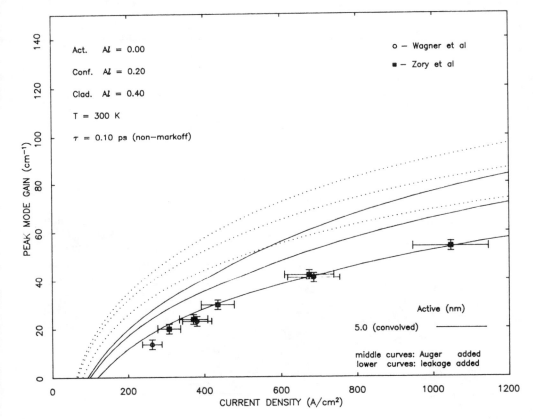

Figure 1. Peak TE mode gain as a function of current density for a structure I GRIN-SCH-SQW laser. The dashed curves, from unconvolved spectral gains, are calculated (in order of decreasing gain) for radiative recombination, radiative plus Auger recombination, and radiative and Auger recombination plus carrier leakage over the potential barriers. The corresponding solid curves come from spectrally convolved G(E). The open circle data are from ref. 17 and the closed squares from ref. 18.

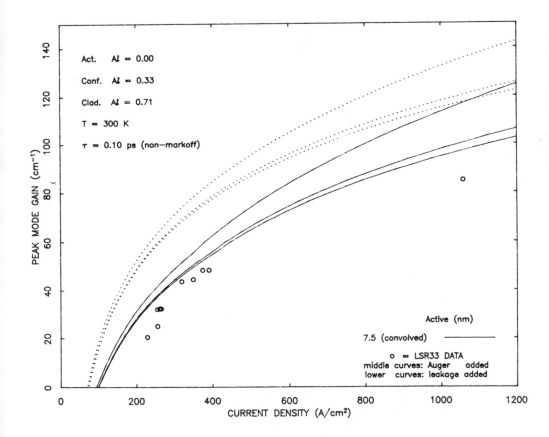

Figure 2. Peak TE mode gain as a function of current density for a structure II GRIN-SCH-SQW laser. The dashed curves, from unconvolved spectral gains, are calculated (in order of decreasing gain) for radiative recombination, radiative plus Auger recombination, and radiative and Auger recombination plus carrier leakage over the potential barriers. The corresponding solid curves come from spectrally convolved G(E).

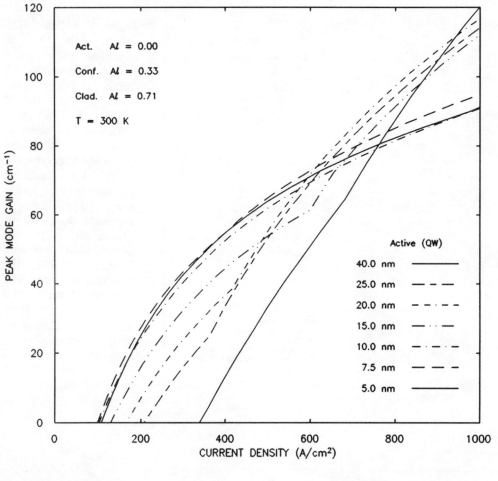

Figure 3. Peak TE mode gain as a function of current density for a structure II GRIN-SCH-SQW laser as a function of quantum well thickness.

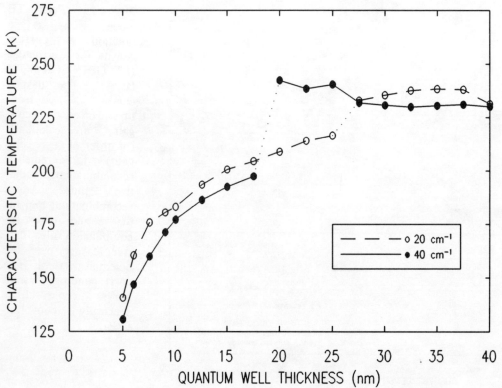

Figure 4. Characteristic temperature of a type-II GRIN-SCH-SQW laser as a function of quantum well thickness at two different threshold gain levels.

Semiconductor laser stabilization by external optical feedback

D.R. Hjelme and A.R. Mickelson

Department of Electrical and Computer Engineering, University of Colorado
Campus Box 425, Boulder, Colorado 80309-0425

R.G. Beausoleil, J.A. McGarvey, and R.L. Hagman

Boeing High Technology Center, P.O. Box 24969, Seattle, Washington 98124-6269

ABSTRACT

We have developed a theory describing the effect of external optical feedback on the steady-state noise characteristics of a single-mode semiconductor laser. This theory is valid for arbitrarily strong feedback and arbitrary external cavity. The general formalism includes relaxation oscillations, and allow us to analyze the effect of feedback on both the laser linewidth, frequency noise, relative intensity noise and the relaxation oscillation sidebands in the field spectrum.

1. INTRODUCTION

For most coherent optical systems applications, the linewidth and frequency stability of regular semiconductor lasers are not sufficient for acceptable system performance. External optical feedback is one of many techniques used to improve the stability and coherence properties of semiconductor lasers. The high sensitivity of these lasers to optical feedback is well known[1], and the presence of feedback strongly affects the linewidth and noise spectra[2]. To aid in the design of optical feedback systems, a general theory describing the effect of feedback on all the spectral properties is needed.

Although several authors have studied the noise properties of semiconductor lasers with external optical feedback, most studies are based on Lang's analysis[1] and are limited to weak feedback from a single mirror and low-frequency fluctuations. Some recent works[3-6] have used more general techniques, extending the analysis to stronger feedback and more general geometries, but are limited only to low-frequency fluctuations.

In this paper, we derive analytical expressions for the noise spectra in semiconductor lasers with generic optical feedback. The calculated spectra involve both the low-frequency spectra resulting in the finite linewidth and the high-frequency spectra exhibiting relaxation oscillation sidebands. The starting point for the analysis is the generalized rate equations first derived in the earlier work by Hjelme and Mickelson[5]. The derivation of these rate equations is outlined in Section 2. In Section 3, we derive the steady-state solutions and their dynamical stability. In Section 4, we linearize the equations around the steady-state solutions. Using perturbation analysis, we treat both the low- and high-frequency fluctuations by splitting the fluctuations into three terms: the low-frequency part and the fluctuations around the two relaxation oscillation satellite peaks in the field spectrum. We derive the analytical formulas for the low-frequency and high-frequency fluctuation spectra. In Section 5, we check the formalism by applying it to the well-known case of a Fabry-Perot cavity semiconductor laser. In Section 6 and 7, we apply the formalism to the diode laser coupled to a single mirror and a high-Q confocal Fabry-Perot cavity respectively.

2. DERIVATION OF RATE EQUATIONS

An accurate treatment of the semiconductor laser that accounts explicitly for the open laser cavity, and thereby the coupling to the outside world, is to integrate the traveling wave equation over the length of the laser. One can do this by assuming that the interaction between the forward and backward propagating waves is negligible except at the mirrors. The geometry under consideration is illustrated in Figure 1, where L is the diode cavity length and r_2 and $r_{\text{eff}}(\omega_0 + \omega)$ are the reflection coefficients seen at the left and right laser facets respectively. The form of $r_{\text{eff}}(\omega_0 + \omega)$ is dependent on the details of the geometry under consideration and is in general straightforward to derive. Later we will derive the reflection coefficient for those systems we consider in detail, but for now we will assume that it exists and is known. The optical field inside the diode cavity will be represented as $\mathcal{E}(t) = \frac{1}{2}(E(t)e^{i\omega_0 t} + E^\star(t)e^{-i\omega_0 t})$, where ω_0 is the lasing frequency. For convenience, the field amplitude $E(t)$ is normalized such that $|E(t)|^2$ equals the photon number in the diode cavity.

The rate equations, including the spontaneous emission noise source, can be derived by considering the build up of spontaneous emission[7]. As the laser oscillations build up, the total field is the sum of the field generated by spontaneous transitions, and subsequently amplified by stimulated emission, in all previous round trips.

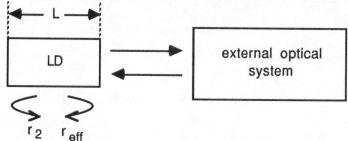

Figure 1: Illustration of the geometry of a laser diode (LD) with generic optical feedback.

With $r_2 r_{\text{eff}} \exp(-j2\hat{k}L)$ simulating the effect of propagating one roundtrip in the cavity, the field can be shown to satisfy the equation

$$[r_2 r_{\text{eff}} e^{-j\hat{k}2L} - 1]\tilde{E} = -\tau \tilde{F} \tag{1}$$

where the tilde indicates the Fourier transform, $\hat{k}$ is the complex wavenumber, τ is the diode cavity round trip time and $\tilde{F}$ is the spontaneous emission noise. Equation (1) describes the fact that the field after one roundtrip in the cavity is equal to itself plus the total contribution of spontaneous emission from the cavity. With $\tilde{F} = 0$, equation (1) has the form of the steady-state lasing condition obtained from a roundtrip analysis of the laser cavity.

To describe the noise characteristics of the laser system, we have to transform equation (1) to the time domain. A linear frequency domain operator can be transformed to the time domain by the relation[5] $\mathcal{F}\{U(\omega_0 + \omega)\tilde{E}(\omega)\} = \hat{U}(\omega_0 - i\partial_t)E(t)$, where $\mathcal{F}\{\ \}$ is the operation of the Fourier transform. The operators in equation (1) are in principle not linear. The wavenumber operator $\hat{k}$ is assumed to be a function of the carrier number N and is therefore implicitly a function of time. By assuming that the time derivatives of N are negligible compared with the time derivatives of E, the operators in (1) can be made to commute with N and therefore act only on E. We can show that this approximation neglects a gain saturation term not considered in this paper. With this approximation, one can transform equation (1) to the time domain by using the correspondence $\omega \leftrightarrow -i\partial_t$. To bring equation (1) into a form similar to the ordinary rate equation, one can write $\hat{k} = k + j\frac{1}{2}\hat{g}$, where k is the wavenumber in the laser medium at transparency and $\hat{g}$ is the complex carrier density dependent gain, and expand the "wavenumber operator" as $k(\omega_0 - i\partial_t) \approx k_N + \partial_\omega k(\omega_0 - \omega_N) - i\partial_\omega k \partial_t$. Here ω_N is the solitary laser cavity resonant frequency closest to the lasing frequency ω_0. The laser cavity roundtrip time is defined as $\tau \equiv 2L\partial_\omega k = 2L/v_g$, where v_g is the group velocity in the laser medium. The generalized rate equation for the optical field can then be expressed as

$$\left[\partial_t - \frac{1}{2}(\hat{\Gamma}_{\text{ex}} - \Gamma_{\text{ex}})\right]E(t) = \left[-i(\omega - \omega_N) + \frac{1}{2}(\hat{G} - \gamma) + \frac{1}{2}\Gamma_{\text{ex}}\right]E(t) + F(t) \tag{2}$$

where we have defined

$$\hat{G} = v_g \hat{g} = (1 + i\alpha)G_N(N - N_{tr}) \qquad (a)$$

$$\gamma = -\frac{2}{\tau}\ln r_2^2 \qquad (b) \qquad (3)$$

$$\hat{\Gamma}_{\text{ex}} = \frac{2}{\tau}\ln\frac{r_{\text{eff}}}{r_2}(\omega_0 - i\partial_t) \qquad (c)$$

where α is the linewidth enhancement factor, $G_N = \partial_N G$, N_{tr} is the carrier number at which the laser material turns transparent and $\Gamma_{\text{ex}}(\omega)$ is the complex number corresponding to the operator $\hat{\Gamma}_{\text{ex}}(\omega_0 - i\partial_t)$. The correlation properties of $F(t)$ can be approximated as $\langle F(t)F^\star(t')\rangle = R\delta(t - t')$, where R is the spontaneous emission rate.

To describe the fluctuations in the high-frequency region, it is essential to include the carrier dynamics. The equation for the total carrier number $N(t)$ is found by integrating the equation for the carrier density over the length of the diode cavity. The resulting rate equation can be written in the well known form

$$\dot{N} = P - N/\tau_c - G|E|^2 \tag{4}$$

where P is the pump term given by the injection current divided by the electron charge, τ_c is the carrier recombination time and G is the real part of $\hat{G}$. In (4), we have neglected a noise source F_N. The spontaneous emission-driven carrier fluctuations make only a small contribution to the intensity noise and frequency noise spectra, so for simplicity we include the spontaneous emission term (noise source) only in the equation for the optical field.

3. STEADY-STATE AND DYNAMICAL STABILITY

In steady state, the operating frequency, field amplitude, and carrier density are found by taking the average of the rate equations. If we denote by ω_s the lasing frequency of the solitary laser ($\Gamma_{ex} = 0$), we can write the steady-state equations in terms of the frequency shift ($\omega_0 - \omega_s$) and the excess gain $\Delta G = (G_0 - G_s)$ as

$$(\omega_0 - \omega_s) = \frac{1}{2}(Im\Gamma_{ex} - \alpha Re\Gamma_{ex}) \qquad (a) \quad (5)$$

$$\Delta G = G_0 - G_s = -Re\Gamma_{ex} \qquad (b)$$

where $\hat{G}_s$ is the gain of the solitary laser and $\hat{G}_0 = (1 + i\alpha)G_N(N_0 - N_{tr})$.

The dynamical stability of the steady-state solutions can be checked by performing a linear stability analysis of equations (2) and (4). The system is found to be unstable when

$$\left(1 - Im\frac{1}{2}\partial_\omega\Gamma_{ex} + \alpha Re\frac{1}{2}\partial_\omega\Gamma_{ex}\right) < 0. \qquad (6)$$

With equations for the mode oscillating frequencies and the excess gain and a criterion for dynamical stability, we are in a position to determine the lasing frequency. Solutions of (5) give the mode spectrum induced around the solitary laser mode, and the lasing mode is the stable solution with the minimum excess gain.

4. NOISE CHARACTERISTICS AND FIELD SPECTRUM

As is usual, we assume that the fluctuations of the optical field and carrier number are small perturbations to the steady-state operating points. This allows us to linearize the rate equations. The presence of the operator $\hat{\Gamma}_{ex}$ in (2) complicates the standard analysis. This operator introduces time constants into the equation that could be long compared to the periods of the relaxation oscillations. For the description of the fluctuations in this high-frequency region, we cannot approximate (2) by a first-order differential equation as is usually done. To avoid these difficulties, we treat the low- and high-frequency fluctuations separately by expanding the optical field, the carrier number and the Langevin noise source as

$$E(t) = A_0(1 + \rho(t))e^{i\phi(t)} + E_{R+}(t)e^{i\omega_R t} + E_{R-}(t)e^{-i\omega_R t} \qquad (a)$$

$$N(t) = N_0 + \Delta N(t) + \frac{1}{2}(N_R(t)e^{i\omega_R t} + N_R^\star(t)e^{-i\omega_R t}) \qquad (b) \quad (7)$$

$$F(t) = F_0(t) + F_+(t)e^{i\omega_R t} + F_-(t)e^{-i\omega_R t} \qquad (c)$$

where $\omega_R = \sqrt{\partial_N G G_0 A_0^2}$ is the relaxation oscillation frequency, $\rho(t)$ and $\phi(t)$ are the slowly varying amplitude and phase perturbations respectively, $E_{R\pm}(t)$ is the complex amplitude of the relaxation oscillations and $\Delta N(t)$ and $N_R(t)$ are the low- and high-frequency carrier number perturbations respectively. The correlation function of $F_i(t)$, $i = 0, \pm$, can be approximated as $\langle F_i(t)F_j^\star(t')\rangle = R\delta(t-t')\delta_{ij}$, $i,j = 0, \pm$.

The relaxation oscillation resonance induces low-intensity sidebands at the frequencies $\omega_0 \pm \omega_R$. Since the values of ω_R are far larger than those of $\Delta\omega_L$, the laser linewidth, the strong optical carrier component at ω_0, and the weak sidebands at $\omega_0 \pm \omega_R$ are well separated from each other in the frequency domain. This means that the relaxation oscillation resonance does not cause any drastic line broadening at the linecenter. We can therefore treat the relaxation oscillation resonance separately from the low-frequency fluctuations as indicated in (7).

To proceed, we must linearize (2) and (4) in terms of the perturbations and then separate the low- and high-frequency fluctuations. To first order, we can do this if we define the new variables

$$A_\pm = E_{R\pm}e^{-i\phi} \qquad (8)$$

It should be noted that the spectra $S_{A\pm}$ (to be defined below) will approximately be the convolution of the spectra at $\pm\omega_R$ and the Lorentzian laser line. If the laser line is much narrower than the relaxation oscillation sidebands, we have the approximate result $S_{A\pm}(\omega) \approx S_{E_{R\pm}}(\omega)$.

Linearizing the equations, and separating the different frequency parts, the resulting equation can be written as

$$\hat{U}(\partial_t)[A_0\rho + iA_0\phi] = \frac{1}{2}G_N(1 + i\alpha)A_0\Delta N + F_0 \qquad (a)$$

$$\hat{U}(\partial_t + i\omega_R)A_+ = \frac{1}{2}G_N(1 + i\alpha)A_0\frac{1}{2}N_R + F_+ \qquad (b) \quad (9)$$

$$\hat{U}(\partial_t - i\omega_R)A_- = \frac{1}{2}G_N(1+i\alpha)A_0\frac{1}{2}N_R^\star + F_- \qquad (c)$$

$$\hat{D}_N(\partial_t)\Delta N = -2G_0 A_0 A_0 \rho \qquad (d)$$

$$\hat{D}_N(\partial_t + i\omega_R)N_R = -2G_0 A_0 (A_+ + A_-^\star)^\bullet \qquad (e)$$

where we for convenience we have defined the operators

$$\hat{U}(\partial_t + i\omega) = (\partial_t + i\omega) - \frac{1}{2}\left[\hat{\Gamma}_{ex}(\omega_0 - i(\partial_t + i\omega)) - \Gamma_{ex}(\omega_0)\right] \qquad (a) \quad (10)$$

$$\hat{D}_N(\partial_t + i\omega) = (\partial_t + i\omega) + 2\Gamma_R \qquad (b)$$

where $2\Gamma_R = (1/\tau_c + G_N A_0^2)$ is the decay rate of the relaxation oscillations of the solitary laser. We have neglected the phase factor $e^{-i\phi}$ in the noise sources $F_i(t)$. This factor has no effect on the second moments needed for the calculation of the noise spectra.

The linear set of equations (9) can be solved in the frequency domain using Fourier analysis techniques. With analytical expressions for the transformed functions, we can find the fluctuation spectra by taking the proper ensemble averages of the absolute value square of the transformed functions. The low-frequency spectra of interest is *the frequency fluctuation spectrum* $S_{\dot{\phi}}(\omega)$ and *the relative intensity noise* RIN $= 4S_\rho(\omega)$ and can be expressed as

$$S_{\dot{\phi}}(\omega) = \langle(i\omega\tilde{\phi}(\omega))(i\omega\tilde{\phi}(\omega))^\star\rangle = \frac{R\omega^2}{A_0^2}\left\{\frac{|H^\star(-i\omega)|^2 + |H(i\omega)|^2}{|D(i\omega)|^2}\right\} \qquad (a) \quad (11)$$

$$\text{RIN} = 4S_\rho(\omega) = 4\langle\tilde{\rho}(\omega)\tilde{\rho}^\star(\omega)\rangle = \frac{4R}{A_0^2}\left\{\frac{|U^\star(-i\omega)|^2 + |U(i\omega)|^2}{|D(i\omega)|^2}\right\} \qquad (b)$$

where we have defined the functions

$$H(i\omega) = U(i\omega) + \omega_R^2(1+i\alpha)/D_N(i\omega) \qquad (a) \quad (12)$$

$$D(i\omega) = U(i\omega)H^\star(-i\omega) + U^\star(-i\omega)H(i\omega) \qquad (b)$$

The central part of the laser lineshape is determined by the noise spectra given in (11). Within this band, the carrier number can adiabatically follow the field amplitude fluctuations and provide gain saturation damping of the amplitude fluctuations. The main contribution to the field spectrum in this frequency band thus comes from the frequency fluctuations. If $S_{\dot{\phi}}(\omega)$ is flat for low frequencies, the central part of the field spectrum can be approximated as

$$S_E(\omega) = \frac{A_0^2 S_{\dot{\phi}}(0)}{\omega^2 + \left(\frac{S_{\dot{\phi}}(0)}{2}\right)^2}. \qquad (12)$$

This is the familiar Lorentzian line with linewidth $\Delta\omega_L = S_{\dot{\phi}}(0)$. The linewidth reduction factor can be written

$$\frac{\Delta\omega_L}{\Delta\omega_0} = \left(1 - Im\frac{1}{2}\partial_\omega\Gamma_{ex} + \alpha Re\frac{1}{2}\partial_\omega\Gamma_{ex}\right)^{-2} \qquad (13)$$

where $\Delta\omega_0 = \Delta\omega_{ST}(1+\alpha^2)$ is the modified Schawlow-Townes linewidth for semiconductor lasers, and $\Delta\omega_{ST} = R/2A_0^2$ is the Schawlow-Townes formula. This result is in agreement with previously derived formulas for the Lorentzian linewidth. It is clear from (13) that the important quantity for linewidth reduction is the frequency derivative of the effective losses in the external optical system. It is also important to note that the term in the bracket in the denominator in (13) is the same as the factor determining the dynamical stability (6). As expected, the linewidth and stability are closely related. It should be noted that the expression (12) for the field spectrum is valid *only* if $S_{\dot{\phi}}$ is flat, and over a frequency range less than the range over where $S_{\dot{\phi}}$ is flat.

Outside this low-frequency regime the field spectrum will deviate from the Lorentzian and is given by $S_E(\omega) \approx S_{A\pm}(\pm\omega + \omega_R)$. These high-frequency field spectra can be expressed in the following form:

$$S_{A+}(\omega) = \langle\tilde{A}_+(\omega)\tilde{A}_+^\star(\omega)\rangle$$

$$= R\left\{\frac{|U^\star(-i(\omega+\omega_R)) + H^\star(-i(\omega+\omega_R))|^2 + |U(i(\omega+\omega_R)) - H(i(\omega+\omega_R))|^2}{|D(i(\omega+\omega_R))|^2}\right\} \qquad (a) \quad (14)$$

$$S_{A-}(-\omega) = \langle \tilde{A}_-(-\omega)\tilde{A}_-^\star(-\omega)\rangle = \langle \widetilde{A_-^\star}(\omega)\widetilde{A_-^\star}^*(\omega)\rangle$$
$$= R\left\{\frac{|U^*(-i(\omega+\omega_R)) - H^*(-i(\omega+\omega_R))|^2 + |U(i(\omega+\omega_R)) + H(i(\omega+\omega_R))|^2}{|D(i(\omega+\omega_R))|^2}\right\} \quad (b)$$

It is instructive to rewrite the two spectra as

$$S_{A\pm}(\pm\omega) = A_0^2\left\{\frac{S_{\dot\phi}(\omega\pm\omega_R)}{(\omega\pm\omega_R)^2} + S_\rho(\omega\pm\omega_R) \pm S_{\rho\phi}(\omega\pm\omega_R)\right\} \quad (15)$$

where the fluctuation coupling spectrum $S_{\rho\phi}$ is easily derived from (14). The form (15) is consistent with Vahala et. al[8]. If the frequency noise is dominating when we approach the linecenter, this formula approaches the tails of the Lorentzian line (12) since $S_E(\omega) \approx A_0^2 S_{\dot\phi}(0)/\omega^2$ for $\omega \gg \Delta\omega_L$. It is clear from the last term in (15) that the field spectrum is not symmetric. The asymmetry is due to the amplitude-phase coupling introduced by both the optical feedback and the α-factor. This asymmetry does not show up in the central part of the field spectrum (12) where we neglected the amplitude fluctuations.

5. SOLITARY LASER DIODE

To check the formalism, we apply the formalism to the well-known case of a Fabry-Perot cavity semiconductor laser. This also provides us with a reference to see the relative effects of the optical feedback in the other cases considered. The fluctuation spectra are found by setting $r_{\text{eff}} = r_2$ in the formulas we have derived. The formulas for the relative intensity noise and the frequency fluctuation spectrum can be shown to reduce to the well known formulas from the literature. The upper part of Figure 2 shows the normalized RIN and $S_{\dot\phi}$, showing the characteristic relaxation oscillation peak. The lower part of Figure 2 shows the various components of the field spectrum. The figure clearly shows how $S_{A\pm}$ approaches the tails of the Lorentzian line at low frequencies, while showing relaxation oscillation resonances at higher frequencies. The coupling spectrum $|S_{\rho\phi}|$ is also shown to peak at the relaxation oscillation frequency.

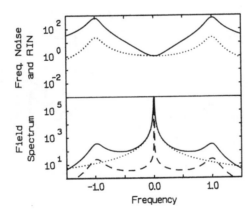

Figure 2: Noise spectra for the solitary laser. The upper two traces show $S_{\dot\phi}/\Delta\omega_0$ (...) and $RIN/(\Delta\omega_{\text{ST}}16\Gamma_R^2/\omega_R^4)$ (——). Lower traces shows S_E (...), $S_{A\pm}$ (——) and $|S_{\rho\phi}|$ (- - -) all normalized to R/ω_R^2. The frequency is normalized to ω_R. $\alpha = 5$, $\Gamma_R/\omega_R = 0.1$, $\Delta\omega_0/\omega_R = 0.01$.

We can obtain simple analytical results for the strength and asymmetry of the sidebands. If we assume $\Gamma_R/\omega_R \ll 1$, we obtain the strength of the relaxation oscillation resonance $S_{A\pm}(0) \approx \alpha^2 R/8\Gamma_R^2$, or relative to the Lorentzian, $S_{A\pm}(0)/S_E(0) \approx (\Delta\omega_0/4\Gamma_R)^2$. First note that the α-factor enhances the relaxation oscillation sidebands with the same factor (α^2) as the linewidth. The relative asymmetry can be approximated as $\approx 8\Gamma_R/\alpha\omega_R$. It also follows that the sidebands are approximately 20–30 dB below the laser line ($\Gamma_R \sim 1$ ns, $\Delta\nu \sim 30$ MHz).

6. LASER COUPLED TO A SINGLE MIRROR

The simplest form of optical feedback is feedback from a mirror placed a distance L_{ex} from the laser. The geometry under consideration here is shown in Figure 3. Here r_2 and r_3 are the amplitude reflection coefficients.

The effective reflection coefficient in this case takes the form

$$r_{\text{eff}} = r_2 \frac{1 + r_3/r_2 e^{-i\omega\tau_{\text{ex}}}}{1 + r_3 r_2 e^{-i\omega\tau_{\text{ex}}}} \tag{16}$$

where $\tau_{\text{ex}} = 2L_{\text{ex}}/c$ is the roundtrip time in the external cavity.

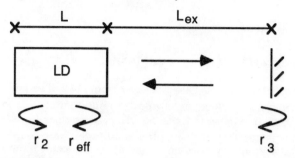

Figure 3: Illustration of the geometry used for a laser with mirror feedback.

Figure 4 shows typical noise and field spectra for this system. In Figure 4(a) we consider a relative short cavity with $\tau_{ex} = 2\pi/\omega_R$ and -20 dB feedback, while in Figure 4(b) we consider a long cavity with $\tau_{ex} = 2\pi/0.25\omega_R$ and -30 dB feedback. The two cases show similar linewidth reduction, but the details of the spectra differs. Most significant is the presense of external cavity resonanses in the spectra for the long cavity. These external cavity modes will eventually grow to become comparable to the central Lorentzian and the laser goes unstable[9]. Since the present theory is based upon a perturbation approach, it is not valid in this unstable regime.

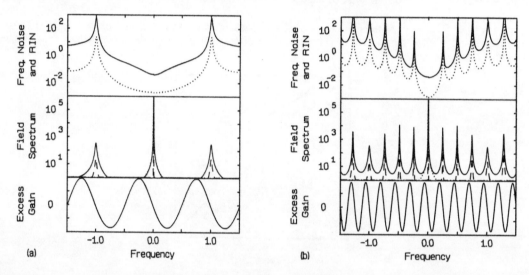

Figure 4: Same as Figure 2, but for a laser with mirror feedback. (a) short cavity and (b) long cavity.

8. LASER COUPLED TO A HIGH Q CAVITY

Resonant optical feedback provides a powerful means for stabilizing laser diodes[10-11]. The basic frequency stabilization system considered here is illustrated in Figure 5. As shown, the confocal Fabry-Perot (CFP) cavity is operated off-axis and has two reflected beams. It is important to note that the two beams have very different characteristics. The beam reflected back to the laser diode, the transmission mode, has the desired characteristic of a power maximum on resonance. In contrast, the other beam, the reflection mode, has a power minimum when the laser frequency matches a cavity resonance. The effective reflection coefficient is straightforward to derive and is found to be

$$r_{\text{eff}} = r_2 \frac{1 + r_{\text{CFP}}/r_2 e^{-i\omega\tau_s}}{1 + r_{\text{CFP}} r_2 e^{-i\omega\tau_s}} \tag{17}$$

where r_{CFP} is the reflection coefficient seen at the input port of the reference cavity,

$$r_{CFP} = k \frac{(1-R_c)\sqrt{R_c}\, e^{-i\omega\tau_c/2}}{1 - R_c^2 e^{-i\omega\tau_c}} \tag{18}$$

where R_c is the reflectivity of the mirrors in the confocal cavity, k represents the coupling factor between the laser mode and the CFP mode, $\tau_c = 4L_c/c$ is the reference cavity roundtrip time, and $\tau_s = 2L_s/c$ is the roundtrip time in the cavity formed between the laser facet and reference cavity input port.

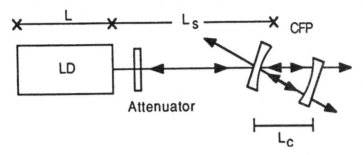

Figure5: Resonant optical feedback locking system.

Figure 6 shows typical noise and field spectra for this system. In Figure 6(a) we consider a cavity with a free spectral range of $\Delta\omega_{FSR} = 3\omega_R$, finess $F = 300$ and -50 dB feedback, while in Figure 6(b) we consider a cavity with $\Delta\omega_{FSR} = 0.25\omega_R$, $F = 25$ and -30 dB feedback. These two cavities have the same resonance width. The first thing to note is the relative narrow range of frequency over which the frequency noise is reduced compared to Figure 4(a). And also note the presense of external cavity resonanses in the spectra for the long cavity. The strength of these resonances varies with the exact relative phases in the system.

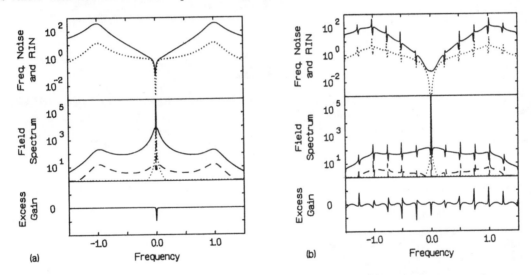

Figure 6: Same as Figure 2, but for a laser with feedback from a cavity. (a) large free spectral range and (b) small free spectral range.

In the weak feedbacklimit we can derive analytical expressions for the frequency noise if the laser operates at the cavity resonance and $\omega_0\tau_s + tan^{-1}(\alpha) = 2m\pi$

$$S_{\dot\phi} \approx \frac{R}{2A_0^2 (kF\tau_c/2F_d\tau)} \frac{1}{T(\omega)} \tag{19}$$

where $T(\omega)$ is the power transmission function of the cavity, normalized to one at the resonance and F and F_d is the finess of the cavity and the diode respectively. From (19) it follows that the we will have strong noise reduction across the cavity resonance width, but if the factor in the denominator is large, the noise reduction bandwidth can be substantially larger than the resonance width. In Figure 7 we have plotted the spectra corresponding to a case were (19) is valid and with parameters $\Delta\omega_{FSR} = \omega_R$, F=100 and -55dB feedback.

10. CONCLUSION

We have derived analytical expressions for the relative intensity noise, frequency noise, and field spectra for semiconductor lasers with generic optical feedback. Applying the formalism to a regular laser diode, we can rederive the well-known spectra for this laser. Two feedback configurations are considered, the standard single mirror feedback and the resonant optical feedback. It is found that if the external cavity mode spacing is larger than the relaxation oscillation frequency, the effective noise reduction bandwidth can be large and no external cavity modes are present. Contrary, when the mode spacing is smaller than the relaxation oscillation frequency, the external cavity modes can be strong.

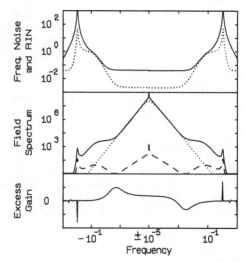

Figure7: Same as Figure 6, but with a different cavity and plotted on a logaritmic frequency scale

REFERENCES

1. R. Lang and K. Kobayashi, "External Optical Feedback Effects on Semiconductor Injection Laser Properties," *IEEE Journ Quant Elect* **QE-16**, pp. 347–355 (1980).
2. L. Goldberg, H. F. Taylor, A. Dandridge, and T. G. Giallorenzi, "Spectral Characteristics of Semiconductor Lasers with Optical Feedback," *IEEE Journ Quant Elect* **QE-18**, pp. 555–564 (1982).
3. E. Patzak, A. Sagimura, S. Saito, T. Mukai, and H. Olsen, "Semiconductor Laser Linewidth in Optical Feedback Configurations," *Elect Lett* **19**, pp. 1026–1027 (1983).
4. R. J. Lang and A. Yariv, "Local-Field Rate Equation for Coupled Optical Resonators," *Phys Rev A* **34**, pp. 2038–2043 (1986).
5. D. R. Hjelme and A. R. Mickelson, "On the Theory of External Cavity Operated Single-Mode Semiconductor Lasers," *IEEE Journ Quant Elect* **QE-23**, pp. 1000–1004 (1987).
6. G. Bjørk and O. Nilsson, "A Tool to Calculate the Linewidth of Complicated Semiconductor Lasers," *IEEE Journ Quant Elect* **QE-23**, pp. 1303–1313 (1987).
7. D. R. Hjelme, Ph.D dissertation, University of Colorado, Boulder CO, (1988).
8. K. Vahala, Ch Harder, and A. Yariv, "Observation of Relaxation Resonance Effects in the Field Spectrum of Semiconductor Lasers," *Appl Phys Lett* **42**, pp. 211–213 (1983).
9. D. Lenstra, B. H. Verbeek, and A. den Boef, "Coherence Collapse in Single-Mode Semiconductor Lasers Due to Optical Feedback," *IEEE Journ Quant Elect* **QE-21**, pp. 674–679 (1985).
10. D. R. Hjelme, A. R. Mickelson, L. Hollberg, and B. Dahmani, "Novel Optical Frequency Stabilization of Semiconductor Lasers," *Topical Meeting on Semiconductor Lasers* and *OSA Tech Digest* **6**, pp. 15–18 (February 1987).
11. B. Dahmani, L. Hollberg, and R. Dullinger, "Frequency Stabilization of Semiconductor Lasers by Resonant Optical Feedback," *Opt Lett* **12**, pp. 876–878 (1987).

Measurement of semiconductor laser linewidth enhancement factor using coherent optical feedback

Ki-Hyun Chung, John G. McInerney and Marek Osiński *

Center for High Technology Materials, University of New Mexico,
Albuquerque, New Mexico 87131

* Currently on leave at the Research Center for Advanced Science
and Technology, University of Tokyo, 4-6-1 Komaba,
Meguro-ku, Tokyo 153, Japan

ABSTRACT

The linewidth enhancement factor α of a semiconductor injection laser is defined to be the ratio of the changes in the real and imaginary parts of the complex susceptibility of the laser medium due to carrier density variations. We have devised a novel method for measuring this parameter by observing the changes in the optical frequency and external quantum efficiency due to coherent optical feedback. The wavelength dependence of α close to the room-temperature gain peak was measured for GaAs/GaAlAs channeled-substrate-planar devices.

I. INTRODUCTION

The asymmetric gain spectrum of a typical III-V semiconductor injection laser results in strong coupling between the real and imaginary parts of the complex susceptibility. The ratio of these changes is known as the linewidth enhancement factor, or α parameter,[1] and it influences many of the static and dynamic properties of these lasers.[2] It affects the spectral linewidth of free-running and external-cavity devices,[3-6] frequency chirping,[7-9] AM-to-FM coupling,[10,11] optical waveguiding and antiguiding,[12] injection locking bandwidth,[13,14] bistability,[15-17] as well as various temporal and spectral instabilities.[18-20]

Many different methods for determining the linewidth enhancement factor have been reported, including measurement of gain and frequency shifts with injection current variations below threshold,[21] measurement of changes in frequency and amplified spontaneous emission spectral width with current variations below threshold,[22] obtaining the ratio of the frequency chirp to the output power of a directly modulated laser,[7,10,11] measuring the product of the output power and temporal width of Gaussian gain-switched pulses,[25] observation of injection locking,[14] and optical frequency instabilities.[19] Despite the pervasive influence of the α parameter, there has been little cross-correlation between these methods, which are performed under a wide range of operating conditions, and which have produced a wide range of values. There is still a pressing need for simpler and more straightforward above-threshold methods for measuring α under well-defined, typical operating conditions. These methods should be cross-correlated and the results compared with recent theories for the linewidth enhancement factor.[24,25]

Here we describe a novel method for measuring α which depends on a few straightforward measurements performed above threshold, under typical operating conditions. The technique avoids the complications of injection current variation or modulation, and all measurements are essentially static. A simple external cavity is set up which coherently reflects a few percent of the output power back into the active region. This coherent optical feedback causes the refractive index and gain to shift, resulting in a different lasing frequency and quantum efficiency. Measurement of these parameters with and without feedback gives the α parameter at that frequency. By temperature-tuning the laser, the temperature dependence of α near the room temperature gain peak can be determined.

II. THEORY

Optical feedback affects the gain spectrum of a semiconductor laser, and hence the output power and frequency are changed from those of the free-running device. The maximum output power of an external cavity laser at a given injection current is attained when the feedback is in-phase, that is when the phase delay due to the round trip in the external cavity is an integral multiple of 2π. The phase of the optical feedback may be varied either by adjusting the oscillating frequency or by controlling the external cavity length. The rate equation for the complex optical electric field $E(t)$ in the presence of coherent optical feedback can be written as[4]

$$\frac{dE}{dt} = i(\omega-\Omega)E(t) + \frac{1}{2}(G-\gamma)(1-i\alpha)E(t) + \kappa E(t-\tau)exp(i\omega\tau) \quad , \tag{2-1}$$

where ω is the optical angular frequency in the presence of feedback, Ω the angular frequency of the free-running laser, G the temporal modal gain and γ the loss rate (reciprocal of the photon lifetime), τ the optical round trip time in the external cavity and α the linewidth enhancement factor. The feedback coupling coefficient κ is defined as

$$\kappa = \frac{(1-R)}{\tau_d}\left[\frac{f_c}{R}\right]^{1/2} \quad , \tag{2-2}$$

where R is the power reflectivity of the internal laser facet, τ_d the optical round trip time in the diode cavity and f_c the fraction of optical power returned to the laser including all coupling, absorption and diffraction losses. The real and imaginary parts of Eq. (2-1) can be separated and written as rate equations for the photon population P and the optical phase ϕ, with $E \approx P^{1/2}exp(-i\phi)$

$$\frac{dP}{dt} = (G-\gamma)P(t) + 2\kappa[P(t)P(t-\tau)]^{1/2}cos[\omega\tau+\delta\phi] \tag{2-3.a}$$

and

$$\frac{d\phi}{dt} = -(\omega-\Omega) + \frac{1}{2}\alpha(G-\gamma) - \kappa\left[\frac{P(t-\tau)}{P(t)}\right]^{1/2}sin[\omega\tau+\delta\phi] \quad , \tag{2-3.b}$$

where $\delta\phi = \phi(t) - \phi(t-\tau)$. In Eq. (2-3.a) we have omitted the negligible spontaneous emission contribution when the laser is operated well above threshold. The rate equation for the carrier population N can be written as

$$\frac{dN}{dt} = \frac{I}{q} - \gamma_e N(t) - GP(t) \quad , \tag{2-3.c}$$

where I is the injection current, q the electron charge, and γ_e the carrier recombination rate (reciprocal of the carrier recombination lifetime).

The steady state behavior of the external cavity semiconductor laser can be analyzed using Eqs. (2-3.a-c), assuming that P, ϕ and N are time-independent. The static solution of the three rate equations is then

$$G-\gamma = -2\kappa\, cos(\omega\tau) \tag{2-4.a}$$

$$\omega-\Omega = \frac{1}{2}\alpha(G-\gamma) - \kappa\, sin(\omega\tau) \tag{2-4.b}$$

$$0 = \frac{I}{q} - \gamma_e N - GP \quad . \tag{2-4.c}$$

By comparison between Eqs. (2-4.a-c) and the steady state solution of the rate equations without feedback ($\kappa = 0$), and assuming negligible changes in the loss rate γ, the feedback-induced gain and frequency changes are found to be

$$G - G_o = \Delta G = -2\kappa \cos(\omega\tau) \qquad (2\text{-}5.\text{a})$$

and

$$\Omega - \omega = \Delta\omega = \kappa\left[\sin(\omega\tau) + \alpha\cos(\omega\tau)\right] \qquad (2\text{-}5.\text{b})$$

respectively, where G_o represents the temporal modal gain of the free-running laser. The photon population in the presence of feedback can be obtained using Eq. (2-4.c), and is given by

$$P = \frac{(I - I_{th})}{q(\gamma + \Delta G)} \,, \qquad (2\text{-}6)$$

where I_{th} is the threshold current with feedback.

The differential (external) quantum efficiency is directly proportional to the slope of the output power/drive current characteristic, and depends on the feedback-induced gain change ΔG. The ratio of the differential quantum efficiencies with and without feedback is then

$$r = \frac{\gamma}{\gamma + \Delta G} \times A \,, \qquad (2\text{-}7)$$

where A is the correction factor due to the altered ratio between the photon population P and the output power from the facet under observation, given by

$$A = \frac{\omega n_o}{\Omega n} \frac{\ln(R_1 R_e)}{\ln(R_1 R_2)} \frac{\sqrt{R_e}}{\sqrt{R_2}} \frac{\left[(1-R_1)\sqrt{R_2} + (1-R_2)\sqrt{R_1}\right]}{\left[(1-R_1)\sqrt{R_e} + (1-R_e)\sqrt{R_1}\right]} \qquad (2\text{-}8)$$

where R_1 and R_2 are the facet reflectivities, R_e the effective reflectivity which can be found from the feedback-induced threshold current reduction [26], n and n_o the refractive indices of the laser medium with and without feedback, respectively. The output is assumed to be collected from mirror 1.

The differential quantum efficiency changes due to external feedback are measured at different values of the feedback phase $\omega\tau$, and hence the coupling coefficient κ is obtained in terms of the photon loss rate γ, which can in turn be found from the feedback-induced threshold current reduction.[29] The required expression for κ is

$$\kappa = -\frac{1}{2}\gamma\left[\frac{1 - r_{in}/A}{r_{in}/A}\right] \,, \qquad (2\text{-}9)$$

where r_{in} represents the quantum efficiency ratio defined by Eq. (2-7) with in-phase feedback, which is established by adjusting $\omega\tau$ to obtain the maximum output power at a given injection current.

Figs. 1.a-c show the calculated optical frequency shift $\Delta\omega$, the gain change ΔG, and the resonant feedback phase $\omega\tau$, for different external cavity lengths. Many external cavity modes, represented by the various curves in Figs.1. a-c, can be seen to coexist with different feedback phases at a given external cavity length. The solid line in Figs. 1.a-c represents the dominant mode having the lowest threshold gain. The number of external cavity modes present depends on the feedback ratio and external cavity length. The maximum possible gain shift is $\Delta G_{in} = -2\kappa$ from Eq. (2-5.a), and corresponds to the in-phase feedback condition (point C in Fig. 1). The optical frequency shift from the free-running condition due to in-phase feedback is given by Eq. (2-5.b) as the product of the coupling ratio κ and the linewidth enhancement factor α. From Fig. 1.a, we see that the output power and optical frequency should vary periodically when the external cavity length is varied over a few wavelengths.

The maximum permissible feedback phase detuning ϕ_{max} is limited by the position of the next external cavity mode (point B in Fig. 1.c). Using Eqs. (2-5.a) and (2-7), we see that

$$\phi_{max} = \cos^{-1}\left[\frac{\gamma}{2\kappa} \frac{1 - r_{out}/A}{r_{out}/A}\right], \qquad (2\text{-}10)$$

where r_{out} is the quantum efficiency ratio under these conditions. The linewidth enhancement factor α can then be found from Eqs. (2-5) to be

$$\alpha = \frac{\delta\Delta\omega/\kappa + \sin(\phi_{max})}{1 - \cos(\phi_{max})}, \qquad (2\text{-}11)$$

where $\delta\Delta\omega$ is the change in the oscillation frequency between points B and C in Fig. 1.b, which can be measured using a Fabry-Perot interferometer or high-resolution monochromator. An alternative expression which may be used to calculate the linewidth enhancement factor is

$$\alpha = \frac{\Delta\omega_{in}}{\kappa} = -\frac{2\pi c}{\lambda^2}\frac{\Delta\lambda_{in}}{\kappa}, \qquad (2\text{-}12)$$

where $\Delta\omega_{in}$ and $\Delta\lambda_{in}$ are the angular frequency and wavelength shifts induced by in-phase external feedback.

III. EXPERIMENTS

Our experiments used several GaAs/GaAlAs channeled-substrate-planar (CSP) double-heterostructure lasers (Hitachi HLP-1400). Each selected device was placed in an external cavity formed by a suitable lens (GRIN-rod, microscope objective or purpose-built laser diode collimator) and an external reflector (HR plane mirror or 1200 line/mm grating) mounted on a translation stage driven by a piezoelectric pusher (PZT). A typical configuration is illustrated in Fig. 2. Neutral density filters were inserted between the lens and reflector to adjust the amount of optical feedback, which was typically a few percent. The range of external cavity lengths used was 8 to 70 mm. A CCD camera was used as an alignment aid, and care was taken to avoid instabilities associated with asymmetric feedback due to tilting of the external reflector.[27,28] The temperature of the laser heat sink was stabilized to within a few millikelvins by a feedback-controlled Peltier device.

Various diagnostics were set up to observe the temporal and spectral behavior of the external cavity laser. For devices on open packages, the beam for these diagnostics is conveniently taken from the free laser facet on the opposite side from the external cavity. For devices mounted in cans or with otherwise restricted access to the free facet, a small beam splitter can be inserted into the external cavity between the lens and reflector. In the latter case, a different correction factor A to that given in Eq. (2-8) must be used. A fast Si p-i-n detector (Antel AR-S2, risetime 40 ps) was used to measure instantaneous output power, while a grating monochromator (Spex 1704, 1 m, f/9, resolution < 0.01 nm) and scanning Fabry-Perot interferometer (Burleigh RC-110, FSR 2 GHz, finesse ≈ 100) were used to monitor optical spectra. The laser was operated above threshold, under typical operating conditions ($< 1.8 \times I_{th}$), in a single longitudinal mode of the diode cavity when free-running. When a plane mirror is used as the external reflector, the cavity length must be adjusted to equal an integral multiple of the optical length of the diode to avoid diode mode hopping. Using a grating external cavity reduces this tendency considerably, although it is more difficult to achieve high coupling efficiencies with this configuration. If there are any kinks in the light-current characteristics, such as those due to transverse mode changes, measurements are performed below the lowest kink, in the fundamental transverse mode.

Light-current characteristics were measured for the isolated diode, and for the external cavity device as a function of feedback phase. The latter parameter was varied by fine-tuning the cavity length via the PZT voltage. Optical spectra and total output power were also measured as a function of feedback phase, whilst preserving single diode mode operation. Typical results are given in Figs. 3 and 4. Fig. 3 shows changes in external quantum efficiency due to feedback: line A represents the free-running laser, line C refers to the maximum power condition (in-phase feedback, when the phase of the returning light differs from the emitted light by an integral multiple of 2π), and line B gives the quantum efficiency corresponding to the maximum permissible detuning from the in-phase condition (ϕ_{max}: point C in Fig. 1.c). The undulations in the light-current characteristics under coherent feedback are due to the changes in optical frequency due to varying injection current. Output power variations as a function of feedback phase at fixed injection current are shown as an inset to Fig. 3. The period of these undulations ϕ_{max} depends on the coupling coefficient κ in accordance with Eq. (2-10). Fig. 4 shows optical spectra for no feedback, in-phase feedback and maximally-detuned feedback. The total wavelength shift $\Delta\lambda_{in}$ due to in-phase feedback was thus measured. Using Eq. (2-9) we obtained the coupling coefficient κ from changes in the external quantum efficiency, and the linewidth enhancement factor α was then calculated using Eq. (2-12). These measurements were reperepeated for various lasing wavelengths selected by tuning the temperature of the laser heat sink between 10 and 40°C. Thus the spectral dependence of α near the room-temperature gain peak is determined.

As illustrated in Fig. 5, the range of α values measured for our CSP lasers was 2.5 to 4.3 between 830 and 850 nm (gain peak 840 nm at 25°C). These values were compared with the results of measurements performed using the method of Henning and Collins,[23] which gave α values from 2.6 to 3.6 across the same wavelength range as those used for our method. The uncertainty in our method, due mostly to possible errors in measuring quantum efficiencies, is $\approx 5-10$ %. Typical values of the coupling coefficient for our method were $\kappa \approx 0.05\gamma$, and the optimum value of the external cavity delay $\tau\ (= 2L_{ext}/c)$ was such that the product $\kappa\tau \approx 2-4$. Lower feedback coupling coefficients lead to larger errors in measuring the quantum efficiency ratios r_{in} and r_{out} and the wavelength shift $\Delta\lambda_{in}$. Using a short external cavity (a few cm) and large κ (f_c a few percent) is advantageous because it is more stable and has a wider single mode oscillation and continuous tuning range than longer, more weakly coupled cavities.

IV. DISCUSSION AND CONCLUSIONS

A simple method for measuring the linewidth enhancement factor α of a semiconductor injection laser has been developed by observing the gain and optical frequency shifts due to coherent external optical feedback. The measured values of α for GaAs/AlGaAs CSP lasers (Hitachi HLP 1400) near the room-temperature gain peak varied from 2.5 to 4.3. In addition to measurement of the linewidth enhancement factor, the external cavity can be used to narrow the spectral linewidth and fine-tune the center wavelength. The tuning range depends on the external cavity length and coupling coefficient (up to 12 GHz tuning was achieved without special AR coating on the laser facet). Also, it is worthwhile to consider a practical limit to the linewidth reduction in an external cavity: the calculated maximum linewidth reduction[3] with a feedback phase of $\omega\tau = -\tan^{-1}\alpha$ overestimates the true limit when the feedback-induced wavelength shift is larger than the external cavity mode spacing. The linewidth reduction is then limited not by $\omega\tau = -\tan^{-1}\alpha$ but by the maximum permissible phase detuning ϕ_{max}, confined by the position of neighboring external cavity modes.

V. REFERENCES

[1] C. H. Henry, "Theory of the linewidth of semiconductor lasers," IEEE J. Quantum Electron., vol. QE-18, pp.259-264, 1982.
[2] M. Osiński and J. Buus, "Linewidth broadening factor in semiconductor lasers - an overview," IEEE J. Quantum Electron., vol. QE-23, pp.9-29, 1987.
[3] R. Lang and K. Kobayashi, "External optical feedback effects on semiconductor injection laser properties," IEEE J. Quantum Electron., vol. QE-16, pp.347-355, 1980.
[4] G. P. Agrawal, "Line narrowing in a single-mode injection laser due to external optical feedback," IEEE J. Quantum Electron., vol. QE-20, pp.468-471, 1984.
[5] K. Kojima, S. Noda, S. Tai, K. Kuyuma, K. Hamanaki, and T. Nakayama, "Long cavity ridge

waveguide AlGaAs/GaAs distributed feedback lasers for spectral linewidth reduction," Appl. Phys. Lett., vol.49, pp.366-368, 1986.

[6] S. Ogita, Y. Kotaki, K. Kihara, M. Matsuda, H. Ishikawa, and H. Imai, "Dependence of spectral linewidth on cavity length and coupling coefficient in DFB laser," Elect. Lett., vol.24, pp.613-614, 1988.

[7] T. L. Koch and J. E. Bowers, "Nature of wavelength chirping in directly modulated semiconductor lasers," Electron. Lett. vol.20, pp.1038-1040, 1984.

[8] R. Linke, "Modulation induced transient chirping in single frequency lasers," IEEE J. Quantum Electron., vol. QE-21, pp- 593-597, 1985.

[9] G. P. Agrawal, "Power spectrum of directly modulated single-mode semiconductor lasers: chirp-induced fine structure," IEEE J. Quantum Electron., vol. QE-21, pp.680-686, June 1985.

[10] J. E. Bowers, W. T. Tsang, T. L. Koch, N. A. Olesen, and R. A. Rogan, "Microwave intensity and frequency modulation of hetero-epitaxial-ridge-overgrown distributed feedback lasers," Appl. Phys. Lett., vol.46, pp.233-235, 1985.

[11] K. Kikuchi and H. Iwasawa, "Measurement of linewidth enhancement factor of semiconductor lasers by modified direct frequency-modulation method," Electron. Lett., vol.24, pp.821-822, 1988.

[12] W. Streifer, R. D. Burnham, and D. R. Scifres, "Symmetrical and asymmetrical waveguiding in very narrow conducting strip lasers," IEEE J. Quantum Electron., vol. QE-15, pp.136-141, 1979.

[13] L. Goldberg, H. F. Taylor, J. F. Weller, "Locking bandwidth asymmetry in injection locked GaAlAs lasers," Electron. Lett., vol.18, pp.986-987, 1982.

[14] C. H. Henry, N. A. Olsson, and N. A. Dutta, "Locking range and stability of injection locked 1.54 μm InGaAsP semiconductor lasers," IEEE J. Quantum. Electron., vol. QE-21, pp.1152-1156, 1985.

[15] N. K. Dutta, G. P. Agrawal, and M. W. Focht, "Bistability in coupled cavity semiconductor lasers," Appl. Phys. Letter., vol.44, pp.30-32, 1984.

[16] J. G. McInerney, L. Reekie, and D. J. Bradley, "Observation of bistable optical effects in a twin GaAs/GaAlAs diode external cavity ring laser," Electron. Lett., vol.20. pp.586-588, 1984.

[17] J. G. McInerney, "Bistable optoelectronic devices," Proc. SPIE, vol.836, pp.244-253, 1987.

[18] J. H. Osmundsen, B. Tromborg, and H. Olesen, "Experimental investigation of stability properties for a semiconductor laser with optical feedback," Electron. Lett. vol.19, pp.1068-1070, 1983.

[19] C. H. Henry and R. F. Kazarinov, "Instability of semiconductor lasers due to optical feedback from distant reflectors," IEEE J. Quantum Electron., vol. QE-22, pp.295-301, 1986.

[20] N. A. Olsson, C. H. Henry, R. F. Kazarinov, H. J. Lee, K. J. Orlowsky, B. H. Johnson, R. E. Scotti, D. A. Ackerman, and P. J. Anthony, "Performance characteristics of a 1.5 μm single-frequency semiconductor laser with external waveguide Bragg reflector," IEEE J. Quantum Electron., vol.24, pp.143-147, 1988.

[21] I. D. Henning and J. V. Collins, "Measurement of the semiconductor laser linewidth broadening factor," Electron. Lett. , vol.19, pp.927-929, 1983.

[22] K. Kikuchi, "Lineshape measurement of semiconductor lasers below threshold," IEEE J. Quantum Electron., vol. QE-24, pp.1814-1817, 1988.

[23] M. Osiński, D. F. G. Gallagher, I. H. White, "Measurement of linewidth broadening factor in gain switched InGaAsP injection lasers by CHP method," Electron. Lett., vol.21. pp.981-982, 1985.

[24] K. Vahala, L. C. Chiu, S. Margalit, and A. Yariv, " On the linewidth enhancement factor α in semiconductor injection lasers," Appl. Phys. Lett., vol.42, pp.631-633, 1983.

[25] L. D. Westbrook, "Dispersion of linewidth-broadening factor in 1.5 μm laser diodes," Electron. Lett., vol.21, pp.1018-1019, 1985.

[26] J. H. Osmundsen and N. Gade, "Influence of optical feedback on laser frequency spectrum and threshold conditions," IEEE J. Quantum Electron., vol.19, pp.465-469, 1983.

[27] J. D. Park, D. S. Seo, J. G. McInerney, and M. Osiński, "Low frequency intensity noise in asymmetric external cavity semiconductor lasers", CLEO'88 Technical Digest, Anaheim, CA, April 25-29, 1988, paper WM10, pp.212-214.

[28] D. S. Seo, J. D. Park, J. G. McInerney, and M. Osiński, "Effects of feedback asymmetry in external-cavity semiconductor laser systems," Electron. Lett. vol.24, pp.726-728, 1988.

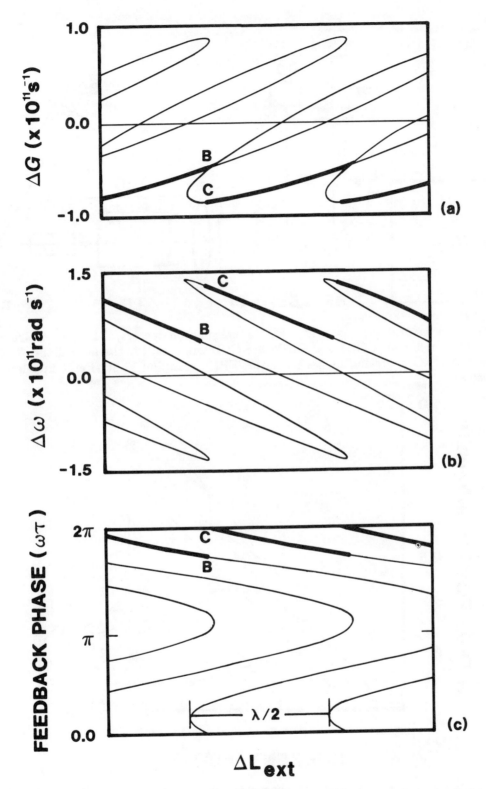

Fig. 1. Theoretical calculations of the gain shift ΔG, frequency shift $\Delta\omega$, and resonant feedback phase $\omega\tau$ versus cavity length change for an external cavity laser with $L_{ext} \approx 8L_d$ (L_d: optical length of the diode cavity) and $\kappa = 0.06\gamma$. B represents the maximum detunable feedback phase ϕ_{max}, while C refers to in-phase feedback.

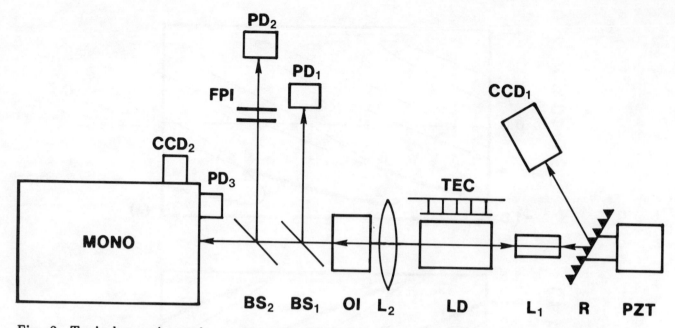

Fig. 2. Typical experimental arrangement. PD1-3 are photodetectors, L1 and L2 are collimating lenses, R the external reflector, CCD1 and CCD2 are CCD cameras, LD the laser diode, TEC the thermoelectric cooler, MONO a grating monochromator, FPI a scanning Fabry-Perot interferometer, and OI an optical isolator.

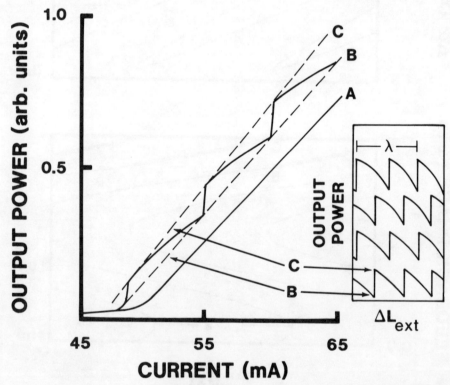

Fig. 3. Output power versus drive current characteristics for a GaAs/GaAlAs CSP laser (Hitachi HLP1400) with $L_{ext} = 8L_d$ and $\kappa = 0.06\gamma$. A: without feedback, B: feedback with maximum detunable phase, C: in-phase feedback. The inset shows the output power dependence on the feedback phase at fixed injection current above threshold.

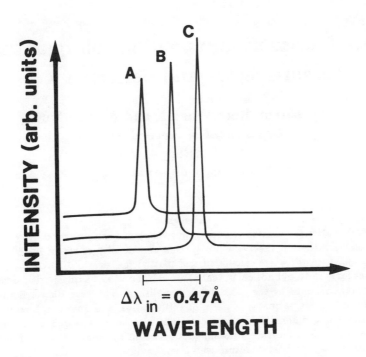

Fig. 4. Feedback-induced shift in oscillation wavelength. A: free-running laser diode (no feedback), B: maximally detuned phase, C: in-phase feedback.

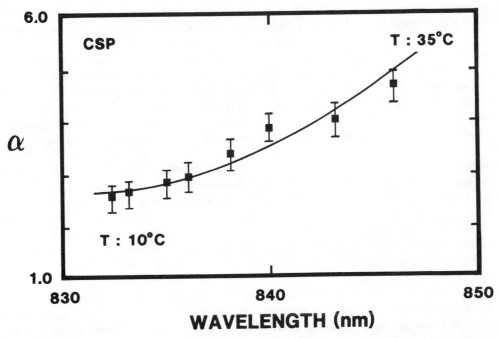

Fig. 5. Linewidth enhancement factor α versus wavelength near room-temperature gain peak for a GaAs/GaAlAs CSP laser (Hitachi HLP1400).

The effects of fabricational variations on quantum wire laser gain spectra and performance

Hal Zarem, Kerry Vahala, and Amnon Yariv
Department of Applied Physics
California Institute of Technology
Pasadena, California 91125

Abstract

The effects of fabricational variations on the gain spectra of quantum wires are calculated within the limits of first order perturbation theory. Gain spectra and density of states for 50Å radius and 150Å radius cylindrical quantum wires are calculated and plotted for several different fabrication tolerances. The wave functions for a finite, cylindrical potential are calculated and a quasi-critical radius, below which the carriers are weakly confined by the potential, is established. This sets a lower limit on quantum wire size. Upper limits on the size of quantum wells, quantum wires, and quantum boxes are also discussed. The threshold current and differential gain of quantum wire lasers and quantum wire array lasers are calculated. These calculations indicate a possible reduction in threshold current of one to two orders of magnitude as compared to the best quantum well lasers to date.

I Introduction

In recent years it has been shown both theoretically and experimentally that quantum well lasers have many advantages over conventional lasers. These advantages, such as ultra-low threshold current [1], narrow linewidth [2,3], reduced temperature dependence of the threshold current[4], and high modulation rate [2,5], are related to the two dimensional nature of the electrons in quantum wells. As the dimensionality is reduced from three to two, the density of states acquires a sharp edge on the low energy side, increasing the number of states near the band edge. When these states are filled the gain spectrum is narrower. This is advantageous since we are generally concerned with peak gain and carriers contributing to gain in other spectral regions are wasted. As the dimensionality is further reduced to one or zero dimensions, giving quantum wires and quantum boxes, the density of states becomes even sharper and narrower. Theoretical investigations of the one dimensional or zero dimensional structures, quantum wires and quantum boxes, have predicted further enhancements in many of these areas [2,4,6]. Gain calculations for quantum wires and quantum boxes predict large reductions in the threshold current. These calculations also indicate that such structures will have a higher differential gain leading to higher modulation rates. There have been several observations of quantum size effects in quantum wires and quantum boxes [7,8,9,10], but these structures are quite difficult to fabricate. Quantum well structures in high magnetic fields have been used to simulate some of these effects [2,11].

The technology used to fabricate quantum wells relies on growth techniques capable of atomic layer tolerances, leading to actual quantum well devices which exhibit nearly ideal properties. Confinement in directions other than the growth direction requires lithographic patterning and the best lithographic techniques have resolutions on the order of ten nanometers. Quantum size effects are extremely sensitive to the dimensions of the confining structure. For these reasons, it is important to consider the effects of fabricational inhomogeneities on quantum wire and quantum dot structures. Variations in the size and shape of quantum wires or quantum dots will smear some of the sharpness out of the density of states of these structures, reducing some of the benefits of lower dimensionality. Inhomogeneities in quantum boxes have been considered recently and it was found that quantum box arrays with realistic fabrication tolerances are not well suited to high gain applications, but they may make possible very low threshold current lasers and may lead to optical amplifiers with improved noise characteristics [12]. A critical radius, below which no bound states exist for the quantum box, was also shown.

In this paper, we investigate the properties of quantum wires, in particular, the effects of inhomogeneities on the density of states function and on gain are examined. The inhomogeneities are treated as a perturbation to an ideal wire and the perturbation energy is calculated to first order. The density of states for an array of wires with different widths is calculated and is used to calculate the gain of such a structure. This is done for cylindrical wires of 50Å radius and 150Å radius with several different degrees of inhomogeneity. The properties of a quantum wire laser are examined and we attempt to answer the question of whether quantum wires with realistic fabrication tolerances can fulfill the expectations of lower threshold currents, and higher modulation rates. The finite barrier quantum wire is studied and a quasi-critical radius is established, below which, the carriers are weakly confined by the wire. Upper limits on the wire radius, determined by the requirement that the energy subbands be separated by an energy greater than $k_B T$, are also discussed.

II Solution to the Two Dimensional Finite Well Problem

A calculation of the electron and hole wave-functions is necessary to obtain the position of the energy subbands. In this paper we have treated the case of a cylindrical wire rather than the, somewhat simpler, rectangular wire employed elsewhere. This potential is chosen since the Schroedinger equation can be separated in the case of a finite cylindrical potential but not for a finite rectangular potential. A proper treatment of the finite potential is necessary to investigate the possibility of a critical radius below which no bound states exist. Such a critical radius has been shown to exist for the quantum box [12]. In this section we calculate the electron and hole wave-functions using the effective mass approximation. Their behavior as the radius of the wire goes to zero is examined.

In cylindrical coordinates the potential takes the simple form

$$V = V(\rho) = \begin{cases} 0 & \text{for } \rho < \rho_0 \\ V_0 & \text{for } \rho \geq \rho_0 \end{cases} \quad (1)$$

For this potential the Schroedinger equation is easily solved, giving

$$\Psi(\rho, \phi, z) = N \begin{cases} J_\nu(k\rho)e^{i\nu\phi}e^{ik_z z} & \text{for } \rho < \rho_0 \\ A K_\nu(\kappa\rho)e^{i\nu\phi}e^{ik_z z} & \text{for } \rho \geq \rho_0 \end{cases} \quad (2)$$

where $J_\nu(k\rho)$ is the Bessel function of order $\nu = 0, \pm 1, \pm 2, \ldots$, and $K_\nu(\kappa\rho)$ is the modified Bessel function. The energy is given by

$$E = \frac{\hbar^2}{2m}(k_{\nu n}^2 + k_z^2) \quad (3)$$

The constants N, A, $k_{\nu n}$, and $\kappa_{\nu n}$ are determined by the normalization, the boundary condition at $\rho = \rho_0$, and the condition

$$k_{\nu n}^2 + \kappa_{\nu n}^2 = \frac{2m}{\hbar^2}V_0 \quad (4)$$

which comes directly from the Schroedinger equation. The radial momentum, $k_{\nu n}$, is a discrete variable whereas the axial momentum, k_z, varies continuously to fill the energy spectrum. In accordance with convention [13], $k_{\nu n}$ is the nth k-value to satisfy the boundary conditions for J_ν. In general there are an infinite number of k-values for each ν. In this treatment, only the first eight k-values are considered. This can be done with no loss of generality since we will only populate the first two or three subbands.

There is no known way to solve for $k_{\nu n}$ analytically but for $V_0 \gg \hbar^2 k_{\nu n}^2/2m$, the boundary condition $J_\nu(k\rho_0) = 0$ applies approximately and the zeros of J_ν are tabulated [13]. As the radius of the wire becomes smaller, the subband energy is pushed up towards the top of the potential well and the above approximation is no longer valid. For small radius wires, the value of $k_{\nu n}$ can be obtained by expanding $J_\nu(k\rho)$ and $K_\nu(\kappa\rho)$ about the origin. These expansions plus the continuity condition at $\rho = \rho_0$ give,

$$k\rho_0 = \left[\frac{2}{\frac{1}{2} - \ln \kappa\rho_0}\right]^{\frac{1}{2}} \quad (5)$$

The intersection of the two curves defined by Eq. 4 and Eq. 5 gives the eigenvalues for k and κ. Analysis of these two equations shows that there always is a bound state for this potential, but there exists a quasi-critical radius given by

$$\rho_c = \frac{1}{2}\sqrt{\frac{\hbar^2}{2mV_0}},\qquad(6)$$

below which the electron or hole is very weakly confined. At this point it becomes improbable that the carrier remains in the wire. For quantum boxes, there exists a strict critical radius below which no bound states exist [12]. The quasi-critical radius for quantum wires is a factor of π smaller than the critical radius for quantum boxes.

III Roughened Cylinders

In this section we treat the case of an imperfect quantum wire. The wire is taken to have hard boundaries with a potential step equal to V_0 but the potential is no longer a function only of ρ_0, but of all three coordinates. We assume that the wire is close enough to cylindrical that the roughness may be treated as a perturbation of the form,

$$W(\rho,\phi,z) = \begin{cases} -V_0 & \text{for } \rho_0 < \rho \leq \rho_0 + \delta\rho(\phi,z) \\ 0 & \text{otherwise} \end{cases}\qquad(7)$$

where $\delta\rho(\phi,z)$ is an arbitrary, nonnegative function of ϕ and z whose magnitude is much less than ρ_0. We further require that $\delta\rho$ vary on a scale which is smaller than the coherence distance of the electron. With this perturbation, the average radius of the cylinder is increased by an amount $<\delta\rho(\phi,z)>_{\phi,z}$ where $<>_{\phi,z}$ denotes a spacial average over the coordinates ϕ and z. It is straightforward to show that, in the limit as V_0 goes to infinity, the application of first order perturbation theory to the ground state gives,

$$<\delta E> \equiv <\Psi_0|W|\Psi_0> = -2\frac{<\delta\rho>_{\phi,z}}{\rho_0}E_{01}\qquad(8)$$

where,

$$E_{01} = \frac{k_{01}^2\hbar^2}{2m} = \frac{x_{01}^2\hbar^2}{2m\rho_0^2}\qquad(9)$$

is the energy of the first subband for the infinite barrier cylinder. To first order, the effect of the roughness is only through a change in the average radius. This implies that, to first order, quantum wires are insensitive to inhomogeneities that do not effect the average radius of the structure. Therefore, a fabrication tolerance of ten angstroms may be quite tolerable if the average radius does not change by more than a few angstroms from wire to wire. This does not apply if the perturbation varies with z on a scale which is large compared to the coherence length of the electron. Sections of the wire which are at least one coherence length apart can be considered as separate wires so that the averaging of $\delta\rho$ should be done for $z_0 < z < z_0 + l_c$ where l_c is the coherence length of the electron. If we assume an intraband scattering time of $2\times10^{-13}s$ [6] and thermal velocity, l_c is on the order of 800Å at room temperature.

Equations 8 and 9 are general results in that they can be shown to hold for quantum wells and quantum boxes as well (with x_{01}^2 replaced by the appropriate value for wells or boxes) [12]. In the case of wells and boxes the confinement energy, E_{10}, is different, however. The confinement energy increases as the number of confined dimensions increases. For this reason, inhomogeneities will affect quantum boxes more severely than quantum wires and, likewise, quantum wires more severely than quantum wells. As the size of the structure is increased the confinement energy decreases, reducing the effect of inhomogeneities. The size can be increased only so far since the subbands must be separated by an energy which is greater than a few k_BT in order for quantum size effects to be realized. For all three low dimensionality structures, the subband energy has a ρ^{-2} dependence. If we define ΔE as the separation between the first and second subbands we can calculate the proportionality constant between ΔE and ρ^{-2}. The results are shown in Table 1 where ΔE is calculated for several values of ρ with $V_0 = \infty$ and using a spherical potential for the quantum box and a cylindrical potential for the quantum wire. In Table 1 and all of the figures and calculations here, values of constants which are appropriate for GaAs are chosen.

From Equation 9 we see that a small change in radius $d\rho$ gives a change in subband energy

$$dE_{01} = -2\frac{d\rho}{\rho_0}E_{01}\qquad(10)$$

which is the same as the result from the perturbation calculation. Comparing Equations 8 and 10 we see that the effect on the subband energy of roughening the cylinders with an average roughness $<\delta\rho>_{\phi,z}$ is equivalent to changing the wire width by $d\rho = <\delta\rho>_{\phi,z}$. It should be noted that Equation 10 is an upper limit since it applies for the case of an infinite barrier; the finite barrier case will produce a smaller shift because of the softer boundaries. In what follows we assume that we have an ensemble of wires with different values of $<\delta\rho>_{\phi,z}$. In accordance with the central limit theorem we assume a Gaussian distribution of wire radii

$$P(\rho) = \frac{1}{\sqrt{2\pi}\delta\rho} \exp\left[\frac{-(\rho-\rho_0)^2}{\delta\rho^2}\right] \tag{11}$$

where ρ_0 is the average wire radius and $\delta\rho$ is the standard deviation of $<\delta\rho>_{\phi,z}$. The length of a typical semi-conductor laser is several hundred times the coherence length of the electron so the gain of a single wire must be obtained by considering the gain of many wires each of length l_c.

IV Gain Spectra

The density of states for an ideal (unroughened) wire of radius ρ_0 is,

$$D(E) = \sum_{l=1}^{\infty} \frac{(m_r/2\hbar^2)^{1/2}}{\pi^2 \rho_0^2} (E - E_g - E_l)^{-1/2} \eta_l \tag{12}$$

where E is the energy of the transition, E_g is the band-gap, E_l is the position of the lth subband (the index l is a combination of the indices n and ν of the previous sections), η_l is the degeneracy of the lth subband ($\eta_l = 1$ for $\nu = 0$, $\eta_l = 2$ otherwise) and $m_r = m_e m_h/(m_e + m_h)$ where m_e and m_h are the masses of the electron and the hole respectively. In all of the calculations here, values of the material parameters which are appropriate for GaAs are used. These values are: $m_e = 0.067, m_h = 0.45, E_g = 1.424$. The subband positions, E_l, are calculated assuming an infinite bandgap discontinuity.

Changing the radius of a wire will affect the gain by moving the subband edge. We obtain a Gaussian distribution of subband energies by combining Equations 10 and 11

$$P(E_l) = \frac{1}{\sqrt{2\pi}\delta E_l} \exp\left[\frac{-(E_l - \overline{E_l})^2}{\delta E_l^2}\right] \tag{13}$$

where δE_l and E_l are related to $\delta\rho$ and ρ through Equations 8 and 9. The bulk density of states for the material is found by integrating Equation 12 over all values of E_l weighted by Equation 13 giving the inhomogeneous density of states,

$$D_{inh}(E) = \sum_{l=1}^{\infty} \frac{1}{\delta E \sqrt{2\pi}} \left(\frac{m_r}{2}\right)^{1/2} \frac{\eta_l}{\pi \rho_0^2 \hbar} \int (E - E_g - E_l)^{-1/2}$$
$$\exp\left[\frac{-(E_l - \overline{E_l})^2}{\delta E_l^2}\right] dE_l \tag{14}$$

The integral in Equation 14 is evaluated numerically and the inhomogeneous density of states is plotted for wires of radius $\rho = 50\text{\AA}$ in Figure 1. The effects of the inhomogeneities are quite dramatic: for $\delta\rho = 2.5\text{\AA}$, which corresponds to a mono-layer variation in radius, the subbands are distinct and the density of states resembles the ideal density of states, whereas, for $\delta\rho = 10\text{\AA}$ all subband structure is washed out and the density of states resembles that of bulk material. As the subbands broaden, their peak value decreases since the area under each curve must be the same. In general, the magnitude of the density of states will be inversely proportional to the radius of the wire if $\delta\rho/\rho$ is kept fixed (this follows directly from Equation 14 when the dependence of E_l and δE_l on ρ_0 is considered). For $\rho = 150\text{\AA}$ the first and second subband are separated by only 18meV. This means that at room temperature there will be substantial filling of the second subband when the first subband is partially filled, leading to increased threshold currents.

The density of states calculations are the basis of the gain calculations to follow. The broadening caused by the inhomogeneities is, in all cases considered here, greater than or equal to relaxation broadening. The gain is therefore given by,

$$G(E) = \frac{E}{\hbar}\sqrt{\mu/\epsilon}\, |d|^2\, D(E)(f_c - f_v) \tag{15}$$

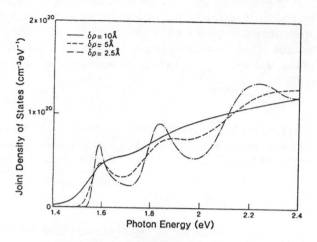

	Well	Wire	Box
$\rho = \rho_0$	$(7.4)\frac{\hbar^2}{2m\rho_0^2}$	$(8.9)\frac{\hbar^2}{2m\rho_0^2}$	$(10.3)\frac{\hbar^2}{2m\rho_0^2}$
$\rho = 50\text{Å}$ cb	168	202	234
vb	25	30	35
$\rho = 100\text{Å}$ cb	42	51	59
vb	6.2	7.6	8.8
$\rho = 200\text{Å}$ cb	11	13	15
vb	1.6	1.9	2.2

cb = conduction band
vb = valence band

Table 1: The separation of the first and second subbands for different size quantum wells, quantum wires, and quantum boxes in GaAs. The parameter ρ is the radius, or, in then case of quantum wells, a half width. When ΔE is smaller than $k_B T$, thermal broadening smears out quantum size effects.

Figure 1: The density of states for 50Å radius quantum wires with three different values of the roughness parameter; $\delta\rho = 2.5\text{Å}$, $\delta\rho = 5.0\text{Å}$, and $\delta\rho = 10.0\text{Å}$.

where ϵ is the dielectric constant of the material, μ is the magnetic susceptibility, f_c and f_v are the Fermi distributions for the conduction and valence bands respectively, and d is the component of the dipole moment parallel to the electric field. A value of $d/q = 4\text{Å}$ has been assumed and any dependence of d on the orientation of the electric field with respect to the wire axis is ignored. The light hole band has also been ignored in the calculation. The overlap of the field with the gain region is not yet accounted for in these plots. As the carrier density is doubled, the peak gain increases almost proportionally, indicating that, even at this high carrier density, the carriers are going predominantly into the first subband. In Figure 2 gain is calculated for the density of states functions of Figure 1, showing the effects of increased inhomogeneities on the gain spectrum. All of the curves are for the same carrier density. Here, the benefits of a sharp density of states function are clear as the peak gain drops by roughly a factor of two when $\delta\rho$ goes from 2.5Å to 10Å. Figure 3 shows the dependence of peak gain on carrier density for these same wires. The gain rises steeply at first, but it begins to level off at around $7\times10^{18} cm^{-3}$ as the first subband becomes full. At a carrier density of roughly $1.3\times10^{18} cm^{-3}$ the gain begins to rise sharply once again. It is at this point that the gain of the second subband exceeds that of the first. This has been observed experimentally in quantum well lasers [14] and it is accompanied by a large change in lasing wavelength. A plot similar to that of Figure 3 but for 150Å radius wires is shown in Figure 4 . For any given carrier density, the gain of a 150Å wire is lower than that of a 50Å wire. This is due to two factors: first, the density of states is smaller for larger wires, and second, the subbands are separated by an energy which is less than $k_B T$ so several subbands are being filled simultaneously.

V Lasing Properties

So far, we have discussed the properties of quantum wires without considering the device in which they are to be imbedded. In this section we consider the modal gain, threshold current, and the modulation rate for a quantum wire laser.

Figure 5 shows a schematic diagram of a quantum wire array laser. The dashed cylinder which envelops the quantum wires represents the optical confinement region and the width of the optical mode in the x and y directions is shown as W_x and W_y. The modal gain is obtained by multiplying the bulk gain for a wire by the confinement factor, which is a measure of the overlap of the optical field with the gain region. Switching to rectangular coordinates and keeping the cylinder axis as the z-axis, the confinement factor is a product of confinement factors for the x and y directions, $\Gamma_x = d/W_x$ and $\Gamma_y = d/W_y$. For a single wire of 50Å radius,

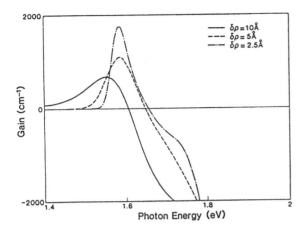

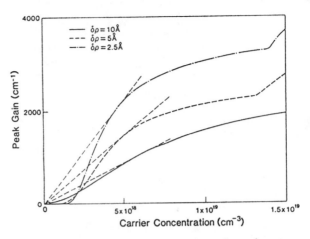

Figure 2: Gain as a function of photon energy for 50Å radius quantum wires with $\delta\rho = 2.5$Å, $\delta\rho = 5.0$Å, and $\delta\rho = 10.0$Å at a carrier concentration of $4 \times 10^{18} cm^{-3}$.

Figure 3: Peak gain as a function of carrier concentration for the quantum wires of Figure 1. The sudden change in slope at high carrier densities is indicative of second quantized state lasing. The point of maximum gain per carrier density is given by the dashed tangent.

$\Gamma_x = \Gamma_y = 0.04$ is a reasonable value [1]. If we take a peak gain of $3000 cm^{-1}$ and the above confinement factors, the peak modal gain is $G_{mode} = 4.8 cm^{-1}$ per wire. This is about enough gain to overcome the distributed losses, so clearly we must employ an array of such quantum wires to make a laser.

The threshold gain is given by,

$$G_{modal,th} = \alpha - \frac{1}{l} \ln R \qquad (16)$$

where α is the distributed loss coefficient for the mode, l is the length of the cavity, and R is the reflectivity of the mirrors. To estimate threshold current densities we assume values of $\alpha = 3 cm^{-1}$, $l = 300 \mu m$, and $R = 0.9$. For these values, $G_{modal,th} = 6.5 cm^{-1}$. To achieve the lowest threshold current, we want to pump the wires to the point of maximum gain per carrier density. This is the point on the peak gain vs. carrier density curve whose tangent intersects the origin. From Figure 3, we see that this occurs at a carrier density of approximately $5 \times 10^{18} cm^{-3}$ for a 50Å radius wire with $\delta\rho = 2.5$Å. At this point, the gain in the wire is approximately $2250 cm^{-1}$. To optimize the structure for low threshold current operation, the number of wires in the array should be chosen such that at threshold they are pumped to this point. With the above confinement factors, a laser with two such wires would have a modal gain of $7.2 cm^{-1}$, which is just above the estimated threshold gain. To arrive at a threshold current, a value of the carrier lifetime must be assumed. The effect of the two dimensional confinement on the carrier lifetime is not known, so bulk the carrier lifetime is used. If we assume a carrier lifetime of $3ns$ [15], and 100 percent injection efficiency, this two wire laser would have a threshold current of approximately $11 \mu A$, which is nearly two orders of magnitude lower than the best quantum well lasers. When the same considerations are applied to a 50Å wire with $\delta\rho = 10$Å, the optimal carrier density is approximately $6.5 \times 10^{18} cm^{-3}$, and a laser containing four such wires would have a threshold current of approximately $33 \mu A$, which is still extremely low. In the case of 150Å radius wires, the confinement factors increase to $\Gamma_x = \Gamma_y = 0.12$. Working backwards, if we assume a modal gain of $6.5 cm^{-1}$ and the above confinement factors, the bulk gain requirement is only $450 cm^{-1}$. One wire can provide this gain and, under the same assumptions as above, the estimated threshold current is $34 \mu A$ for the cases of $\delta\rho = 15$Å and $\delta\rho = 30$Å (here, the effects of thermal broadening exceed those of the inhomogeneities so both $\delta\rho = 15$Å and $\delta\rho = 30$Å wires behave the same at room temperature). It is clear that the threshold current does not suffer much as the fabrication tolerance requirements are relaxed.

The modulation bandwidth is determined by the relaxation oscillation corner frequency,

$$f_c = \frac{1}{2\pi} \left[\frac{G' P_0}{\tau_p} \right]^{1/2} \qquad (17)$$

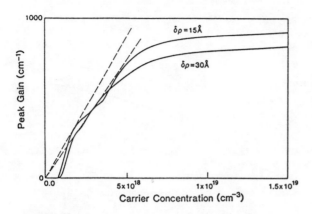

Figure 4: Peak gain as a function of carrier concentration for $\rho = 150 Å$ quantum wires. The point of maximum gain per carrier density is given by the dashed tangent.

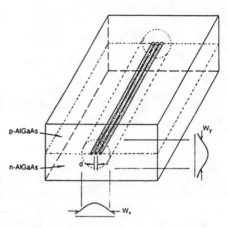

Figure 5: A schematic of a quantum wire array laser. The width of the optical mode is given by W_x and W_y and the wire diameter is d. The confinement factor is given by the relation $\Gamma_i = d/W_i$.

where $G' = dG/dn$ is the differential gain, P_0 is the steady state photon density in the cavity, and τ_p is the photon lifetime [16]. Due to the sharpened density of states function, the differential gain for quantum wires should be higher than for bulk material. The differential gain can be found from Figures 3 and 4. For the $50 Å$ radius wires, the maximum differential gain is, $dG/dn = 1.0 \times 10^{-15} cm^2$ and $2.2 \times 10^{-16} cm^2$ for $\delta\rho = 2.5 Å$ and $10 Å$ respectively. This is to be compared to a value of $dG/dn = 2.0 \times 10^{-16} cm^2$ for bulk GaAs, and $dG/dn = 5.0 \times 10^{-16} cm^2$ for quantum wells [2] The differential gain for the $150 Å$ wires, as calculated from Figure 4, is close to the bulk value. We see that the modulation bandwidth of the well fabricated wire is greater by a factor of $\sqrt{5}$ than that of a laser with a bulk active layer, but that for more realistic fabrication tolerances the increased bandwidth disappears.

VI Conclusion

We have calculated the gain spectra of quantum wires accounting for fabricational inhomogeneities. The inhomogeneities were treated as a perturbation and it was found that to first order, the component of the perturbation which varies quickly compared to the coherence length of the carrier is averaged out and has no effect if the wire radius is chosen so that the roughness function has zero average. This indicates that the gain in quantum wires is somewhat insensitive to small scale inhomogeneities. An ensemble of wires with differing widths was considered and a bulk density of states and gain were calculated from this. According to these calculations, quantum wires with realistic fabrication tolerances are advantageous for low threshold laser applications but unless they are fabricated with atomic layer precision, they will not display a large enhancement in modulation bandwidth.

The wave functions for quantum wires have been examined using a finite cylindrical potential and we found a quasi-critical radius, below which, the carriers are not confined by the potential, although, in a strict sense, the state is a bound state. This puts a lower limit on the radius of quantum wires. An upper limit on the wire size is given by the requirement that the subbands be separated by an energy greater than $k_B T$ and the effects of increasing the size and changing the number of quantized dimensions were tabulated for two, one, and zero dimensional structure.

As a result of these calculations, it is concluded that quantum wire lasers with realistic fabrication tolerances are promising structures for reduced threshold current. Reductions of one to two orders of magnitude over the best quantum well lasers are possible. Such large reductions in threshold current could open new realms of applications for semiconductor lasers.

Two of us (H.Z. and A.Y.) would like to acknowledge the support of ONR and DARPA. One of us (K.V.) would like to acknowledge the support of ONR.

References

[1] P. L. Derry, A. Yariv, K. Y. Lau, N. Bar-Chaim, and J. Rosenberg, "Ultralow-Threshold Graded-Index separate-confinement Single Quantum Well Buried Heterostructure (Al,Ga)As Lasers With High Reflectivity Coatings," *Appl. Phys. Lett.*, vol. 50, pp. 1773-1775, 1987.

[2] Y. Arakawa, K.Vahala, and A.Yariv, "Dynamic and Spectral Properties of Semiconductor Lasers With Quantum-Well and Quantum-Wire Effects," *Surf. Sci.*, vol. 174, pp.155-162, 1986.

[3] P. L. Derry, T. R. Chen, Y. H. Zhuang, J. Paslaski, M. Mittelstein, K. Vahala, and A. Yariv, "Spectral and Dynamic Characteristics of Buried Heterostructure Single Quantum Well (Al,Ga)As Lasers," *Appl. Phys. Lett.*, vol. 53, pp.271-273, 1988.

[4] Y. Arakawa and H. Sakaki, "Multidimensional quantum well laser and temperature dependence of threshold current," *Appl. Phys. Lett.*, vol. 40, pp. 939-941, 1980.

[5] K. Uomi, T. Mishima, and N. Chinone, "Ultrahigh Relaxation Oscillation Frequency (up to 30GHz) of Highly P-Doped GaAs/GaAlAs Multiple Quantum Well Lasers," *Appl. Phys. Lett.*, vol. 51, pp. 78-80, 1987.

[6] M. Asada, Y. Miyamoto, and Y. Suematsu, "Gain and the Threshold of Three-Dimensional Quantum-Box Lasers," *IEEE Journal of Quantum Electron.*, vol. QE-22, pp. 1915-1921, 1986.

[7] P. M. Petroff A. C. Gossard, R. A. Logan, and W. Wiegman, "Toward Quantum Wires: Fabrication and Optical Properties," *Appl. Phys. Lett.*, vol. 41, pp.635-638, 1982.

[8] K. Kash, A. Scherer, J. M. Worlock, H. G. Craighead, and M. C. Tamargo, "Optical Spectroscopy of Ultrasmall Structures Etched From Quantum Wells," *Appl. Phys. Lett.*, vol. 49, pp.1043-1045, 1986.

[9] J. Cibert, P. M. Petroff, G. J. Dolan, A. C. Gossard, and J. H. English, "Optically Detected Carrier Confinement to One and Zero Dimension in GaAs Quantum Well Wires and Boxes," *Appl. Phys. Lett.*, vol. 49, pp.1275-1277, 1986.

[10] H. Temkin, G. J. Dolan, M. B. Panish, and S. N. G. Chu, "Low-Temperature Photoluminescence From InGaAs/InP Quantum Wires and Boxes," *Appl. Phys. Lett.*, vol. 50, pp. 413-415, 1987.

[11] K. Vahala, Y. Arakawa, and A. Yariv, "Reduction of the Field Spectrum Linewidth of a Multiple Quantum Well Laser in a High Magnetic Field — Spectral Properties of Quantum Dot Lasers," *Appl. Phys. Lett.*, vol. 50, pp.365-367, 1987.

[12] K. Vahala, "Quantum Box Fabrication Tolerance and size Limits in Semiconductors and Their Effect on Optical Gain," *IEEE Journal of Quantum Electron.*, vol. QE-24, pp. 523-530, 1988.

[13] Abromawitz and Stegun, *Handbook of Mathematical Functions*, National Bureau of Standards, 1972.

[14] M. Mittelstein, Y.Arakawa, A. Larsson, and A. Yariv, "Second Quantized State Lasing of a Current Pumped Single Quantum Well Laser," *Appl. Phys. Lett.*, vol. 49, pp.1689-1691, 1986.

[15] H. C. Casey, Jr. and M. B. Panish, *Heterostructure Lasers* (Academic Press, New York, 1978).

[16] K. Y. Lau, N. Bar-Chaim, I. Ury, C. Harder, and A. Yariv, "11-GHz Direct Modulation Bandwidth GaAlAs Window Laser Operating at Room Temperature," *Appl. Phys. Lett.*, vol. 45, pp. 316-318, 1984.

Design of Multi Quantum Well Lasers
for Surface Emitting Arrays

J.Z. Wilcox, W.W. Simmons, G.P. Peterson, J.J. Yang,
M. Jansen, and S.S. Ou

TRW S&TG
One Space Park, R1/2178, Redondo Beach, Ca 90278

ABSTRACT

A quantum well (QW) gain model was developed and was applied to optimization of surface emitting diode laser arrays. To increase output power density per unit surface area, short cavity lengths must be considered. We show how the maximum power density and power efficiency requirements lead to multiple wells; the performance is limited by gain saturation associated with QW subband filling at increased threshold gain requirements in short cavity lasers.

1. INTRODUCTION

Quantum well (QW) lasers (Figure 1) have the potential of tayloring the emission wavelength and increasing the efficiency of diode laser based systems as a result of quantization of the transition levels and high gain. For surface emitting (SE) diode laser arrays, the additional requirement is for maximum output power density (p_{out}) per unit surface area. The power efficiency (η) is maximized by decreasing the threshold current density (j_{th}); this is obtained by increasing the laser length (L). On the other hand, the emitted p_{out} and the differential (slope) efficiency are maximized by decreasing the L. This leads to optimization of L. In addition, because the local threshold gain (g_{th}) is high in thin wells (causing rapid well filling, Figure 2, gain saturation, Figure 3, and nonradiative loss of carriers), j_{th} increases very rapidly (nearly exponentially) with increased g_{th} requirements in thin-well, short-cavity lasers. Therefore, relatively small design changes may produce large effects in device performance, requiring careful optimization. Specifically, we show in this paper how an increase in the optical mode confinement ($\Gamma = N_z \Gamma_{SQW}$, where N_z is number of wells in the active layer, and Γ_{SQW} is the confinement factor into a single QW) reduces well filling; and therefore, reduces optimum L and increases maximum p_{out} and η.

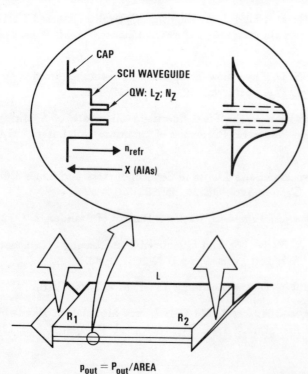

Figure 1. Surface emitting quantum well laser with a separate confinement heterostructure waveguide.

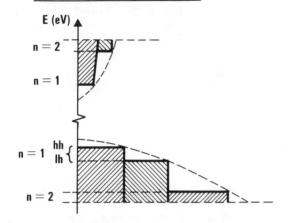 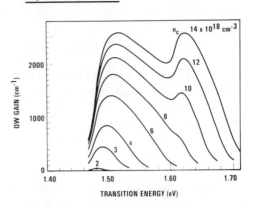

Figure 2. Band filling and spectral gain in a 70A GaAs well with a 20% AlAs barrier.

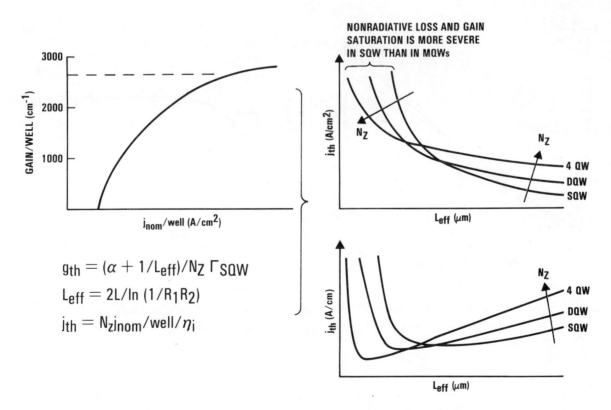

$$g_{th} = (\alpha + 1/L_{eff})/N_Z \Gamma_{SQW}$$
$$L_{eff} = 2L/\ln(1/R_1 R_2)$$
$$j_{th} = N_Z j_{nom}/well/\eta_i$$

Figure 3. (a) Gain-current relation in a single well, and (b) threshold currents in MQW lasers (70A well, 20%-60%, 2000A thick SCH waveguide).

2. QUANTUM WELL GAIN MODEL

To accomplish the optimization, we have developed[1] a QW gain model by extending the formalism that appears in Agrawal and Dutta[2]. The QW levels are calculated by solving the Schrodinger equation for a particle in a finite potential well. The gain is calculated by summing over all QW sub-bands, the k-momentum conservation has been relaxed by broadening the transition line by a Lorentzian with lifetime 7×10^{-14}s, and we took into account nonradiative loss of carriers due to the presence of L valleys in the conduction band,[2,3] Auger recombination processes,[2,4] and leakage current.[3] To reduce the g_{th} required from a single QW (SQW) (and thus avoiding an unnecessary increase in j_{th} caused by gain saturation in short L, SQW lasers), we consider multiplicity of QWs (MQW) in the active layer. All quantities are temperature dependent.

3. RESULTS

Using the model, spectral gain (Figure 2), lasing frequencies, gain-current and j_{th} vs. L relations (Figure 3) were determined for a number of QW structures, and used with threshold gain and power balance equations to optimize MQW lasers for maximum n and p_{out}. (Note that the gain-current relation follows a near semi-logarithmic form, $g = bj_o \ln(j/j_o)$ where b is the gain-current coefficient and j_o is nominal current at transparency for a single well).[5-8] The j_{th} is determined by combining the gain-current curve with $j_{th} = N_z j_{nom}/\eta_i$ and $g_{thr} = (\alpha + 1/L_{eff})/N_z \Gamma_{SQW}$, where α is distributed optical loss coefficient, $L_{eff} = 2L/\ln(1/R_1 R_2)$ is the laser effective length, N_z is number of QWs, Γ_{SQW} is modal confinement factor for a single quantum well (which depends on SCH-QW thickness t_g, concentrations x_{Al}, and thickness L_z, see Figure 1). The result is schematically demonstrated in Figure 3. Note that because of the gain saturation associated with band filling at increased g_{th} requirements in short lasers, the increase in j_{th} at short L_{eff} is more rapid, and its onset occurs at longer lengths in SQW than in MQW lasers; it is this j_{th} increase that will eventually limit power efficiency of densely packed, surface emitting lasers with short L_{eff}.

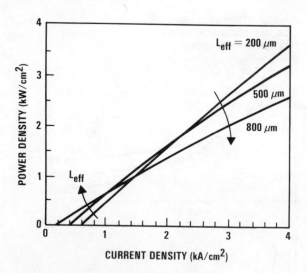
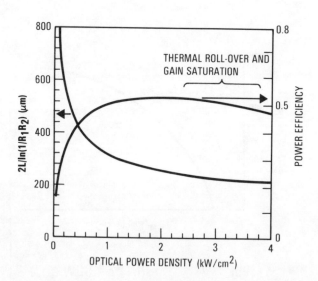

Figure 4. (a) Power output curves for the same MQWs as in Figure 3 with the laser effective length $L_{eff} = 2L/\ln(1/R_1 R_2)$ as a parameter, and (b) optimum L_{eff} and maximum efficiency as a function of output power density per unit surface area.

Figure 4a shows the basis for optimization of L_{eff} (the example shown is for double, DQW, lasers) in an example calculation for lasers structures consisting of 70Å thick GaAs MQWs incorporated into a 20%-60% GaAlAs separate confinement heterostructure (SCH) waveguide. The single well $\Gamma_{SQW}=0.03$. The curves were calculated self consistently for a temperature rise (the increase in j_{th} with T was modeled as $j_{th} \sim \exp(T/T_0)$ where $1/T_0 = 1/T_1 + 1/T_2$, T_1 is a characteristic temperature at transparency, and $1/T_2 \sim g_{th}$)[9] associated with thermal resistance $\theta = 12°C\text{-}cm^2/W$ (corresponding to an effective θ experienced by a 600 usec pulse for the laser mounted with the epi-side down). Note that depending upon the required p_{out}, the efficiency is maximized by different L_{eff}'s that depend upon p_{out}. The optimum L_{eff} and η are shown as functions of p_{out} in Figure 4b. The optimum L_{eff} decreases with p_{out} increasing; the efficiency first increases until it reaches a local maximum at some p_{out}, after which it decreases; the decrease being the result of both the usual thermal rollover and the increase in j_{th} associated with gain saturation at short L_{eff}'s. Figure 5 compares the parametrized (i.e. maximized for specific p_{out} by adjusting L_{eff}) efficiencies for SQW, DQW, and 4QW lasers. At low p_{out}, long SQW lasers have lower j_{th}, resulting in higher η for SQW than for MQW lasers. At high p_{out}, the increase in j_{th} associated with gain saturation in short QW lasers causes the efficiency to decrease more rapidly, its onset occuring at lower p_{out}, for SQW than for MQWs. This gives an η that has a local maximum at some p_{out} value that increases with the number N_z of QW increasing. Note also that the maximum is wider (and slightly higher) for MQWs than for SQW; the relative extend of the latter effect depends upon the actual values of α and Γ_{SQW}. In our example calculation, $\Gamma_{SQW}=0.03$ and (room temperature) $\alpha = 5 cm^{-1}$. Reducing the local threshold gain required from a single well by other means such as by increasing the Γ_{SQW} by grading the refractive index in GRIN-SCH structures, or by optimizing the SCH waveguide thickness and increasing the Al concentration in the cladding layers, will produce changes in η and p_{out} that are qualitatively similar to those produced by increasing the multiplicity of QWs. Reducing the α will increase the differential efficiency η_d in long L lasers; causing the peak efficiency of low N_z lasers (peaking at low p_{out}) to approach the peak efficiency (occuring at high p_{out}) of high N_z lasers.

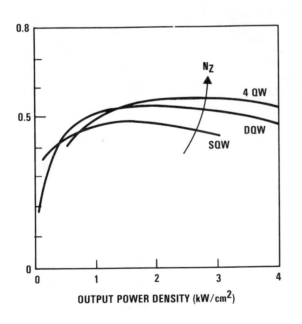

Figure 5. The parametrized efficiencies as a function of output power density per unit surface area for $N_z=1$, 2, and 4 MQWs.

4. SUMMARY AND CONCLUSION

In summary, we have developed a QW gain model, and applied it to optimization of surface emitting MQW diode laser arrays. We find that for a given MQW structure, the efficiency is maximized by different $L_{eff}=2L/\ln(1/R_1R_2)$, which depends on the surface density p_{out} emitted from the array; and that with the p_{out} increasing, this efficiency first increases until it reaches a local maximum after which it decreases because of the thermal roll-over and the rapid increase in j_{th} associated with gain saturation at short laser lengths. The value of p_{out} at which the parametrized efficiency reaches its local maximum is higher for MQWs than for SQW; and depending upon the value of the confinement factor Γ_{SQW}, distributed absorption loss α, and the characteristic temperature T_1, the maximum may be higher for MQWs than for SQW. The maximum predicted efficiencies for $N_z>4$ are about 55% at $p_{out}=3kW/cm^2$. The results of this investigation are being applied to design and fabrication of 2-D surface emitting arrays.

REFERENCES

1. J.Z.Wilcox,S.S.Ou,J.J.Yang,and M.Jansen, Electron.Lett. 24,1218(1988)
2. G.P.Agrawal and N.K.Dutta, Long Wavelength Semiconductor Lasers (Van Nostrand Reinhold, New York, 1986), pp.372-409.
3. A.R.Reisinger,P.S.Zory,and R.G.Waters,IEEE J.Quantum Electron.QE-23,993(1987)
4. M.Takeshima,J.Appl.Phys.58,3846(1985)
5. P.W.A.McIlroy,A.Kurobe,and Y Uematsu,IEEE J.Quantum Electron.QE-21,1958(1985)
6. A.Kurobe,H.Furuyama,S.Naritsuka,N.Sugiyama,Y.Kokubin,and M.Nakamura,IEEE J.Quantum Electron.QE-24,635(1988).
7. S.R.Chinn,P.S.Zory,and A.R.Reisinger,IEEE J.Quantum Electron.,Nov.1988
8. J.Z.Wilcox,S.S.Ou,J.J.Yang,and M.Jansen,J.Appl.Phys.64, Dec 1,1988
9. J.Z.Wilcox,S.S.Ou,J.J.Yang,and M.Jansen,Appl.Phys.Lett. 53,2272(1988)

Leaky-guided channeled substrate planar (LCSP) laser with reduced substrate radiation and heating

S. J. Lee, R. V. Ramaswamy,
Electrical Engineering, University of Florida
Gainesville, Florida 32611
and L. Figueroa
Boeing Electronics High Technology Center
Seattle, Washington 98124-6269

ABSTRACT

A new semiconductor laser design, the leaky-guided channeled substrate planar (LCSP) laser is presented. The analysis, by using the effective index method in the complex domain, shows that the LCSP structure provides better lateral mode stability than either gain guided or positive index step structures. The LCSP structure with reduced heating and strong lateral coupling effect may be more useful for high power linear array lasers.

1. INTRODUCTION

Recently there have been increasing interests in leaky-guided semiconductor laser structures. Botez et al. fabricated leaky-mode coupled array lasers and their devices showed very stable array modes with diffraction limited output [1, 2]. However, previous studies on leaky-mode structures have been somewhat limited. Some of the earlier studies were too general and may not be directly applicable to semiconductor laser geometries [3, 4].

In this paper, we propose a new semiconductor laser structure, as schematically shown in Figure 1. The structure has a buffer layer in the region outside the channel. The buffer layer has two effects. One is to minimize the optical radiation into the substrate. If the buffer layer index n_4 is smaller than the effective index (which also depends on n_4), the mode will be damped in the buffer layer. Consequently, the transverse mode cannot penetrate significantly into the substrate with a reasonable choice of buffer layer index and thickness. In the CSP laser [5], significant substrate radiation occurs in the region outside the channel, and leads to a preferential higher local temperature rise over the channel shoulder as a result of the band to band absorption and heating [6,7]. Another important effect of the buffer layer is to vary the effective index in the region outside the channel. In general, the effective index increases if we choose the buffer layer index n_4 slightly higher than the lower cladding layer index n_3, otherwise the effective index decreases (when $n_4 < n_3$) or a leaky mode results (when n_4 is too high) with significant substrate radiation as in the conventional CSP lasers. In the LCSP laser, the buffer layer index n_4 is chosen slightly higher than the lower cladding layer index n_3, and the region outside the channel will have a higher effective index than the region inside the channel. This effective index step will give the structure the effect of leaky-guiding in the plane parallel to the junction.

Due to the lateral optical leakage as a result of the negative effective index step, the LCSP laser will have a two-lobed far field beam with somewhat increased threshold current density. However, the lateral optical leakage combined with reduced mode loss outside the channel will provide strong coupling between elements in a linear array geometry [1, 2]. In the array geometries using the CSP type element [8], the coupling effect is minimized because the field intensity is very small between elements as a result of higher mode loss due to the significant substrate radiation.

2. ANALYSIS

For the analysis, we have used the effective index method in the complex domain. The complex effective index method is especially useful for the analysis of structures such as CSP laser with a transverse leaky mode (large imaginary part of the effective index) [5] and the LCSP structure with a lateral leaky mode [9, 10]. It may be difficult to separate the complex effective index (resulting from either the structure itself or the injected gain) into real and imaginary parts and to consider them independently. In the complex effective index method, the complex effective indices are determined by solving a transverse mode characteristic equation by assuming either gain or loss. After that the lateral mode structure with complex effective indices are solved directly in the complex domain.

In order to consider the current spreading effect, the current density profile estimated by Yonezu [11] has been sliced into seven sections using a stair-case approximation as shown in Figure 2. The active layer gain $g(y)$ is related to the current density $J(y)$ by [12]

$$g(y) = 45 \frac{J(y)}{D} - a_0 \qquad (1)$$

where the active layer thickness D is in μm, $J(y)$ is in kA/cm^2 and a_0 is the background absorption coefficient at lasing wavelength which we assume a value $a_0 = 190$ cm^{-1}. The gain induced refractive index change Δn_c is related to the gain change Δg by

$$\Delta n_c = \alpha \Delta g = \alpha \frac{g(y) + a_0}{2k} \qquad (2)$$

where the parameter α, which may be geometry dependent [13, 14], is assumed to $\alpha = -6.2$ [15]; $k = 2\pi/\lambda$ is the free space propagation constant, λ is the wavelength. For each layer, the complex refractive index n^* is defined by

$$n^* = n + j(a - g) \qquad (3)$$

where n, a and g are the the real refractive index, loss and the injected gain respectively in each layer. The transverse mode characteristic equation is solved in the complex domain to obtain the complex effective index $n_{ex}(y)$. The transverse mode loss A_x or transverse mode gain G_x is defined by

$$A_x = -G_x = 2k \text{Im}(n_{ex}(y)) \qquad (4)$$

In the CSP laser (TB = 0 μm), the transverse mode loss is very high in the region outside the channel, because of the significant substrate radiation. This substrate radiation is analogous to prism output coupling in dielectric optical waveguides. In the case with a buffer layer, the mode analysis is more difficult. In general, there are two modes which are variations of the even modes and odd modes in the twin-channel wave guides [16]. However, the even type mode is the principal mode which has a much higher coupling (to the mode inside the channel) coefficient (~0.95) [17] than the odd type mode when the buffer layer index is relatively low ($n_4 < 3.45$). In this case, the effect of the odd type mode which is distorted relative to the inside mode is negligible. As shown in Figure 3, the complex effective indices for the principal modes are plotted for three buffer layer indices n_4 = 3.37, 3.40, 3.43. Here we fix the lower cladding layer index at n_3 =3.40. When the buffer layer thickness TB > 1 μm, both the real part and the imaginary part of the complex effective indices become saturated. However, the larger buffer layer index gives larger real part of the effective index. Thus if we assume the buffer layer thickness TB > 1 μm, the structure with each buffer layer index corresponds to a gain guided ($n_4 = n_3 = 3.40$, no index step), positive step ($n_4 = 3.37 < n_3 = 3.40$) and negative step ($n_4 = 3.43 > n_3 = 3.40$) structure respectively. When the buffer layer thickness TB = 0, all the three cases become identical to the CSP structure with a larger mode loss in the region outside the channel.

The seven layer lateral mode characteristic equation with complex transverse mode effective indices are solved directly in the complex domain. The overall mode gain G is defined by

$$G = -2k\,\text{Im}(n_{ey}) \quad (5)$$

where n_{ey} is the effective index for the lateral mode. The threshold is achieved when the mode gain is equal to the output mirror loss. The transverse complex effective index at threshold are plotted in Figure 4 and Figure 5 for the CSP and the LCSP structure respectively. It is noted that the CSP laser has a very stable and large imaginary step of the complex effective index, even though the real part changes significantly due to the gain induced refractive index change Δn_c. This large imaginary step is the direct result of the significant substrate radiation in the region outside the channel. However, in the LCSP laser with negligible substrate radiation, the imaginary step is relatively small because it is given primarily by the injected gain step. Similarly, either in the positive step structure or the gain guided structure, the imaginary step is relatively small as in the LCSP structure.

We speculate that the imaginary step of the complex effective index is very important in stabilizing the lateral mode. The CSP lasers have very stable lateral modes as shown in Figure 6(a) without being affected significantly by the gain induced refractive index change Δn_c. Even though the LCSP structure is not as stable as the CSP structure, The LCSP lasers have better lateral mode stability than either the gain guided lasers or the positive step structures.

3. SUMMARY

The LCSP structure may be fabricated in an inverted geometry as in the LCSP laser [18] using either MBE or MOCVD technology. We have tried to grow

LCSP type structure using liquid phase epitaxy by applying selective growth and melt-etch scheme. Figure 7 shows a SEM cross-sectional picture of a grown sample. As a preliminary test, the light vs. current characteristic was measured as shown in Figure 8. Pulsed threshold currents for the devices are in the range of 80 ~ 100 mA. The LCSP structure may be useful for the linear array lasers. As already demonstrated by Botez et al., leaky-mode coupled array lasers have very stable modes with diffraction limited output. The reduced heating effect due to the negligible substrate radiation will help the LCSP type array lasers to increase the output power.

4. REFERENCES

[1] D. Botez, L. Mawst, P. Hayashida, G. Peterson, and T. J. Roth, "High-power diffraction-limited-beam operation from phase-locked diode-laser arrays of closely spaced 'leaky' waveguides (antiguides)," Appl. Phys. Lett., vol. 53, pp. 464-466, Aug. 1988.

[2] L. Mawst, D. Botez, T. J. Roth, G. Peterson, and J. J. Yang, "Diffraction-coupled, phase-locked arrays of antiguided, quantum-well lasers grown by metal organic chemical vapor deposition," Elect. Lett., vol. 24, pp. 958-959, July 1988.

[3] R. W. Englemann and D. Kerps, "Leaky modes in active three-layer slab waveguides, IEE Proc., vol. 127, pp. 330-335, Dec. 1980.

[4] T. Tamir and F. Y. Kou, "Varieties of leaky waves and their excitation along multilayered structures," IEEE J. Quantum Electron., vol. QE-22, pp. 544-551, Apr. 1986.

[5] T. Kuroda, M. Nakamura, K. Aiki, and J. Umeda, "Channeled-substrate-planar structure $Al_xGa_{1-x}As$ lasers : an analytical waveguide study," Appl. Opt., vol. 17, pp. 3264-3267, Oct. 1978.

[6] S. Todoroki, M. Sawai, and K. Aiki, "Temperature distribution along the striped active region in high power GaAlAs visible lasers," J. Appl. Phys., vol. 58, pp. 1124-1128.

[7] S. Todoroki, "Influence of local heating on current-optical output power characteristics in $Ga_{1-x}Al_xAs$ lasers," J. Appl. Phys, vol. 60, pp.61-65, July 1986.

[8] D. Botez and J. C. Connolly, "High power phase locked arrays of index guided diode lasers," Appl. Phys. Lett., vol. 43, pp. 1096-1098, Dec., 1983.

[9] S. J. Lee and L. Figueroa, "Modified channeled substrate planar (CSP) lasers with lateral leaky mode behavior," in Proc. Topical Meet. Semiconductor lasers, Albuquerque, NM, Feb. 1987, pp. 128-131.

[10] S. J. Lee, L. Figueroa, and R. V. Ramaswamy, "Leaky-guided channeled substrate planar (LCSP) laser with reduced substrate radiation and heating," accepted for publication in IEEE J. Quantum Electron..

[11] H. Yonezu, I. Sakamura, K. Kobayashi, T. Kamejima, M. Ueno, and Y. Nannichi, "GaAs-$Al_xGa_{1-x}As$ double heterostructure planar stripe laser," Japan J. Appl. Phys., vol. 12, pp. 1585-1592, Oct. 1973.

[12] J. K. Butler and D. Botez, "Mode characteristics of nonplanar double-heterojunction and large-optical-cavity laser structures," IEEE J. Quantum Electron., vol. QE-18, pp. 952-961, June 1982.

[13] M. Osinski and J. Buus, "Linewidth broadening factor in semiconductor lasers - an overview," IEEE J. Quantum Electron., vol. QE-23, pp. 9-29, Jan. 1987.

[14] S. S. Lee, L. Figueroa, and R. V. Ramaswamy, "Variations of linewidth enhancement factor and linewidth as a function of laser geometry in (AlGa)As lasers," accepted for publication in IEEE J. Quantum Electron..

[15] C. H. Henry, R. A. Logan, and K. A. Bertness, "Spectral dependence of the change in refractive index due to carrier injection in GaAs lasers," J. Appl. Phys., vol. 52, pp. 4457-4461, July 1981.

[16] L. Figueroa, T. L. Holcomb, K. Burghard, D. Bullock, C. B. Morrson, L. M. Zinkiewicz, and G. A. Evans, "Modeling of the optical characteristics for twin channel laser (TCL) structures," IEEE J. Quantum Electron., vol. QE-22, pp. 2141-2149, Nov., 1986.

[17] R. Chinn and R. J. Spiers, "Calculation of separated multiclad-layer stripe geometry laser modes," IEEE J. Quantum Electron., vol. QE-18, pp. 984-991, June 1982.

[18] J. J. Yang, C. S. Hong, J. Niesen, and L. Figueroa, "High-power single longitudinal mode operation of inverted channel substrate planar lasers," J. Appl. Phys., vol. 58, pp. 4480-4482, Dec. 1985.

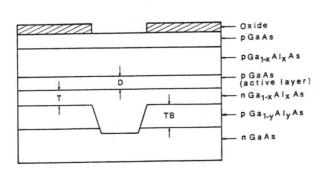

Fig. 1 The schematic diagram of LCSP structure.

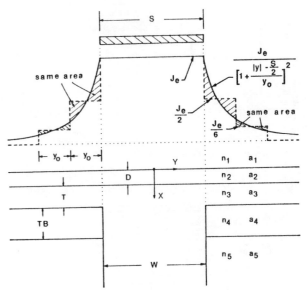

Fig. 2 The simplified geometry and approximated stair-case current density profile.

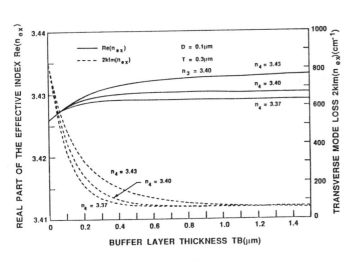

Fig. 3 The complex effective index in the region outside the channel.

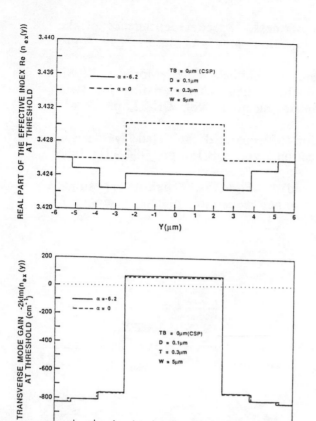

Fig. 4 The complex effective index distribution at threshold (CSP).

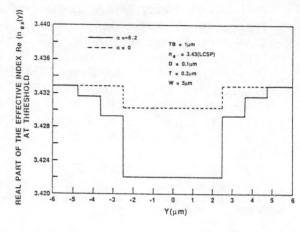

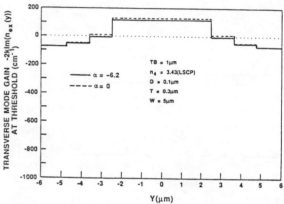

Fig. 5 The complex effective index distribution at threshold (LCSP).

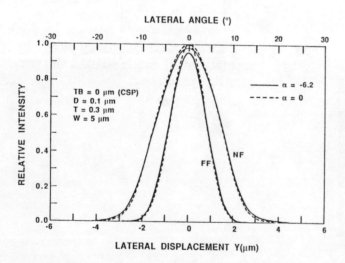

Fig. 6(a) The lateral mode fields (CSP).

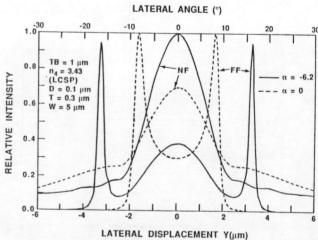

Fig. 6(b) The lateral mode fields (LCSP).

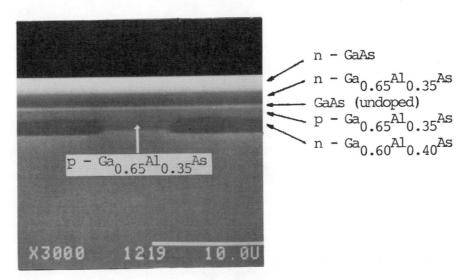

Fig. 7 The SEM cross-sectional view of a grown sample.

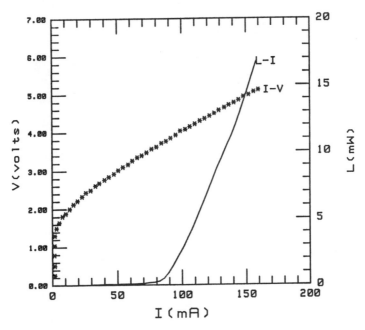

Fig. 8 The light-current characteristics.

LASER DIODE TECHNOLOGY AND APPLICATIONS

Volume 1043

SESSION 4

Low Threshold and High Frequency Lasers

Chair
James N. Walpole
Lincoln Laboratory/Massachusetts Institute of Technology

Invited Paper

Short Pulse and High Frequency Signal Generation in Semiconductor Lasers

K.Y. Lau

Columbia University, Dept. of Electrical Engineering, New York, N.Y. 10027

1. Introduction

The field of high speed semiconductor lasers has undergone substantial advances since the first demonstration of a laser with modulation bandwidth beyond 10GHz[1]. Much of the present understanding on the high speed modulation of semiconductor lasers comes from a small signal analysis of the laser rate equations, which is basically a book-keeping of the rate of supply, annihilation and creation of carriers and photons inside the laser cavity and describes laser dynamics in a most basic manner. The resulting small signal bandwidth is given by the now standard formula [1]

$$2\pi B = \sqrt{\frac{AP_o}{\tau_p}} = \sqrt{\frac{1}{\tau_p \tau_{stim}}} \tag{1}$$

where B is the relaxation oscillation frequency of the laser which is commonly taken to be the nominal bandwidth, A is the differential optical gain, P_o is the average photon density in the laser cavity, and τ_p is the photon lifetime and τ_{stim} is the stimulated carrier lifetime. While the initial development of high speed lasers and the basic verification of the parameter dependence of bandwidth given by Eq. (1) was in the short wavelength devices, the considerably more attractive properties of single mode fibers at 1.3 - 1.55µm provide impetus for development of high speed sources in this range. The present state of the art is exemplified by the demonstration of a 16GHz bandwidth (-3dB)[2] contricted mesa laser and a 22GHz bandwidth vapor phase regrown buried heterostructure laser[3], both at 1.3µm at operating cw at room temperature. These capabilities are well beyond those required by standard telecommunication, which has moved only recently into the lower Gbit/sec range. However, they make possible many new applications in microwave signal transmission and processing, where fiber-optic techniques have received only limited use despite its tremendous advantage in loss and bandwidth, mainly due to a lack of high speed optoelectronic components in the tens of gigahertz regime.

On a parallel front, there has been substantial progress in using laser diodes for picosecond pulse and microwave/millimeter wave signal generation. Picosecond optical pulse sources are major tools for studying ultrafast physical and chemical phenomena. A compact and reliable semiconductor picosecond laser source is highly desirable, especially for instrumentation applications such as picosecond optical sampling for non-invasive characterization of high speed electronic curcuits. Demonstrated methods of picosecond pulse generation from a laser diode include mode-locking and gain/Q switching. So far, the shortest pulses from a laser diode are generated by passive mode-locking, using defects inside the laser medium as the saturable absorber. Gain switching is a very simple technique of producing short pulses from a laser diode, although the pulse width seldom falls much below 20ps unless a saturable absorber is introduced into the cavity.

2. Mode-locking

Mode locking is achieved by introducing a mechanism inside the laser cavity to cause the longitudinal modes to interact with one another thereby locking them in phase[4]. A means of doing so (active mode-locking) is to modulate the gain or loss of the laser at a frequency equal to the frequency spacing between longitudinal modes, so that each mode is driven by the modulation sidebands of its neighbors. A saturable absorber placed in the laser cavity can achieve the same effect (passive mode-locking), though this is more appropriately described in the time domain. The typical length of a semiconductor laser is approximately 300μm and the intermodal frequency spacing is beyond 100GHz. It is highly unlikely that the gain of the laser can be modulated, either actively or passively, at these frequencies, so that almost all mode-locking configurations of semiconductor lasers use an external cavity[5] to reduce the intermodal frequency spacing to below a few gigahertz, well in the range of the direct modulation bandwidth of the laser. A standard configuration for active mode-locking is shown in Fig. 1.

Figure 2 illustrates the various schemes of mode-locking of a laser diode. The basic geometry is that shown in Fig. 1, with the device coupled to an external cavity. For active mode-locking one starts with a well behaved (non-aged, undamaged) laser diode, which is antireflection coated (AR) on the inner crystal facet(the one facing the external reflector). If no (or imperfect) AR coating is applied, the resulting three-mirror cavity configuration will lead to undesirable effects for active mode-locking. The requirement on the removal of residual reflectivity is stringent for complete locking of the modes[6].

For passive mode-locking, one starts with a laser which is degraded or damaged to a certain extent. These lasers often exhibit self-pulsation, which is understood as an undamped relaxation oscillation, or repetitive Q-switching, due to the presence of saturable absorption centers in these lasers. Anti-reflection coating is applied to one facet (which would suppress lasing and hence self-pulsation), and feedback is provided by an external reflector to achieve the conventional passive mode-locking geometry. If the AR coating is not perfect, one can expect the optical beam to experience multiple bounces within the laser diode cavity and the resultant mode-locked pulse could contain periodic substructures with a period equal to the round trip time of the laser diode. On the other hand, if an uncoated self-pulsing laser is coupled to an external reflector, a large variety of effects have been observed : for weak external feedback, the self-pulsation frequency is pulled to a harmonic of the reciprocal round trip time of the external cavity[7]. Since the width of the optical pulses emitted by self-pulsating lasers can be as short as 10ps[8], the result is very similar to passive mode-locking, but it is debatable whether this is mode-locking in the conventional sense. The optical pulses obtained this manner is certainly not transform limited. If a strong feedback is applied to a self-pulsing laser, then bifurcation, pulsation period doubling and chaos can result[8,9]. These are certainly not the desirable regimes for short pulse generation.

3. Gain/Q switching

The first indication that very short optical pulses can be generated by a directly modulated laser, with the optical pulse width being considerably shorter than the electrical drive pulse, was the observation of relaxation ocillation when turning on a laser from below threshold[10]. When biased above threshold, relaxation oscillation can sometimes be observed but at a much suppressed level. The potential for actually ultilizing this technique was realized when the exact pulsewidth was measured by streak camera and optical autocorrelation to be around 20ps[11-13], comparable to that obtained by actively mode-locking. The attractiveness of this technique is its simplicity. The shortest pulses that can be generated by gain switching is related to the strength of relaxation oscillation and therefore depends on laser structure. The standard gain-switching arrangement is to bias a laser below threshold (or not biased at all) and driving it with a comb generator, which is capable of delivering 70ps long electrical pulses of up to 20V into 50Ω. The idea is to excite the first spike of relaxation oscillation, and terminates the electrical pulse before the onset of the second spike. Subsequently, it was discovered that single pulses can be generated simply by modulating a laser diode biased below threshold with a large amplitude sine wave[14-16]. The idea here is again to catch the first spike of relaxation oscillation without exciting the subsequent ones. The conditions are decidedly more restrictive in this scheme since it requires an appropriate combination of modulating current, bias current and relaxation oscillation strength and frequency.

Complementing the gain switching technique is the Q-switching technique, which is actually more common amoung other laser systems due to the difficulty in providing fast gain modulation. The cavity Q is raised to a high level by an intracavity element, so that the laser can be pumped to a very high gain level without lasing. The Q is abruptly lowered and the laser suddenly finds itself with a huge amoung of excess gain, and responds by emitting a short intense pulse that dissipates (preferably) all of the excess gain. Q-switching has been implemented in quaternary semiconductor lasers by a monolithically integrated modulator[17]. Modulation is effected by shifting the bandedge through Franz-Keldish effect from an applied (reverse biasd) electric field . For the modulation to be effective, the lasing wavelength must be below the bandgap of the modulator material to begin with. Since the modulator and laser are fabricated monolithically out of the same chip and hence have exactly the same material composition, heavy doping by Zn diffusion is applied in the laser section in order to (1) shift the bandgap to lower energies and (2) introduce bandtail in which lasing occurs. Q-switching was observed at repetition rates exceeding 10GHz, the pulse width observed was detector limited to approximately 50ps. The exact pulse width was not measured. Q-switched lasers was also implemented in GaAs multi-quantum well lasers[18]. Carrier induced band shrinkage was used to lower the lasing frequency down to below the absorption edge of (intrinsic) modulator section. Pulses as short as 18ps was obtained at 3GHz repetition rate[18].

References

1. K.Y. Lau and A. Yariv, "Ultra high speed semiconductor lasers", IEEE J. Quant. Electron., **QE-21**, 121-138 (85)

2. J.E. Bowers, B.R. Hemmenway, A.H. Gnauck and D.P. Wilt, "High speed InGaAsP constricted mesa lasers", IEEE J. Quant. Electron., **QE-22**, 833-844 (86)

3. R. Olshansky, W. Powazinik, P. Hill, V. Lanzisera and R.N. Lauer, "InGaAsP buried heterostructure laser with 22GHz bandwidth modulation efficiency", Electron. Lett., **23**, 839 (87).

4. A.E. Siegman, **Lasers**, University Science Books Press, Mill Valley, Calif. 1986.

5. J.P. Van der Ziel, "Mode locking of semiconductor lasers", **Semiconductor and semimetals**, Vol. 22, Part B, Chp. 1, Academic Press 1985.

6. T. Kobayashi, A. Yoshihawa, A. Morimoto, T. Aoki and T. Sueta, 11th International Quant. Electron. Conf., Boston 1980.

7. L. Figueroa, K.Y. Lau and A. Yariv, "Intensity self-pulsations in GaAlAs injection lasers operating in an external cavity", Appl. Phys. Lett., **36**, 248-250 (1980).

8. K. Otsuka and H. Kawaguchi, "Theory of optical multistability and chaos in a resonant type semiconductor laser amplifier", Phys. Rev. A, **28-5**, 3153-3155 (1984).

9. Y.C. Chen, H.G. Winful, and J.M. Liu, "Subharmonic bifurcation and irregular pulsing behavior of modulated semiconductor laser", Appl. Phys. Lett., **47**, 208-210 (1985).

10. T. Ikegami and Y. Suematsu, "Large signal characteristics of directly modulated semiconductor injection lasers", Electron. Comm. Japan, **53B**, 69-75 (1970).

11. T. Kobayashi, A. Yoshihawa, A. Morimoto, T. Aoki and T. Sueta, 11th International Quant. Electron. Conf., Boston 1980.

12. P.L. Liu, T.C. Daman and D.J. Eilenberger, Picosecond phenomena meeting, North Falmouth, Mass., 1980.

13. C. Lin, P.L. Liu, T.C. Damen, D.J. Eilenberger and R.L. Hartman, "Simple picosecond pulse generation scheme for injection lasers", Electron. Lett., **16**, 600-602 (1980).

14. H. Ito, H. Yokoyama, S. Murata and H. Inaba, "Picosecond optical pulse generation from an RF modulated AlGaAs DH diode laser", Electron. Lett., **15**, 738-740 (1979); IEEE J. Quant. Electron., **QE-17**, 663-670 (1981).

15. J. Auyeung, "Picosecond optical pulse generation at GHa riate by direct modulation of a semiconductor laser", Appl. Phys. Lett., **38**, 308-310 (1981).

16. J.P. Van der Ziel and R.A. Logan, "Generation of short optical pulses in semiconductor lasers by combined DC and microwave current injection", IEEE J. Quant. Electron., **QE-18**, 1340-50 (1982).

17. D.Z. Tsang, J.N. Walpole, S.H. Groves, J.J. Hsieh and J.P. Donnelly, "Intracavity loss modulation of GaInAsP diode lasers", Appl. Phys. Lett., **38**, 120-122 (1980); D.Z. Tsang, J.N. Walpole, Z.L. Liau, S.H. Groves and V. Diadiuk, "Q-switching of low threshold buried heterostructure diode lasers at 10GHz", Appl. Phys. Lett., **45** 204-206 (1984).

18. Y. Arakawa, A. Larsson, J. Paslaski and A. Yariv, "Active Q-switching in a GaAs/GaAlAs multi-quantum well laser with an intracavity loss modulator", Appl. Phys. Lett., **45**, 204 (1984).

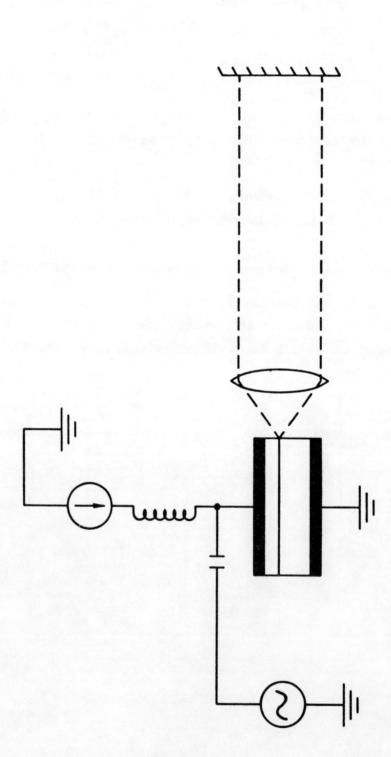

Fig. 1 Schematic diagram of active mode-locking of a semiconductor laser

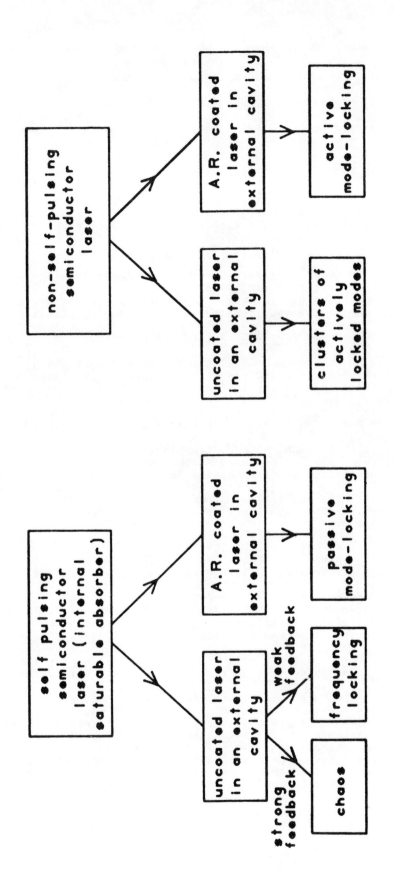

Fig. 2 Regimes of mode-locking of a semiconductor laser

Invited Paper

Laser based optoelectronic integrated circuits for
communications.

R. M. Ash, R. C. Goodfellow, A. C. Carter

Plessey Research Caswell Ltd, Caswell, Towcester,
Northants, NN12 8EQ, England.

ABSTRACT

Performance advantages and cost reductions are expected from the introduction of optoelectronic integrated circuit technology. A common technology base for different functions and applications will permit the fabrication of a wide range of different OEICs.

1. INTRODUCTION

This paper is intended to give a flavour for some of the applications and technologies that Plessey is currently working on in the laser based Optoelectronic Integrated Circuit (OEIC) field. Much of the technology is common to several different devices and applications, making an overall strategy for the development of OEICs attractive.

2. RATIONALE FOR OEIC

It is expected that both performance advantages and cost reductions will follow from smaller circuit size, fewer bondwires and hence reduced parasitic inductances and capacitances. This reduction in interconnections (both electrical and optical) will result in increased reliability and mechanical stability. Furthermore, new functions and architectures are expected to result, with devices which were too large or unstable to consider in discrete form being implemented with relative ease in OEICs.

Cost reduction will follow through the reduction in the number of critical optical alignments and the consequent simplification of packaging. One common OEIC process will allow several different devices to be fabricated in parallel (for example all the lasers on one OEIC will be fabricated at one time). A common technology base for different functions and applications will permit the fabrication of OEICs with widely differing applications in the same process run (even on the same wafer). Both of these factors will lead to cost savings and yield enhancement.

3. APPLICATIONS FOR OEICs

Two applications of current interest within Plessey for OEICs are outlined below.

A terminal for a bidirectional link for the Customer Access Connection is shown in figure 1. In this example an OEIC is coupled to the fiber port and contains a wavelength duplexer, a DFB laser and its associated power monitor diode. Within the same package are a silicon driver circuit for the laser and a silicon receiver IC which, in this implementation, is coupled to a PIN photodiode which is not part of the main OEIC. The critical fiber to optical device interfaces are reduced to one (at the input/output port) since the alignment of the waveguide to the PIN diode is relatively coarse.

A second example of an integratable component is shown in figure 2. The polarization diversity coherent receiver needs polarization splitters, 3dB couplers, photodetectors, a laser with external cavity, monitor photodiode and control electronics. The only component which is not readily integratable at present is the isolater, which is needed to overcome the reflection sensitivity of the laser. Work is therefore required to develop lasers which are less sensitive to reflections before integration of this whole receiver is possible. It will not be cost effective to integrate all the electronic components indicated here, but the front end receivers will probably benefit from integration.

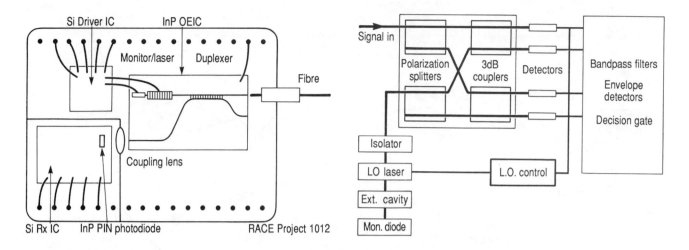

Figure 1. Partially integrated bidirectional CAC terminal

Figure 2. Coherent polarization diversity receiver.

4. TECHNOLOGY EVOLUTION

The technologies for many OEIC devices are already in place. During the 1970's epitaxial growth, dry processing and IC processes were extensively investigated. Quantum well technology, which is becoming increasingly important in laser, detector and waveguide fabrication, first emerged at this time.

In the 1980's we have seen the development of many of the building blocks needed for integration. Lasers, amplifiers, waveguides, switches, modulators and InP based electronics have all been the subject of extensive development in their discrete forms.

Looking forward, the 1990's will see realizations of the first commercially applicable OEICs for optoelectronic communication systems. High performance receivers, complex multi-section lasers and signal processing and routing devices will also emerge during the next decade.

5. LASERS FOR INTEGRATION

Some of the features needed for an integratable laser are low threshold current and high temperature operation (for use without thermoelectric coolers and with simple drive circuitry), tuneability and narrow linewidth for coherent communication systems and efficient waveguide coupling for maximum system performance. In addition to the above a simple (and high yield) process is required to allow good overall OEIC performance.

Figure 3 shows a buried ridge DFB laser which is ideally suited to integration. This structure fabricated by Plessey and others (eg ref.1) is fabricated by growing a source wafer with buffer, active region and a thin InP or quaternary cladding layer. In the DFB variant a grating is added, prior to mesa etching to form the active region waveguide and overgrowth with an InP waveguide and a GaInAs cap layers. Proton implantation is used to reduce parasitic currents and capacitance prior to metallization. The simple current confinement technique (utilizing the difference in bandgap between active and blocking junction diodes) allows reliable operation to greater than $90^\circ C$. Low series resistance ($\approx 3\Omega$) and low capacitance ($\approx 10-20pF$) gives adequate high speed operation for communications systems at least to 2.4Gbit/s.

A first step towards integration is shown in figure 4 - a laser is integrated with a monitor photodiode formed by forming facets using a dry etch technique (ref.2). Some performance degradation results owing to the imperfect mirrors, but there are significant advantages: lower assembly costs for the complete packaged laser module, self alignment (or deliberate angling) of the monitor diode and the possibility of probe testing the lasers on wafer.

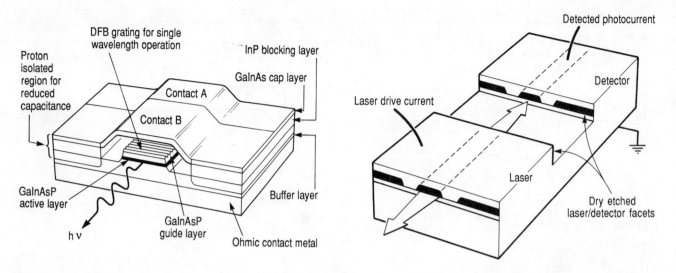

Figure 3. Buried ridge DFB laser.   Figure 4. Integrated laser and monitor photodiode.

Figure 5 shows two devices with more complex integration functions. The integrated passive cavity DFB has an extra (unpumped) cavity to reduce the linewidth of the laser. The example shown here gave a linewidth of 8MHz for a total cavity length of 3.5mm. The multisegment tuneable DBR also shown has an active region, a phase control region and a tuning region with a grating reflector.

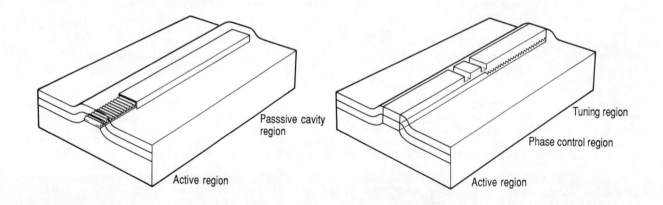

Figure 5. Integrated passive cavity DFB and Multisegment tuneable DBR

A simpler version of this device is shown in figure 6, and has two sections, both with an integral grating. Wavelength tuning is possible by altering the ratio of the currents in the front and back regions of the cavity. The tuning range for this simple structure is 1.14nm, with a linewidth less than 25MHz over this range, as the current fraction through the back region is changed from 0% to 45% of the total 140mA drive current. A similar device can operate as a (non-tuneable) DFB with an integral monitor diode. The tracking of the monitor current with output power is shown in figure 7, together with the light current characteristics for the device. Coupling to the monitor diode is high in this design since the waveguide is not broken between the two regions.

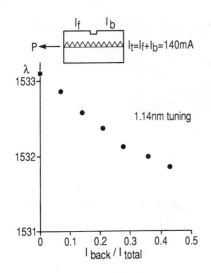
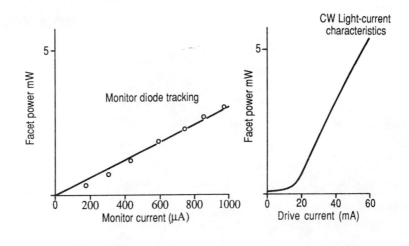

Figure 6. Two section DFB tuneability

Figure 7. Monitor diode tracking and light current characteristics

An essential feature of OEICs will be the efficiency of coupling between lasers and waveguides. Two approaches for coupling are shown in figure 8. The bundle integrated guide or BIG structure is simple to fabricate but has the disadvantage that the waveguide layers extend over the laser active region. The butt jointed structure is more difficult to fabricate, requiring selective area epitaxy, but has the advantage of allowing separate optimisation of the waveguides over the active and waveguiding regions. In general for low loss waveguides low doped material is required, whereas for lasers a low series resistance is desirable which means that highly doped cladding regions are needed.

A micrograph of a test structure for butt coupling is shown in figure 9. The waveguide and active regions are slightly misaligned in this example giving rise to a non-planar surface. A flat surface is desirable for subsequent photolithography steps which will define the laser and waveguide dimensions.

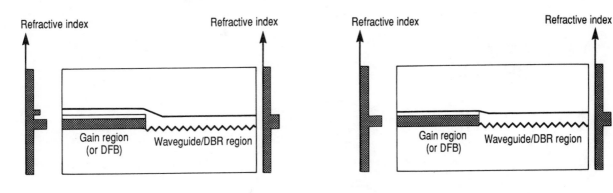

Figure 8. Laser waveguide coupling schemes

6. WAVEGUIDES

An essential requirement for complex OEICs is a low loss and versatile waveguide technology which is integratable with lasers and detectors. Losses of 0.5dB/cm are readily achieved in InP based waveguides with wavelength multiplexer (grating, Mach-Zehnder or coupler) technologies all being available. Corner reflectors, another useful addition for complex OEICs in which routing of the signals around the chip is required have been fabricated using dry etch techniques to form mirrors on the end of waveguides. Test structures used are shown in figure 10 with straight guides and 2 and 4 reflection optical paths. Excess losses were 3dB and 9dB for two and four reflection paths respectively (ref.3).

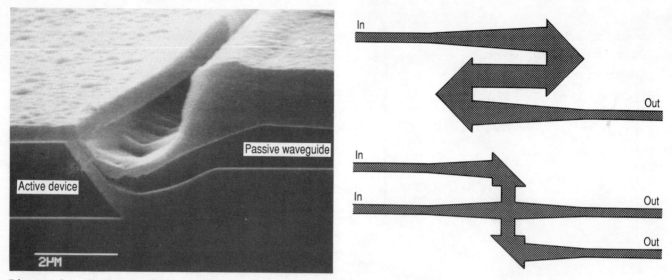

Figure 9. Butt coupling test structure.   Figure 10. Waveguide corner reflector test structures.

Switching technology is being developed for routing signals at high speed on OEICs. An example of a switch in the GaAs/AlGaAs materials system is shown in figure 11. Advanced airbridge technology is used to minimise bond pad parasitics to give very high speed operation. The latest devices fabricated similar to this but with push-pull electrical drive give 13GHz operation (ref.4). Similar technology in the InP materials system for integration with long wavelength components is under development.

7. DETECTORS

The last optically active devices required for OEIC implementation are photodetectors. Performance requirements vary from low speed, moderate efficiency devices for power monitor applications through to very low dark current, low capacitance and high quantum efficiency detectors for high speed, low noise receivers. As in all the previous components waveguide coupling is a highly desirable feature.

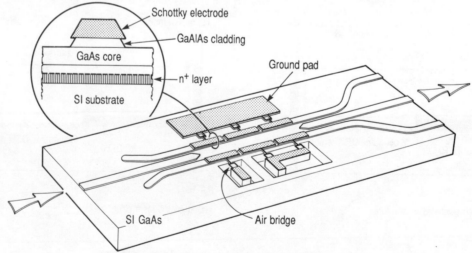

Figure 11. GaAs high speed modulator.

An early integration concept is shown in figure 12. A high performance (0.02pF, 20ps) p-i-n photodiode is flip-chip bonded onto a high impedance GaAs MESFET amplifier chip. (ref 5). This structure has the potential of very high performance but has the disadvantage of not being waveguide coupled. A development of the above concept is shown in figure 13 in which a GaInAs p-i-n diode is recessed into a GaAs substrate (ref.6) on which a GaAs MESFET amplifier could subsequently be fabricated. A variable pitch superlattice grading structure is required to relieve the strain caused by the lattice constant difference between GaAs and GaInAs. The photodiode performance was good with a dark current of <1nA at 20v bias and a capacitance of only 0.5pF for a 100μm diameter device.

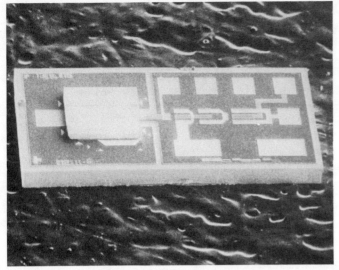
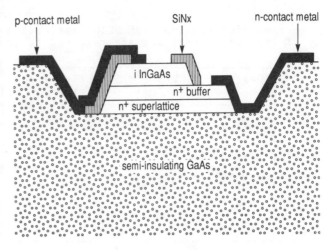

Figure 12. P-i-n diode flip-chip bonded onto a GaAs MESFET IC front end amplifier.

Figure 13. GaInAs P-i-n recessed into a GaAs substrate.

8. ELECTRICAL INTERFACE AND DRIVE

The capacity to fabricate laser drivers and controllers, amplifiers, receivers and control electronics for optical switches is desirable. These circuits will in general require transistors, resistors and possibly capacitors.

Some of the options for a transistor technology are heterojunction bipolar transistors, AlInAs FETs or HEMTs. Our work has concentrated on HBTs (eg ref.7) since they are a compact vertical structure which is readily integratable with other devices. An example of an HBT circuit (made in GaAs/GaAlAs) is shown in figure 14. This is capable of providing current drive for a laser of 100mA and has a -3dB bandwidth of 5GHz. Figure 15 shows the electrical input and optical output signals when using this device to modulate a laser at 2Gbit/s NRZ.

Similar circuits have been made in InP/GaInAs HBTs. These devices have an f_T of 6.5GHz and have 16μm emitters.

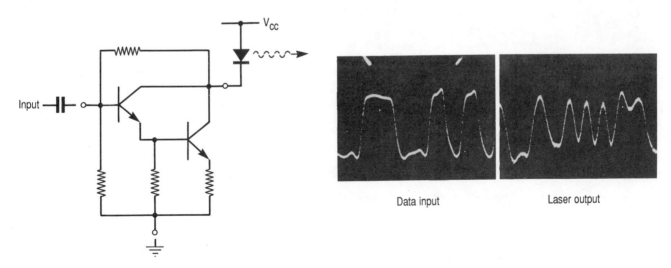

Figure 14. Circuit of HBT laser driver.

Figure 15. Modulation of a laser at 2Gbit/s using the HBT driver.

9. CONCLUSIONS

The technologies required for OEIC fabrication are well advanced. Table 1 below shows how many of the same techniques are required to form the different components for an OEIC process.

Device	Selective Area Epitaxy	III-V Dry Etch	Multi-level Metals	Quantum Wells
Lasers	✓	✓		✓
Waveguides	✓	✓		✓
λ Multiplexers		✓		✓
Detectors	✓	✓		✓
Electrical	✓	✓	✓	

Table 1. Technology commonality.

The use of OEICs for a wide variety of communications and signal processing applications will follow the development of the discrete components and technologies described above. The first generation of OEICs are being designed now.

10. ACKNOWLEDGMENTS

The authors would like to thank all those from the Plessey team contributing to the above work and acknowledge the support of Central Engineering GPT and the EEC under the RACE project (1012) for some of the work on OEICs.

11. REFERENCES

1. M. Razeghi et al, Appl. Phys. Lett. 46 (2), p131-3, 15 January 1985.
2. P. Williams et al, Elec. Lett. 22 p472, 24 April 1986.
3. E. Drummond, SIOE Cardiff 1988.
4. R. Walker, ECOC 88 proceedings vol.1 p565-568, September 1988.
5. R. S. Sussmann et al, Elec. Lett. 21 p593-5, 4 July 1985.
6. P. D. Hodson et al, Elec. Lett. 23 p273, 28 March 1985.
7. P. J. Topham et al, ESSCIRC, Manchester, Sept. 1988.

High Performance 1.3 µm Buried Crescent Lasers and LEDs for Fiber Optic Links

R. J. Fu, E. Y. Chan and C. S. Hong

Boeing Electronics High Technology Center
P. O. Box 24969, MS 7J-05
Seattle, Wa 98124

ABSTRACT

Self-aligned Buried Crescent Heterostructure (BCH) semiconductor lasers and LEDs have been sucessfully developed as superb light sources for fiber optic communications. The fabrication and performance characteristics of these InGaAsP/InP lasers and LEDs are described. For lasers, the threshold currents as low as 10 mA and differential quantum efficiencies as high as 50% are achieved. For LEDs, the output powers at 150 mA are higher than 1 mW. Good far field patterns are obtained in both the LEDs and lasers. Measured I-V, L-I, spectrum and far field patterns are presented.

1. INTRODUCTION

InGaAsP/InP semiconductor lasers and LEDs are the devices of choice for fiber optic communication systems that take advantage of the low loss at 1.3 µm and 1.55 µm wavelengths and zero characteristic dispersion of silica fibers at 1.3 µm emitting wavelength. For single mode fiber optic systems used for long haul telecommunication or higher bit rate (>1 Gbit/sec) applications, lasers are the ideal source to be considered. While, for many local area networks and low bit data rate communication applications, LEDs are the preferred source. Various types of InGaAsP diode lasers have been studies previousely [1-8]. Among them the Buried Crescent (BC) Structure lasers and the Buried Heterostructure (BH) diode lasers are most promising due to their superior characteristics such as low threshold current and stable single transverse mode. In this work, the performance characteristics and device structure for Buried Crescent lasers and LEDs are discussed.

2. FABRICATION

The structure for both lasers and LEDs are Buried Crescent Heterostructure (BCH) grown on a V-grooved n-type InP substrate. Figure 1 shows the schematic diagram of the BCH laser. Figure 2 shows the SEM cross section photograph of the as-grown wafer. Our InGaAsP/InP BCH lasers are fabricated by liquid phase epitaxy (LPE). Current blocking layer is formed and V-shape channels are chemically etched prior to the LPE growth. By carefully controlling the degree of supercooling of the growth solution, it is possible to produce a crescent-shaped active region completely surrounded by InP layers which have a lower refractive index and higher energy gap. The higher energy gap provides a potential barrier to lateral carrier diffusion while the lower refractive index forms the index-guided mechanism that gives the better optical confinement. Thus the BCH incorporating a current blocking layer results in low threshold current and high quantum efficiency performance. Epitaxial layers grown on the V-shape channelled n-type InP substrate are: a buffer layer of n-InP to remove surface defects; an InGaAsP active layer with the energy gap that will emit light at 1.3 µm; a p-doped InP cladding layer; and a p+-doped InGaAsP layer for electrode contact. A broad-area ohmic metallization of AuZn/Au and AuGe/Ni/Au were used for the p and n contact of the wafer, respectively. The wafer was then cleaved into individual chips for testing. For the fabrication of high power LEDs, BCH is also used. In order to suppress the lasing action, the rear mirror is destroyed by chemical etching and the reflectivity of the front mirror is reduced to less than 1% by anti-reflective (AR) coating of quarter wavelength thickness of Si_3N_4. By utilizing the BCH design, we achieved high power and good far field LEDs.

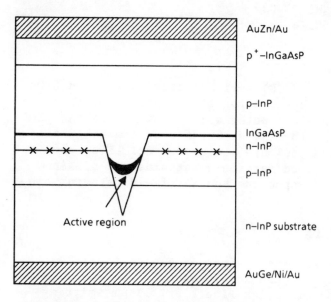

Figure 1. Schematic Cross Section of Buried Crescent Laser Structure

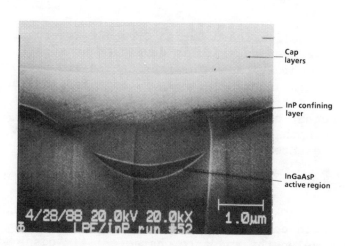

Figure 2. SEM Cross Section of Buried Crescent Laser Structure

3. PERFORMANCE

Laser diodes

The I-V and L-I characteristics for the device with 300 µm cavity are shown in Figure 3. The series resistance is about 5 ohms. Typical threshold currents are in the range of 10 to 20 mA and differential quantum efficiencies are about 40 to 50%. Linear L-I characteristics up to 10 mW were observed for these lasers. L-I characteristic curves versus temperature for 1.3 µm laser are shown in Figure 4. It is well known that the threshold current of InGaAsP/InP DH laser is strongly affected by temperature changes. The far field emission pattern is shown in figure 5. An almost circular beam with divergent angle of 28° in the direction parallel to junction plane and 36° in the direction perpendicular to junction plane was measured. The optics for coupling the circular beam into single mode fiber is simpler than that for elliptical beams. The emission spectrum of the device at the power level of 3 mW is shown in Figure 6. A dominant longitudinal mode with a 12 dB side-mode-suppression-ratio was observed. The integrity of the current blocking junction was preliminarily tested when we operated the laser at high power levels. A pulse power as high as 50 mW was obtained without observing negative slope (dL/dI) efficiency.

Edge emitting LEDs (EELEDs)

An L-I characteristic curve for 1.3 µm LEDs (or SLDs) is shown in Figure 7. The output power from the device is greater than 1 mW at 150 mA drive current and 23°C. It is at least two times higher than typical edge emitting LEDs. Figure 8 shows the spectrum for this 1.3 µm EELED. The spectral width of such devices is about 30 nm. The far field pattern of the EELED is as good as the BCH laser and will warrant high coupling efficiency for both single mode and multimode fibers.

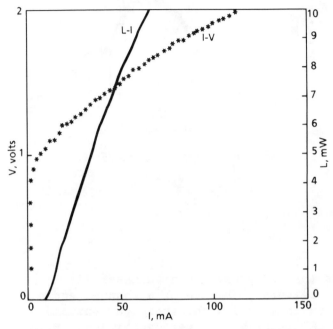

Figure 3. Light-Current and Current-Voltage Curves of BC Lasers

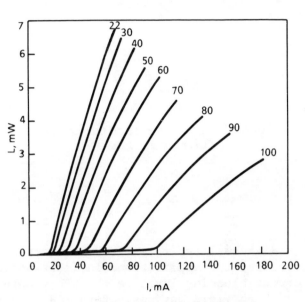

Figure 4. Light-Current Curve Versus Temperature of BC Laser

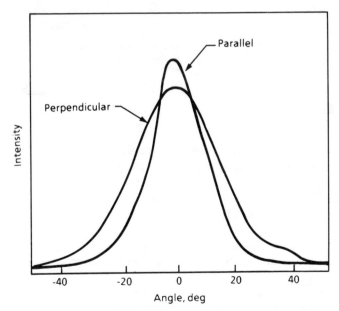

Figure 5. Far-Field Pattern of BC Laser In Both Directions

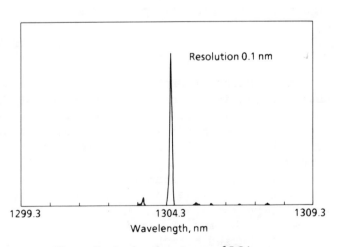

Figure 6. Lasing Spectrum of BC Laser

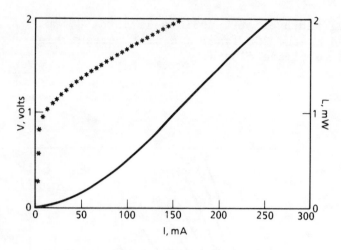

Figure 7. Light-Current and Current-Voltage Curves of BC LEDs

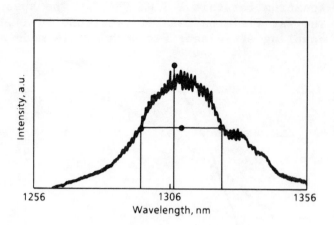

Figure 8. Spectrum of BC EELED

4. SUMMARY

High quality, reliable BCH lasers and LEDs (or SLDs) have been successfully developed for applications in fiber-optic transceivers. The use of a channel and a current blocking layer in the LPE growth results in very low threshold current and very high yield devices. Both BCH lasers and LEDs show high power capability. High coupling efficiency should be expected from the good far field pattern. All these characteristics make the BCH devices (both lasers and LEDs) very suitable for fiber optical communication systems.

5. ACKNOWLEDGEMENT

The authors would like to thank Dr. C. Tang for material characterization, Dan Booher and Andy Burnett for the photolithography and metalization works and Dr. L. Figueroa for his encouragement and support.

6. REFERENCES

1. M. Hirao, A. Doi, S. Tsuji, M. Nakamura and K. Aiki, "Fabrication and characterization of narrow stripe InGaAsP/InP buried heterostructure lasers," J. Appl. Phys., vol. 51, pp. 4539-4540, Aug. 1980.
2. I. Mito, M. Kitamura, K. Kaede, Y. Odagiri, M. Seki, M. Sugimoto and K. Kobayashi, "InGaAsP planner buried heterostructure laser (PBH-LD) with very low threshold current," Electron. Lett., vol. 18, pp. 2-3, 1982.
3. I. Mito, M. Kitamura and K. Kobayashi, "Double-channel planar buried-heterostructure laser diode with effective current confinement," Electron. Lett., vol. 18, pp.953-954.
4. H. Ishikawa, H. Imai, T. Tanahashi, K Hori and K. Takahei, "V-grooved substrate buried heterostructure InGaAsP/InP laser emitting at 1.3 µm wavelength," IEEE J. Quantum Electron., vol. QE-18, pp. 1704-1711, Oct. 1982.
5. E. Oomura, T. Murotani, H. Higuchi, H. Namizaki and W. Susaki, "Low threshold InGaAsP buried crescent laser with double current confinement structure," IEEE J. Quantum. Electron., vol. QE-17, pp. 646-650, May, 1981.

6. R. Hirano, E. Oomura, H. Higuchi, Y. Sakakibara, H. Namizaki and W. Susaki, "Low threshold current 1.3 μm InGaAsP burried crescent lasers," Japan. J. Appl. Phys., vol. 22, suppl. 22-1, pp.231-234, 1983.

7. M. Oron and N. Tamari, "High power single mode InGaAsP lasers fabricated by single step liquid phase epitaxy," Appl. Phys. Lett., vol. 42, pp. 139-141, Jan. 1983.

8. K. Kishino, Y. Suematsu and Y. Itaya, "Fabrication and lasing properties of meas substrate buried heterostructure GaInAsP/InP lasers at 1.3 μm wavelength," IEEE J. Quantum Electron., vol. QE-16, pp. 160-164, Feb. 1980.

LASER DIODE TECHNOLOGY AND APPLICATIONS

Volume 1043

SESSION 5

Novel Semiconductor Laser Applications I

Chair
Luis Figueroa
Boeing Electronics High Technology Center

Diode Laser Radar System Analysis and Design for High Precision Ranging

Michael de La Chapelle, J. Doyle McClure, Edward J. Vertatschitsch,
Raymond G. Beausoleil, James G. Bull and John A. McGarvey

Boeing Electronics Company, High Technology Center, P.O. Box 24969, Seattle, WA 98124-6269

Abstract

Laser radar (ladar) performance parameters such as range accuracy, estimation time and target range are analyzed as a function of the component parameters that comprise the system. Design tradeoffs and performance comparisons are evaluated for two popular ladar system designs: intensity modulated(IM)/direct detection(DD) and frequency modulated(FM)/coherent detection(CD). The comparison includes practical discussions of modulation, signal processing and component performance. The analysis begins by presenting accurate signal to noise ratio (SNR) equations that include the often omitted phase noise and intensity noise terms. Next, the SNR is related to the range accuracy, estimation time and modulation frequency or bandwidth via the Cramer-Rao lower bound (CRLB) for optimal processing. The results of the analysis are used to identify critical component design and performance issues for precision IM/DD and FM/CD ladar systems.

Introduction

High performance aerospace systems require advanced ladar sensors for a variety of functions such as remote/robotic vision and inspection, high precision metrology for space system configuration control, as well as range imaging for aircraft guidance, control, navigation, and threat detection/recognition. These applications all demand depth and lateral accuracy which is not possible from conventional RF radars.

The emphasis of this paper is on ranging accuracy of the order 10^{-3} cm, target ranges of 10-100 m, and data rates of 10-1000 pixels/sec. The moderate operating range requirement allows the use of semiconductor diode laser sources with CW output power levels of less than 1 Watt. These sources are best suited for the aerospace flight environment because of their high efficiency, small size, rugged construction, low cost and high reliability. In addition, the extremely large modulation bandwidth of these devices makes it possible to simultaneously meet the tough resolution and data rate requirements.

Pulsed modulation is not generally used for ultra high accuracy ladars operating at moderate range for two important reasons:
  (1) It is impractical to measure pulse arrival times to sub picosecond accuracies in the receiver.
  (2) The sensitivity is low for short pulse measurements because of the limited energy content of the pulses and the necessity for wide instantaneous receiver bandwidth.

To avoid these problems, the laser source can be frequency or intensity modulated and the frequency or phase of the detected signal can be measured at the receiver.

The scope of this analysis is limited to two particular ladar systems that are fundamentally different in design and performance. One uses an intensity modulated (IM) source and a direct detection (DD) receiver and the other uses a frequency modulated (FM) source and a coherent detection (CD) receiver, as shown in Figures 1a and 1b. The direct detection system has a laser source that is intensity modulated by a continuous wave (CW) radio frequency (RF) signal which also serves as the local oscillator (LO) for mixing with the direct detected optical return signal. The measured phase difference, $\delta\theta$, between the transmit and receive signal is proportional to the target range as given by, $R = c\,\delta\theta\,/\,4\pi f_0$. The range measurement becomes ambiguous when the phase exceeds 2π radians which corresponds to a target range of $c/2f_0$, where f_0 is the modulation frequency.

The coherent system employs a frequency modulated laser diode that is linearly tuned as a function of time to produce a "chirped" signal. The chirp rate is $\dot{f} = B/T$ where B is the chirp bandwidth and T is the chirp duration. The heterodyne detector output is the difference frequency, f_{if}, between the transmit and receive signals, which is proportional to target range as given by, $f_{if} = \dot{f}\tau$, where $\tau = 2R/c$ is the round trip time delay to the target.

The question of which method yields better system performance is very complex and is strongly dependent on the performance of the constituent components. Both systems have demonstrated their utility for high resolution ranging. ERIM has developed an IM/DD ladar under contract from the US Postal Service for automatic package sorting.[1] The system has .004" range accuracy at a maximum range of three feet while operating at a measurement rate of 1 MHz. Digital Optronics Corp. has developed a commercial FM/CD ladar with .0015" range accuracy at a maximum range of 15 feet while operating at a measurement rate of 0.5 Hz.[2]

The purpose of this paper to present a preliminary analysis of ladar performance for the competing systems of FM/CD and IM/DD, to make performance comparisons, and to draw conclusions from the results. R.J. Keyes of Lincoln Laboratory has written a good review paper with the same purpose.[3] However, his emphasis was on ladar systems with less precision. Consequently, he neglected noise terms (such as phase noise) that are very important in the analysis of high precision ladars with diode laser sources. Furthermore, he did not extend the analysis to include tradeoffs between range accuracy, SNR and measurement time.

The results of the analysis are strongly dependent on a few assumed component performance parameters (especially for the laser diode source) that are uncertain or unknown due to lack of published data. For this reason, some of the results are presented for a range of component parameter values. The large number of parameters in the analysis and the brevity of the paper do not permit a comprehensive analysis of how each component parameter affects the overall system performance. Instead, we concentrate on the most important component parameters that limit system performance. The baseline component parameter values presented in Table 1 are our best estimate of achievable performance. A section has been included to describe component performance uncertainties and to identify necessary topics of component research and development.

SNR Analysis

The classic laser radar signal to noise ratio (SNR) analysis that is common in the literature does not account for the non ideal performance of the laser source.[4] Accounting for the excess intensity noise and phase noise of laser diode sources is essential for an accurate analysis of high precision ladar system performance. Laser phase noise must be considered in the FM/CD analysis when the desired frequency resolution is small compared to the laser linewidth.[5] For this condition, the laser phase noise is often the dominant noise source that limits the SNR, as will be demonstrated in the following analysis. This paper presents equations and plots of S/N_0, where S is the photodetector signal power and N_0 is the one sided noise power spectral density. S/N_0 can be regarded as the SNR out of the photodetector in a 1 Hz bandwidth.

The general form of the S/N_0 equations are given below.

$$(S/N_0)_{CD} = \frac{\text{signal}}{\text{shot noise + thermal noise + intensity noise + phase noise}} \tag{1}$$

$$(S/N_0)_{DD} = \frac{\text{signal}}{\text{shot noise + thermal noise + intensity noise}} \tag{2}$$

The complete S/N_0 equations corresponding to these forms appear in Table 1 along with a list of parameter definitions.

The shot noise term includes the effects of solar background radiation, received and LO powers, as well as the detector dark and leakage currents. The excess intensity noise term is derived from intensity fluctuations in the laser diode output power.[6] The phase noise contribution arises from the power spectrum of the photocurrent produced by optically heterodyning the LO and the delayed-return ranging laser fields.[5] The detected RF power spectrum for a laser with fluctuations which result in a Lorentzian field spectrum is a coherent "delta function" signal centered on a modified Lorentzian phase noise "pedestal." The Fourier spectrum of the phase noise "pedestal" is sufficiently uniform over the receiver bandwidth of interest that for high-precision ranging measurements it can be approximated as a white noise source.

Typical amplitudes of the various noise sources in the FM/CD and IM/DD ladar systems are shown in Figures 2 and 3 for the assumed 10 kHz laser linewidth. The laser phase noise dominates the other noise terms at all target ranges for the FM/CD ladar. In contrast, the IM/DD ladar is shot noise limited at all target ranges. The variation of the signal power with range is also plotted in figures 2 and 3. The target is assumed to be a diffuse scatterer with a reflectivity of 10%. Targets can of course have reflectivities varying from nearly 0 to 100%, with low reflectance targets producing a relatively greater degradation of S/N_0 in IM/DD systems and higher reflectance targets producing a larger improvement in S/N_0 for IM/DD. As the equations of Table 1 indicate, there is $1/r^2$ signal power dependence for FM/CD ladar and $1/r^4$ signal power dependence for IM/DD ladar. This explains the advantage of FM/CD ladar for long range target detection. The total value of S/N_0 for IM/DD and FM/CD ladar systems (see Figure 4) can be determined by taking the ratio of the signal curve to the dominant noise curve in Figures 2 and 3. Notice that the S/N_0 values for both systems are approximately equal at short target ranges with FM/CD having an increasing advantage at target ranges beyond 30 meters, for the assumed system parameters.

The plots were generated assuming a baseline set of parameters given in Table 1 for the laser diode transmitter and photodiode receiver. These parameters correspond to commercially available components for the IM/DD case. For the FM/CD case, a 100 mW single mode laser was assumed to be line narrowed to 10 kHz and linearly chirped over a 10 GHz bandwidth. These assumption are based on anticipated component developments in the next one to two years.

Evaluation of the relative advantages and disadvantages of FM/CD over IM/DD ladar for different applications is difficult because the question is very dependent on laser technology. Figure 5 shows plots of S/N_0 for IM/DD and FM/CD ladar as a function of range for laser power levels of 10 mW, 100 mW and 1W. Notice that S/N_0 of the FM/CD system saturates at 100 mW for a laser linewidth of 10 kHz. There is no performance improvement for using lasers of greater than 100 mW power when the linewidth exceeds 10 kHz. The S/N_0 saturation power can be increased by employing narrower linewidth lasers. The IM/DD S/N_0 does not saturate at high powers and therefore has larger S/N_0 values over the entire plotted range for a 1 Watt laser. However, it is not known whether the beam quality of available high power broad stripe lasers is adequate for ladar applications (see discussion below). The saturation of S/N_0 with increasing source power in the FM/CD ladar is caused by the laser phase noise. Figure 6 shows how S/N_0 increases with decreasing linewidth. This plot clearly depicts the need for development of laser line narrowing techniques for FM/CD ladar.[5]

Receiver design is very important in direct detection systems. The SNR is maximized by achieving shot noise limited operation. This is accomplished by using high gain, low noise APDs and/or high impedance preamplifiers. Large m (avalanche gain) and R_0 (photodetector load resistance) values have the effect of decreasing the thermal noise relative to the shot noise as seen in the S/N_0 equations of Table 1. The m=150 value assumed in this analysis is consistent with the performance of the best commercial Si APDs at 2 GHz. The APD alone did not provide enough gain to achieve shot noise limited detection so a high input impedance (5 kΩ) preamplifier (such as a transimpedance amplifier) was included to reduce the thermal noise.

Coherent detectors normally operate in the shot noise limit because of the presence of a strong LO signal. For the high resolution ranging problem, where the receiver frequency resolution is small compared to the laser linewidth, phase noise is the dominant noise source. In both cases, the dominant shot or phase noise cannot be reduced by employing a high gain APD or high impedance preamplifier. Instead, the best receiver performance can usually be derived from a simple PIN photodiode operating into a 50 Ohm load.

Measurement Time

SNR is not the best figure of merit for evaluating ladar system performance because it does not account for such factors as the modulation bandwidth or frequency of the signal and the time required to make the range estimate, all of which are important for determining range accuracy. It is well known that extremely high range accuracy can be achieved with very low SNR given enough measurement time. Therefore, simply specifying the range accuracy and/or the SNR for a particular ladar system does not provide a useful figure of merit for its performance. A new figure of merit for high resolution ladars is proposed that will permit useful comparisons between systems.

The Cramer-Rao lower bound (CRLB) (which is the mean square error achievable in an optimal receiver) was used to derive an expression for the minimum time required to estimate the frequency of the FM/CD ladar heterodyne detector output in the presence of noise.[7] In a similar manner, the minimum time required to estimate the RF phase of the photodetector output was derived for the IM/DD ladar processor. These equations are shown in Table 1.

The estimation time equations have a inverse dependence on S/N_0 and an inverse squared dependence on modulation bandwidth or frequency. Therefore, the modulation bandwidth is actually more important than the SNR in evaluating system performance, which is a fact generally not emphasized in the field of ladar design. The form of the estimation relations suggests that, $\delta t \times \delta r^2$, be adopted as a figure of merit for high precision ladars, where δt is the measurement time and δr is the range accuracy. The consequence of the estimation relations is that even though FM/CD and IM/CD have approximately the same S/N_0 for the baseline component parameters over a target range out to 100 m, FM/CD is theoretically capable of much higher data rate operation because of the ability to chirp the laser over a much greater bandwidth than the high power IM/DD laser source can be intensity modulated (see discussion below).

The $1/(S/N_0)$ dependence of these equations means that it takes longer to estimate the range to a given accuracy at long target ranges where S/N_0 is small. This fact is demonstrated by the plot of Figure 7 showing increasing estimation time with range given a required range accuracy of 10 μm for both FM/CD and IM/DD ladars. The estimation time for direct detection exceeds that of coherent detection at all target ranges. The difference is a factor of two at 30 meters and a factor of ten at 100 meters when a 10 GHz chirp is employed for the FM source and a 2 GHz modulation frequency is used for the IM source. A second FM/CD curve is plotted to illustrate the performance leverage achieved by chirping over a larger bandwidth. It is important to note that chirp bandwidth limitations on high power line narrowed lasers are unknown (see discussion below). Also, there is little information on high frequency modulation limitations of directly modulated high power lasers. Despite these uncertainties, the high frequency modulation characteristics of diode lasers make them especially suitable as optical sources for high precision ranging.

Intensity Modulation

There are many different types of intensity modulation that can be considered. The simplest, CW intensity modulation, is very popular for applications in which relative rather than absolute range measurement is required. However, range ambiguities can be resolved at the cost of extra measurement time by switching modulation frequencies.[8]

Very wide modulation frequency (18 GHz) laser diodes have recently become commercially available although their output power is low (<15 mW). The maximum frequency of intensity modulation for high power broad stripe laser diode sources is not known. There is unpublished data suggesting a bandwidth of at least 2 GHz for a commercially available 100 mW device. It is in principle possible to externally modulate the intensity of a laser source over an extremely wide bandwidth. The problem has been that wide bandwidth (up to 30 GHz) external modulators such as those fabricated from $LiNbO_3$ and GaAs have high insertion loss and are limited to low power operation. Given the practical limitations on present day component performance, it is advantageous for reasons of system performance and cost to operate at less than 2 GHz where high gain APDs and high power laser sources can be employed.

Signal Processing

As discussed earlier, the target range is proportional to the phase of the I/Q demodulated output in the direct detection system of Figure 1a, while the range is proportional to the frequency at the output of the detector in the chirped system of Figure 1b. In order to eliminate DC offset drifts in the IM-CW direct detection system, the signal is offset using a digitally generated tone synchronous with and a submultiple of the sampling rate. An FFT is performed and the phase of the frequency component corresponding to the offset tone is used to estimate target range.

There exist a number of techniques for estimating the frequency of a received signal as necessary for the FM/CW system. Maximum likelihood estimation (MLE) is asymptotically efficient (that is, the mean square error approaches that predicted by the CRLB for sufficiently large SNR).[7] If the signal is coherently demodulated (in-phase and quadrature-phase components), and then digitally sampled, the optimal estimate of the frequency, $\hat{\omega}$, is that value of ω which maximizes:

$$\left| \sum_1 z_i \exp(j\omega t_i) \right|^2 \qquad (3)$$

where z_i is the data signal sampled at time, t_i. Several techniques exist for this maximization, the simplest of which is to use a padded FFT (although algorithms with fewer digital computations exist under certain conditions, they are beyond the scope of this summary). The data set is padded with zeroes to a time duration equivalent to the inverse of the desired frequency accuracy. Since the padding occurs in the digital hardware only, no additional "real time" is required. The magnitude squared of the FFT of the data sequence is computed and the maximum located. The frequency corresponding to the maximum is proportional to the range estimate. For this problem, the maximum likelihood frequency estimator provides the minimum mean square error for a given SNR compared to other estimator approaches. For a very low SNR, all estimation approaches will yield very poor estimates of frequency. The SNR for which an efficient estimator is within 1 dB of the CRLB of the mean square error is referred to as the threshold SNR. This is generally considered to be the minimum usable SNR. MLE results in the lowest threshold SNR when compared to other estimators. These factors may increase the range, reduce the signal power requirements, and/or relax the noise performance requirements of the hardware.

Component Parameter Uncertainties

Uncertainties in the performance of laser diode sources for IM/DD and FM/CD are listed below:

IM/DD

(1) High quality, narrow-stripe, single-mode laser diodes are commercially available to about 50 mW power levels. High quality broad-stripe lasers in the 100 mW to 1 W range are becoming commercially available, but are not generally single mode. It is expected that beam quality will be a problem for intensity modulated broad stripe lasers. There may be RF phase front variations in the beam for large modulation depth that produce a degradation in system performance.[9]

(2) The intensity noise of high power, broad-stripe diode lasers arising from spontaneous emission, mode competition, etc. is unknown, especially for the condition of large signal modulation. This parameter can limit the system SNR at the shorter target ranges.

(3) The highest achievable modulation frequencies of high power, broad-stripe lasers are not yet established. The fundamental limit on frequency modulation is the laser relaxation oscillation frequency. Other bandwidth limiting factors such as package parasitics can in principle be eliminated by better packaging and/or impedance matching.[10]

FM/CD

(1) It is unknown whether high power, broad-stripe laser diodes can be stabilized to linewidths of less than 10 kHz. Linewidth reduction has been achieved by the use of external optical cavities and/or electrical feedback.[5,11,12] External cavity stabilization may be subject to vibrational noise.

(2) Whether line-narrowed, high power diode lasers can be linearly chirped at the fast 1 kHz rates required for some high precision imaging applications has not been determined.[13] Furthermore, there is no information on the degree of linearity possible for high speed chirps.

(3) The maximum bandwidth of a repetitive high rate chirp produced by a line-narrowed laser has not been investigated. This parameter may be limited by laser or external cavity modes.

Conclusions

o This paper has presented a comparative analysis of FM/CD and IM/DD diode laser radars, as applied to high precision ranging measurements, in terms of the many component and application parameters that govern their performance.

o The results indicate that such ladars, based on lasers operating at 10-100 mW power levels, have the potential to achieve ranging accuracies of order 10^{-3} cm at operational ranges of 10-100 m or more, operating at data rates of 10-1000 pixels/sec or higher.

o The extremely high chirp bandwidth possible with coherent FM diode lasers provides the potential for much greater performance with FM/CD ladar than is currently attainable from IM/DD ladars operating at comparable power levels. For low laser power and/or long operational range, coherent detection also provides SNR advantages relative to direct detection.

o These advantages for the FM/CD approach require much higher laser coherence levels (narrower linewidth) and the means to simultaneously provide rapid wideband linear frequency modulation. These requirements have not been demonstrated.

o IM/DD ladars based on diode lasers operating at 100 mW to 1 W power levels also have the potential to provide high range accuracy and data rates for longer operational ranges of interest. The relative simplicity and lower cost of the required components for the IM/DD ladar makes this approach attractive for lower performance ladars using lasers with less than 100 mW power.

o Advanced laser development and evaluation will be required to demonstrate the higher performance levels for both IM and FM laser radars indicated in this study. These developments are being pursued by our group at the Boeing Electronics-HTC.

References

[1] K.G. Wesolowicz and R.E. Samrson, "Laser radar range imaging sensor for commercial applications," in Laser Radar II, Proc. SPIE 783, 152-161 (1987).

[2] "Eagle 3515-203 Technical Information Paper for a Precision Measurement System Based on Coherent Laser Radar" Product literature from Digital Optronics, Herndon, VA (1988).

[3] R.J. Keyes, "Heterodyne and nonheterodyne laser transceivers," Rev. Sci. Instrum. 57(4), 519-528 (1986).

[4] E. Brookner, Radar Technology, Chapter 24, Artech House Inc., Dedham, MA, (1977).

[5] R.G. Beausoleil, J.A. McGarvey, R.L. Hagman and C.S. Hong, to be published.

[6] K.Y. Lau and A. Yariv, "Ultra-High Speed Semiconductor Lasers," IEEE Journ. Quant. Elec. 21(2), 121-138 (1985).

[7] H.L. Van Trees, Detection, Estimation, and Modulation Theory, Part 1, John Wiley, New York, 1968.

[8] M.I. Skolnik, Introduction to Radar Systems, Second Ed., Chapter 3, McGraw-Hill, New York (1980).

[9] Private correspondence with W.D. Sherman of Boeing Aerospace.

[10] M. de La Chapelle, J.J. Gulick and H-P. Hsu, "Analysis of low loss impedance matched fiber-optic transceivers for microwave signal transmission," in High Frequency Optical Communication, Proc. SPIE 716, 120-125 (1986).

[11] M. Fleming and A. Mooradian, "Spectral Characteristics of External-Cavity Controlled Semiconductor Laser," IEEE J. of Quantum Elec., QE-17, 44-59(1981).

[12] M. Ohtsu and N. Tabuchi, "Electrical Feedback and its Network Analysis for Linewidth Reduction of a Semiconductor Laser," IEEE J. of Lightwave Tech. LT-6(3), 357-369 (1988).

[13] G. Economou, R.C. Youngquist and D.E.N. Davies, "Limitations and Noise in Interferomic Systems Using Frequency Ramped Single-Mode Diode Lasers," IEEE J. of Lightwave Tech. LT-4(11), 1601-1608 (1986).

FM-CW	IM-CW
$\delta t \, \delta r^2 = \dfrac{3c^2}{4\pi^2 (S/N_o) B^2}$	$\delta t \, \delta r^2 = \dfrac{c^2}{16\pi^2 (S/N_o) f_0^2}$

(a) Estimation relations

FM-CW	$\dfrac{m^2 r^2 P_R P_{LO} e^{-2\pi \Delta f t}}{e F_M m^2 [r(P_R + P_{LO} + P_B) + I_L + I_D] + \dfrac{2 K_B T}{R_o} + m^2 r^2 (P^2_{LO} + P^2_R) \text{RIN} + \dfrac{m^2 r^2 P_R P_{LO}}{\pi \Delta f} [1 - e^{-2\pi \Delta f t}(1 + 2\pi \Delta f t)]}$
IM-CW	$\dfrac{\tfrac{1}{2} (m P_R r M)^2}{e F_M m^2 [r(P_R + P_B) + I_L + I_B] + \dfrac{2 K_B T}{R_o} + (m r P_R)^2 \text{RIN}}$

(b) S/No (dB · Hz)

$P_R = \dfrac{P_o \varepsilon_a^2 \varepsilon_o^2 \rho}{\pi} \left[\dfrac{d_r}{R}\right]^2$	$P_B = \dfrac{\pi}{32} \, \rho \, \varepsilon_a \varepsilon_o H \, l_f \, \dfrac{d_s^2 \, d_r^2}{R^2}$

(c) Optical power relations

Constants
- K_B — Boltzmann's Constant — 1.38E-23 J/K
- c — Speed of light — 3.00E+08 m/s
- e — Electron charge — 1.60E-19 C

Environmental Parameters
- ε_a — One way atmospheric trans. — 1.00E+00
- T — Temperature — 3.00E+02 K
- H — Background irradiance — 1.00E-01 W/cm² μm

Target Parameters
- ρ — Target reflectance — 1.00E-01

Common Component Parameters
- l_f — Optical filter width — 1.00E-02 μm
- R_o — PD load resistance — 5.00E+03 Ohms
- d_s — Diameter of spot on target — 3.00E-01 cm

System Performance Parameters
- δr — Range accuracy — 1.00E-05 m

Laser Parameters		FM	IM
P	Average laser power	1.00E-01 W	5.00E-02 W
P_{LO}	Local oscillator power	1.00E-03 W	
RIN	Relative Intensity Noise	1.00E-16 1/Hz	1.00E-14 1/Hz
Δf	FWHM laser linewidth	1.00E+04 Hz	

PD Parameters		FM	IM
m	PD avalanche gain	1.00E+00	1.50E+02
F_M	PD avalanche noise	1.00E+00	5.00E+00
I_L	PD leakage current	0.00E+00 A	0.00E+00 A
I_D	PD dark current	5.00E-10 A	5.00E-10 A
r	Detector responsivity	4.50E-01 A/W	4.50E-01 A/W

Modulation Parameters		FM	IM
B	Laser chirp bandwidth	1.00E+10 Hz	
f_0	Modulation freq		2.00E+09 Hz
M	Modulation index		1.00E+00

Optics Parameters		FM	IM
d_r	Receiver aperature diameter	5.00E-02 m	5.00E-02 m
ε_o	One way opticl trans	5.00E-01	5.00E-01

(d) Analysis parameters

Table 1. Laser Radar Performance Relations and Design Parameters

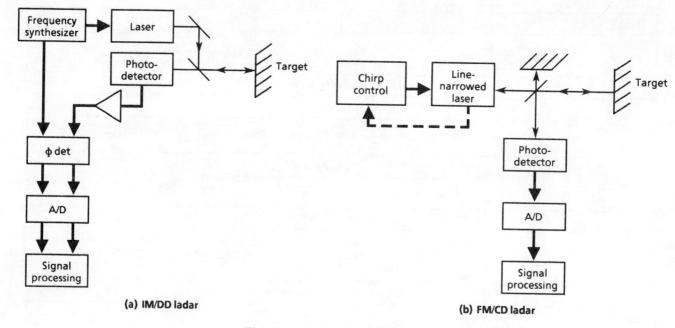

Figure 1. Ladar Block Diagrams

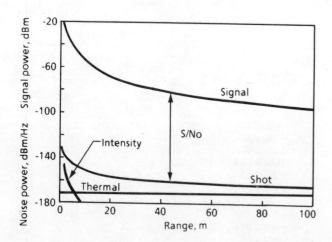

Figure 2. Ladar Signal and Noise Power Versus Range (IM/Direct Detection)

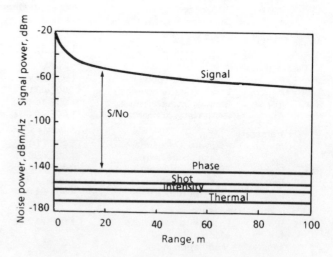

Figure 3. Ladar Signal and Noise Power Versus Range (FM/Coherent Detection)

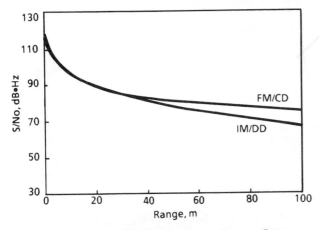

Figure 4. Ladar S/No Versus Target Range (IM/DD Versus FM/CD)

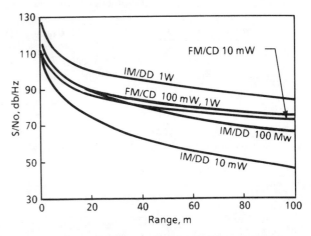

Figure 5. Ladar S/No Versus Target Range (IM/DD Versus FM/CD)

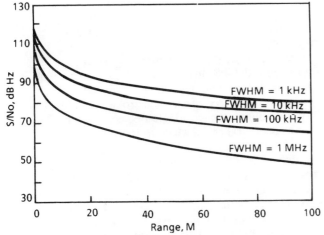

Figure 6. Ladar S/No Versus Range – Coherent FM Detection

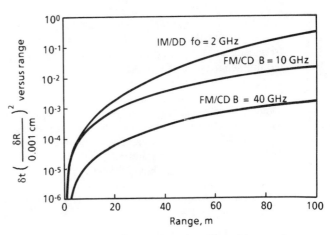

Figure 7. Ladar Estimation Time Versus Range (FM/CD Versus IM/DD)

Compound-cavity lasers for medium range lidar applications

D. A. Cohen, Z. M. Chuang, E. M. Strzelecki, and L. A. Coldren

Department of Electrical and Computer Engineering
University of California, Santa Barbara, California 93106

K. Y. Liou, and C. A. Burrus

AT&T Bell Laboratories
Holmdel, New Jersey 07733

ABSTRACT

Coupled-cavity tunable-single-frequency diode lasers are used in conjunction with an electronically tunable external cavity to increase the range of a coherent lidar system. Three-terminal DFB lasers and cleaved-coupled-cavity lasers are used which allow continuous wavelength tuning over a range greater than 2Å by direct modulation of the injection current. This tuning range results in a distance resolution of less than a centimeter, without signal averaging or other enhancement techniques. By using an electrooptic waveguide phase modulator in the external cavity we have maintained a narrowed laser linewidth while simultaneously tuning the solitary laser. We have achieved a coherence length of 50 meters, a tuning range of 40 GHz, and a simultaneous tuning range-coherence length product of 750 GHz-m.

1. INTRODUCTION

Narrow linewidth tunable-single-frequency lasers are needed for coherent communications, spectroscopy, interferometric sensor systems, and coherent light detection and ranging (lidar). This last application may be useful for robotic sensing, high resolution surface profiling, and fault detection in optical fibers. Presently, optical time domain reflectometry (OTDR), a form of incoherent lidar, is widely used for fault detection, but most OTDR techniques lack the resolution required for short range fiber systems such as might be installed in aircraft and ships. Optical frequency domain reflectometery (OFDR) using the frequency modulated continuous wave (FMCW) technique, can provide high resolution, but stringent requirements are placed on the laser light souces: continuous wavelength tunability over several Angstroms is required, and laser linewidths of the order of one megahertz are needed to obtain system ranges beyond one hundred meters. Additionally, tuning speed is important for lidar systems used in servo control loops, and some environments may place demands on system reliability. Monilithic tunable-single-frequency lasers have demonstrated an adequate tuning range, but have linewidths of 20-100 MHz, which restricts the range of a coherent system. Conversely, diode lasers used in conjunction with external cavities have demonstrated linewidths of tens of kilohertz, which would yield ranges above one kilometer; however, while these compound-cavity lasers have shown very wide discontinuous tunability, their range of continuous tuning has been limited. Some have also suffered from poor mechanical stability and inherently slow tuning. We have addressed these problems by using an electrooptic waveguide phase modulator in an external cavity with a tunable DFB laser operating at 1.3 microns to achieve continuous tunability over more than forty gigahertz (2.4 Å) while maintaining a linewidth below 7 megahertz, and have demonstrated a coherence length-tuning range product of more than 750 GHz-m. Furthermore, this compound-cavity laser does not have the inherent speed and reliability limitations of previously reported devices.

2. FMCW LIDAR

The FMCW technique has been described elsewhere[1,2]; we apply it to an all-fiber Michelson interferometer, as shown in Figure 1. We consider the simplest case of a linearly ramped optical frequency,

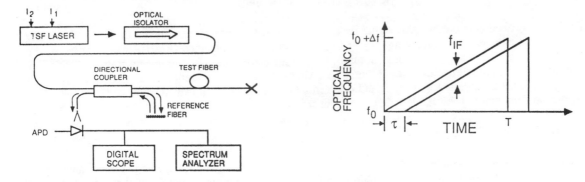

Figure 1. FMCW lidar

which in practice can be achieved by applying a sawtooth bias current to one section of a two-section semiconductor laser. During the sweep time T_s the laser angular frequency f is changed by Δf from the initial value f_0. Part of the signal is delayed by time $\tau = nL/c$ due to the path imbalance L in the interferometer, where n is the refractive index of the medium. After reflecting from the discontinuity in the test fiber, and from the mirrored end of the reference fiber, light at two different optical frequencies arrives at the square law detector and interferes, producing a heterodyne signal f_{IF} given by

$$f_{IF} = \tau \, \Delta f / T_s = nL\Delta f / cT_s. \tag{1}$$

If the tuning excursion of the laser is known and f_{IF} is measured, the distance to the fiber fault may be deduced. In the time domain, the number of cycles in the sinusoidal burst occurring during time $T_s - \tau$ is

$$N = f_{IF}(T_s - \tau) \cong nL\Delta f/c. \tag{2}$$

It has been assumed here that $\tau \ll T_s$. During the flyback time of the laser's tuning ramp, a heterodyne signal at a different (generally higher) frequency occurs, and would normally be gated out prior to signal analysis.

The spectrum of this heterodyne signal has been analyzed [3], and its character depends on the ratio of the path length to the coherence length of the laser, $L/L_c = \tau/\tau_c$. The spectral power density $S(\omega)$ is given by

$$S(\omega) \propto P_1 P_2 \frac{\tau_c}{1 + (\omega - \omega_{IF})^2 \tau_c^2} [1 - \exp(-\tau/\tau_c) \{ \cos(\omega - \omega_{IF})\tau + \frac{\tau}{\tau_c} \frac{\sin(\omega - \omega_{IF})\tau}{(\omega - \omega_{IF})\tau} \}] +$$

$$P_1 P_2 \exp(-\tau/\tau_c)(T_s - \tau) \frac{\sin^2[(\omega - \omega_{IF})(T_s - \tau)/2]}{(\omega - \omega_{IF})^2[(T_s - \tau)/2]^2} \tag{3}$$

where P_1 and P_2 are the optical powers in the two interferometer arms, $\omega_{IF} = 2\pi f_{IF}$, and τ_c is found from the time-average of the phase noise, $|\tau|/\tau_c = \langle(\phi(t) - \phi(t-\tau))^2\rangle$. The first term in (3) is the phase noise which arises due to the finite linewidth of the source. The second term is the inherent IF signal spectrum that arises due to the finite extent of the IF burst. The measured spectrum from the repetitive signal actually consists of lines separated by $2\pi/T_s$ under the envelope represented by this term. For $\tau \ll \tau_c$, the spectrum is as in Figure 2a. The inherent bandwidth limits the ability to separate two closely spaced frequency components, and thus limits the ability to distinguish between two closely spaced reflections. The FWHM of the center peak, Δf_{IF}, is approximately $1/T_s$. By inverting (1) and differentiating, we have

$$\Delta L = (cT_S/n\Delta f)(\Delta f_{IF}) = c/n\Delta f. \tag{4}$$

If only one reflection is present, this signal bandwidth does not present a fundamental limit in determining the center frequency; signal averaging may be used to obtain resolutions much greater than afforded by the FWHM of the IF signal. In the time domain, the distance resolution is limited by how well one can determine the number of cycles in the IF burst. If a simple zero-crossing method is used, this limit may be one cycle. Substituting this for N in (2) and differentiating, we find again that $\Delta L = c/n\Delta f$. However, for $\tau \ll \tau_c$, the IF signal will be stable enough to measure N to subcycle accuracy, and the resolution will be somewhat better than this "transform limit." This corresponds to measuring f_{IF} to an accuracy better than the FWHM of the IF spectrum.

Thus for the best distance-sensing resolution, a large tuning range is required. Very large tuning ranges have been achieved in lasers that tune by mode-hopping or a combination of continuous tuning and mode hopping. In these cases, the IF spectrum is cluttered with harmonics of the mode-hopping frequency. Such a spectrum is shown in Figure 3. In the time domain, even if the heterodyne frequency is the same from mode to mode, phase discontinuities appear in the sinusoidal burst and so the error in measuring N is multiplied by the number of mode hops that occur, and the resolution is degraded.

For the case of $\tau \ll \tau_c$, the signal-to-noise-ratio (SNR) of the system is determined by the amplitude of the center lobe of the heterodyne signal, and the instrumental noise floor. However, as τ approaches τ_c, this amplitude decreases and the phase noise of the laser begins to appear as an FM noise floor in the spectrum, as in Figure 2b. A narrow bandwidth filter must be used to separate the desired IF signal from the phase noise if a high-resolution measurement is desired, but in this case the decreasing IF amplitude results in a decreasing SNR. When the receiver bandwidth is much less than the laser linewidth, the SNR decreases exponentially as a function of τ/τ_c, or equivalently, SNR is proportional to $\exp[-L/L_c]$. Thus, a narrow linewidth is required for long range. When a very long time delay is used so that $\tau \gg \tau_c$, the phase noise term dominantes, and the spectrum becomes purely Lorentzian, as in Figure 2c; τ_c can be easily found from the 3-dB bandwidth. The coherence length is a good measure of the range of a lidar system; for a typical laser linewidth of 30 MHz, the range is then ~ 3 meters in air.

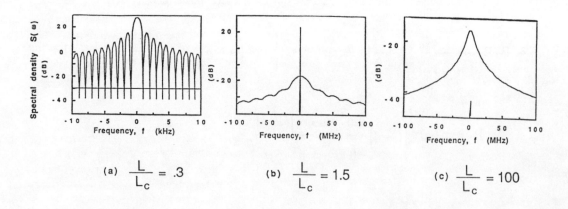

Figure 2. Heterodyne Signal Spectra for three different target distances.

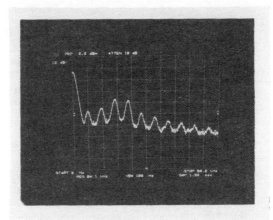

10 dB/div (Vert.)

0-50 KHz (Hor.)

Figure 3. Output spectrum showing deleterious effects of mode hopping.

3. SOURCES

Diode lasers are attractive because they may be tuned by direct modulation of the injection current, they are reliable, small, and relatively inexpensive. Special laser structures have been designed for optimized tunability, including cleaved-coupled cavity lasers and multielectrode DFB lasers. These have recently been reviewed by Kobayashi.[4] While these lasers are continuously tunable over ranges above 100 GHz, their coherence length is generally limited to 1-10 meters. It is well known that using an external optical cavity can significantly improve the coherence of diode lasers, and such methods have been used to achieve linewidths as low as 10 kilohertz. The simplest geometry is a fixed reflector, but because the cavity length is not tuned, as the laser is tuned the wavelength must cross the external cavity mode boundaries, and so the range of continuous tuning is limited to the external cavity mode spacing, $c/2l_{ext}$, where l_{ext} is the external cavity length. The tuning rate df/dI is reduced (chirp reduction), and the laser tunes by a combination of continuous tuning and mode hopping. As noted earlier, this reduces the resolution achievable in a lidar system. If the external reflector is mounted on a piezoelectric translator, the cavity length may be tuned synchronously with the laser; this shifts the mode boundary along with the laser wavelength and allows the compound cavity laser to tune as far as the solitary laser. The required change in the external cavity optical path length, $\Delta n l_{ext}$, is given by $(\Delta n l_{ext}/n l_{ext})=\Delta\lambda/\lambda$, where $\Delta\lambda$ is the change in the lasing wavelength λ. However, the PZT is nonlinear, and the tuning rate is limited to a few kilohertz by the PZT bandwidth. Also, external cavities formed with bulk optics may not be stable enough in practical environments. Alternatively, the optical path length may be tuned by incorporating an electrooptic material in the external cavity and varying the index of refraction n (by applying an electric field), rather than varying the length. Electrooptic waveguide phase modulators fabricated on lithium niobate substrates are available commercially with bandwidths above a gigahertz and may be obtained with a fiber-pigtail to allow compact, robust packaging with a laser.

4. EXPERIMENTAL

The laser diode used in this work was a two-section distributed feedback (DFB) laser made by fabricating separate contacts on a conventional DFB laser.[5] The electrically-isolated sections may then be pumped separately, and the Bragg wavelength of the gratings may be varied by individually modulating the injection currents. In our work, the laser was tunable over nearly 4 Å by varying one injection current from 5 mA to 45 mA; the laser linewidth was approximately 30 MHz at 3 mW power output from one facet, but increased to 80 MHz at low powers, partly due to the proximity to a mode boundary of the solitary laser at 5 mA.

The phase modulator was purchased from Crystal Technology Inc. (Palo Alto, Ca.), and was fabricated by diffusing a titanium waveguide into a $LiNbO_3$ substrate, and depositing electrodes along the side of the waveguide, as shown in Figure 4. The total crystal length was 5 cm, and the electrodes were 4.5 cm long. The facet nearest to the laser was cut at a ten degree angle to eliminate multiple reflections inside the waveguide, and also to prevent reflections from the front facet from returning to the laser. The absence of

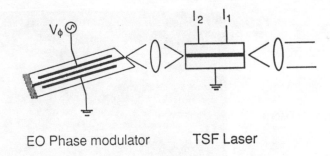

Figure 4. Electrooptically-tuned external cavity laser.

this parasitic cavity meant that the air space between the laser and the phase modulator did not itself require tuning. The facet furthest from the laser was metallized to provide a reflectivity of 90 percent. The voltage required to cause a 2π phase shift for a round trip in the waveguide was only 2 volts, and since the maximum safe voltage for the device was greater than +- 90 volts, nearly one hundred waves of phase shift was available. However, since the power supply we used was unipolar, we were only able to obtain fifty waves of phase shift. With a ten centimeter total cavity length, this still provided a tuning range of 2.4 Å.

The laser and external cavity were operated open-loop by applying tuning ramps to each. Because the laser did not tune linearly, the tracking between the lasing wavelength and the external cavity mode was not perfect, and eventually a mode hop would occur. It was found that mode-hopping could be easily observed as fluctuations in the optical power, and this provided a convenient method to observe the tracking between the laser and external cavity. The tuning range was obtained by measuring the heterodyne frequency in the interferometer when the path imbalance was known (50 cm). The laser coherence length was monitored by splitting the optical power and using a second fiber interferometer with a 6.4 km path imbalance to observe the Lorentzian phase noise spectrum. This allowed measuring the tuning characteristics and the coherence properties simultaneously, under dynamic tuning conditions.

A total tuning range without mode hopping of 2.4 Å (40 GHz) was obtained. The laser tuning was markedly nonlinear at the edges of the tuning ramp due to the thermal time constant of the laser and laser heat sink. It was found necessary to gate out the first 500 μsec to eliminate the effects of this nonlinear

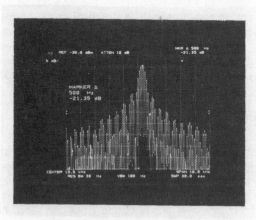
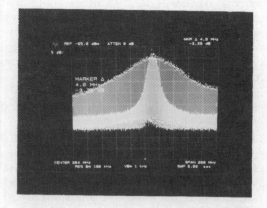

L = 0.5 m

5 dB/div (Vert.)
14-24 KHz (Hor.)

L = 6.4 km

5 dB/div (vert.)
164-364 MHz (Hor.)

Figure 5. Spectra with synchronous tuning

region from the signal spectrum. The heterodyne signal spectrum for a fiber length of 50 cm is shown in Figure 5a. The tuning range was 17 GHz, and the burst period T was 2 msec. The FWHM is found to be transform-limited at 500 Hz. This places an upper limit on the nonlinearity in the tuning ramp: from (1) the fractional tuning error $\Delta(\Delta f)/\Delta f$ equals the fractional error in the signal $\Delta f_{IF}/f_{IF}$. Since the experimental fractional error is less than the 500 Hz transform limit, and the center frequency is 19.3 KHz, the fractional nonlinear tuning must be less than 2.6%. When the burst length was increased to include the nonlinear portion at the beginning of the ramp, a broad low-frequency tail would appear in the spectrum, as expected from the reduced tuning rate during the thermal turn-around time. Figure 5b shows that the linewidth was mainatined at 4 GHz while the laser was tuned. The background trace shows the linewidth of the laser without the external cavity.

The best laser linewidth obtained <u>while tuning the laser</u> was two megahertz, which represents an improvement over the solitary laser by a factor of fifteen. However, this improvement could only be achieved for a tuning range of 4 GHz. Optimum linewidth reduction requires that an accurate phase condition be maintained in the external cavity, but the nonlinear tuning of the laser makes this difficult to achieve. Even when the tracking is adequate to prevent mode-hopping, it may not provide the best linewidth reduction. As the tuning range increases, the tracking becomes poorer. The linewidth increased to 6 megahertz at the extreme tuning range of 40 GHz. It should be noted that this is a result of the nonlinear properties of the laser, and not a fundamental limitation of the approach. The results over a range of tuning are shown in Figure 6, where the linewidth has been converted to coherence length in air and plotted on the horizontal axis. The tuning range for which this coherence length was obtained is plotted on the left, and the resolution $\Delta L = c/n\Delta f$ corresponding to this tuning range is plotted on the right.

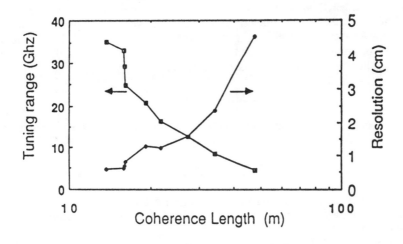

Figure 6. Tuning and coherence results.

4.DISCUSSION

We have demonstrated a ten-fold improvement in coherence under dynamic, continuous tuning using an external cavity. Other authors have achieved thousand-fold improvements, but their results were not obtained over wide tuning ranges or under dynamic conditions. More importantly, they were obtained by using a high-Q external resonator to provide frequency-selectivity. Tunable filters have been integrated onto lithium niobate substrates for this purpose[6], and linewidths below 100 KHz have been reported over discontinuous tuning ranges of 70 Å, although the continuous tuning range was limited to 1 GHz. It is reasonable to expect that by combining a similar filter with the phase shifter reported here that such linewidths could be obtained with continuous tuning over 40 GHz.

The nonlinear tuning response of the laser diode led to tracking difficulties which caused poor coherence, as well as mode-hopping and a broadened signal spectrum in extreme cases. Tuning linearity becomes critical when very high resolution is required. An obvious approach to improving the linearity is to use feedback control to linearize the laser response, and continue with open-loop tracking between the laser and the external cavity. To this end, we have used an auxiliary all-fiber Mach-Zehnder interferometer and a phase-locked-loop as a frequency discriminator to provide a feedback signal to the laser tuning current. Such a technique has been unsuccessfully attempted to stabilize the tuning of a lidar system using a solitary laser, but it was not intended as a means to improve the tuning linearity.[7] Our initial tests were with a C^3 laser that was exhibiting a +- 15% nonlinearity; when the feedback loop was closed, the nonlinearity was reduced to below +- 2.5%, which was the limit of our measurement accuracy. A second approach to improving the linearity, as well as the tracking, is to use a linearly-tuned external cavity, such as is provided with the EO phase modulator, and to lock the laser wavelength to the external cavity mode. This might be achieved with a feedback control loop that senses when the lasing wavelength is drifting away from the optimum phase. It has been shown that the optical power can be used as a control signal for such a loop under static conditions[8], but because the power fluctuations due to a phase mismatch are small compared to the power fluctuations that result from the tuning current ramp, we have not yet obtained closed-loop control. More advanced lasers that achieve tuning without power fluctuations may ease the problem.

5. SUMMARY

Tunable single frequency lasers with tuning ranges of greater than 2 Å and linewidths on the order of a megahertz are required for coherent detection systems including lidar. We have approached these goals by using an electrooptically-tuned external cavity in conjunction with a two-section 1.3 micron DFB laser, and have demonstrated that the coherence improvement can be maintained while tuning continuously over a significant range. To our knowledge, this is the first time such simultaneous tuning and coherence improvement have been reported. We have obtained a minimum linewidth of two megahertz, which corresponds to a coherence length in air of fifty meters, and we have obtained a maximum tuning range of forty gigahertz. While we have not simultaneously obtained the maximum coherence length and tuning range, we have obtained a coherence length-tuning range product of more than 750 GHz-meters. We believe that this combination of continuous tuning and coherence length compares well with the best results obtained to date with either monolithic or external cavity lasers.

6. ACKNOWLEDGEMENTS

This work was supported by the Boeing Electronics Company, and Tektronix Corporation under a UC-Micro grant.

7. REFERENCES

1. D. Uttam and B. Culshaw, "Precision time domain reflectometry in optical fiber systems using a frequency modulated continuous wave ranging technique," IEEE J. Lightwave Technol., vol. LT-3, pp. 971-977, (1985).
2. S. A. Kingsley and D. E. N. Davies, "OFDR diagnostics for fiber / integrated optic systems and high resolution distributed fiber optic sensing," Fiber Optic and Laser Sensors III Conf. Proc, SPIE vol. 566, pp. 265-275, (1985).
3. E. M. Strzelecki, D. A. Cohen, and L. A. Coldren, "Investigation of tunable single frequency diode lasers for sensor applications," IEEE J. Lightwave Technol., vol. LT-6, pp. 1610-1618, (1988).
4. K. Kobayashi and I. Mito, "Single frequency and tunable diode lasers," IEEE. J. Lightwave Technol., vol. LT-6, pp. 1623-1633, (1988).
5. N. K. Dutta, A. B. Piccirilli, T. Cella, and R. L. Brown, "Electronically tunable distributed feedback lasers," Appl. Phys. Lett., vol. 48, pp. 1501-1503, (1986).
6. F. Heismann, R. C. Alferness, L. L. Buhl, G. Eisenstein, S. K. Korotky, J. J. Veselka, L. W. Stultz, and C. A. Burrus, "Narrow-linewidth, electro-optically tunable InGaAsP-Ti:LiNbO3 extended cavity laser," Appl. Phys. Lett., vol. 51, pp. 164-166, (1987).
7. G. Economou, R. C. Youngquist, and D. E. N. Davies, "Limitations and noise in interferometric systems using frequency ramped single-mode diode lasers," IEEE. J. Lightwave Technol., Vol. LT-4, pp. 1601-1608, (1986).
8. L.A. Coldren, K.J. Ebeling, R.G. Swartz, and C.A. Burrus, "Stabilization and optimum biasing of dynamic-single-mode coupled-cavity lasers," Appl. Phys. Lett., vol. 44, pp. 169-171, (1984).

UTILIZING GaAlAs LASER DIODES AS A SOURCE FOR FREQUENCY MODULATED CONTINUOUS WAVE (FMCW) COHERENT LASER RADARS

Anthony R. Slotwinski
Digital Signal Corporation
8003 Forbes Place
Springfield, VA 22151
(703) 321-9200

Francis E. Goodwin
Digital Signal Corporation
8003 Forbes Place
Springfield, VA 22151
(703) 321-9200

Dana L. Simonson
Digital Signal Corporation
8003 Forbes Place
Springfield, VA 22151
(703) 321-9200

ABSTRACT

This paper describes the development of a Coherent Laser Radar utilizing a Frequency Modulated (FM) GaAlAs laser diode as an optical source. Both metrology (low speed, high accuracy) and vision (high speed, low accuracy) systems have been developed. Characteristics of presently available laser diodes important to this application are discussed, including coherence length, modal and tuning properties, and the effect of back reflected light on the laser diode's performance. Techniques to overcome current laser limitations are presented. These include an electronic linewidth narrowing scheme to enhance the coherence length of the source laser and thus the ultimate range of the radar, and the use of tuning linearization electronics. Finally, the impact of future laser diode technology, such as electronically tunable lasers, is discussed with respect to this application.

1.0 INTRODUCTION

The solution of many machine vision and automated manufacturing problems is simplified by the use of quickly acquired, accurate 3-dimensional data. For example, the ability of a machine to select and sort components in a factory environment or of an autonomous vehicle to avoid obstacles can be greatly enhanced by the use of a 3-D vision system. A precision 3-D measurement system can significantly reduce the labor intensive inspection time required for the testing of large precision structures, such as microwave antennas and aircraft surfaces.

While 3-D imaging laser radar systems using pulsed or amplitude modulated sources and direct detection have been demonstrated and reported by others [1,2], the use of a frequency modulated (FM) GaAlAs laser diode source in a coherent mixing arrangement offers unmatched speed and precision advantages. The principle is similar to that of FMCW microwave radars.

2.0 CLR DEVELOPMENT

2.1 Concept Summary

The FMCW laser radar developed by Digital Signal Corporation [3,4] uses the relatively large tuning range of injection laser diodes to achieve greater precision than available with other techniques. As shown in Figure 1, the optical frequency of the laser is swept linearly as a function of time. This signal is

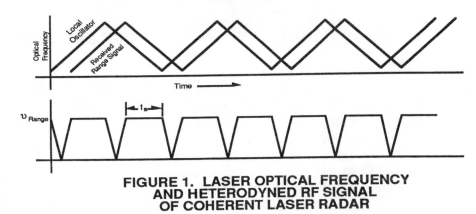

FIGURE 1. LASER OPTICAL FREQUENCY AND HETERODYNED RF SIGNAL OF COHERENT LASER RADAR

divided and used both as a local oscillator and as the signal to be transmitted. After being time delayed by the round trip transit time to the target, the received signal is mixed with the optical local oscillator on a photodetector. The resultant beat frequency is equal to the sweep rate of the optical signal multiplied by the time delay between the received signal and the local oscillator. Since this time delay is proportional to target distance, the RF beat frequency will be proportional to target distance.

Due to the short wavelength of the laser compared to a microwave source, a proportionally small frequency deviation results in a large beat frequency. For example, at an optical wavelength of 830 nm, a shift in wavelength of only 1 Angstrom (0.1 nm) results in a frequency shift of 43 GHz. This frequency modulation is accomplished by modulating the laser's injection current thereby thermally tuning the laser wavelength.

written:

$$\phi = \frac{2\pi}{\lambda}R = \frac{2\pi f}{c}R \quad (1)$$

As the source frequency changes over the interval Δf, the phase in the path changes by:

$$\Delta\phi = \frac{2\pi\Delta f}{c}R \quad (2)$$

The number of interference counts N detected is $\Delta\phi/\pi$. Solving for range R,

$$R = \frac{c}{2\Delta f}N \quad (3)$$

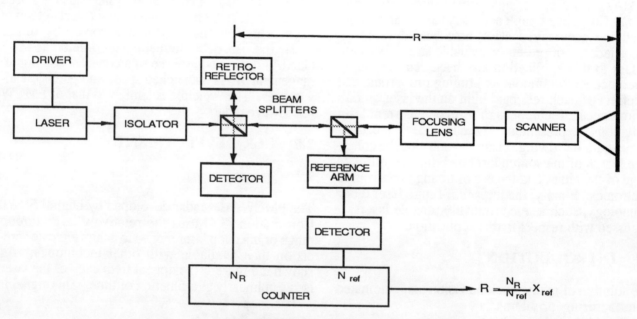

**FIGURE 2
COHERENT LASER RADAR BLOCK DIAGRAM**

The FMCW coherent laser radar (CLR) is illustrated in block diagram form in Figure 2. The FM source produces a continuous beam of optical radiation which is directed at the target as well as at the detector, interference beats are detected as the frequency is swept over the interval Δf. The rate of these beats is a function of the range as well as the magnitude of the sweep frequency rate. Referring to the block diagram of Figure 2, the phase over the path R can be

The precision of the measurement is determined by the uncertainty in counting N. With an averaged quantization error of 1/2,

$$\delta R = \frac{c}{4\Delta f} \quad (4)$$

Assuming a precision measurement of the frequency interval Δf, a single channel technique is valid. However, in an FMCW laser radar, the precise measurement of Δf is impractical.

Where high accuracy is important the laser radar uses a precisely known reference length to eliminate the need for direct measurement of the optical frequencies. A reference arm, consisting of a fiber optic Mach Zehnder interferometer, located within the radar optics housing and temperature regulated for stability, provides information to the counter necessary to make the range computation.

Figure 2 also illustrates the incorporation of the reference arm. In this system the reference signal and the ranging signal are counted separately, and the range is computed from:

$$R = \frac{N_r}{N_{ref}} X_{ref} \quad (5)$$

where X_{ref} is the reference path length.

Provided that the reference length is known precisely, the measurement precision achievable from the reference channel method is comparable to that of a single channel method with known Δf.

2.2 Current Capabilities

The time-precision product for the coherent laser radar is given by:

$$dR(\tau)^{3/2} = \frac{cR}{4\pi^{1/2}(d\nu/dt)d} \left[(NEP)_h \frac{\sigma}{P_L \rho} \right]^{1/2} \quad (6)$$

where :
- dR = measurement precision
- τ = measurement time
- R = target range
- dv/dt = laser frequency sweep rate
- d = antenna lens aperture
- $(NEP)_h$ = heterodyne noise equivalent power
- σ = threshold SNR
- P_L = laser power
- ρ = target reflectivity
- c = speed of light

A graph of the theoretical capability of the current CLR is given in Figure 3. Indicated in the graph is the operating point for the 3-D vision system which utilizes a 3.8 μsec laser chirp waveform to produce 262,144 measurement/sec with a 4 mm resolution. This system utilizes a facet wheel line scanner and a galvanometer frame scanner to produce a 256 x 256 pixel frame at 4 frames/sec.

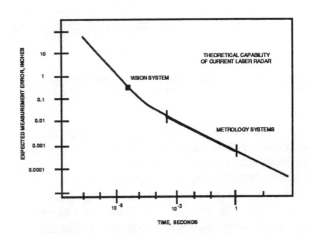

FIGURE 3 LASER RADAR PRECISION/TIME TRADEOFFS

In the case of the high precision metrology system, the laser is chirped at a rate of 10 KHz. To produce high accuracy measurements, multiple measurements are averaged. This averaging is indicated by the change in slope of the graph. The current implementation of the CLR metrology system achieves an RMS accuracy of 25 μm in a 0.1 sec measurement time. This is exclusive of the search time needed for the system to acquire a lock on a target via a linear translating autofocus unit. A 2-axis scanning mirror arrangement is used to position the beam at the target area of interest.

3.0 LASER DIODE PARAMETERS LIMITING SYSTEM PERFORMANCE

There are several parameters of currently available laser diode devices which limit the performance of the CLR. Of primary importance are coherence length, FM tuning, and sensitivity to back reflected light.

3.1 Coherence Length

Coherent implementation affords the Laser Radar significant advantages, but it also introduces a limi-

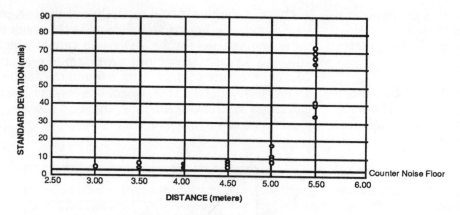

FIGURE 4. SYSTEM ACCURACY AS A FUNCTION OF DISTANCE

tation on the distances at which it can operate. To achieve coherent mixing the delay time between the target beam and the local oscillator needs to be less than the coherence time of the laser source. This means that the target distance must be less than one-half the coherence length. The effect of coherence length on system accuracy is shown in Figure 4. The figure shows the standard deviations of eight sets of 25 measurements taken with a CLR implemented using a Hitachi HL8314 laser diode as the source and a frequency counter-based receiver. The rapid decay of system performance after reaching a coherence limited range is a function of the interaction of the laser radar signal to laser phase noise ratio and the 12 dB SNR limit of the counter-based receiver.

3.2 Laser Mode Structure and FM Tuning

The coherent aspects of the CLR dictates that the source device remain in a single longitudinal mode

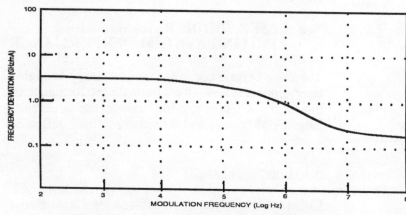

FIGURE 5. CHANNELED SUBSTRATE PLANAR LASER FREQUENCY DEVIATION RESPONSE

as it is being frequency modulated. Typically, currently available devices are limited to ~100 GHz tuning between mode hops at low modulation frequencies. Since it is the thermal tuning mechanism that is utilized to modulate the source, the thermal time constant (~1 μsec) of the devices limits both the degree and the linearity of the tuning. Figure 5 shows a typical frequency tuning response of a Hitachi HL8314 laser diode. The development of a laser drive waveform to linearly frequency modulate the laser at the measurement rates of the CLR must take in account both the laser's frequency deviation response and phase response [5, 6]. Laser drive waveforms have been developed which tune the laser over a 25 GHz range with no more than ± 150 KHz deviation from linear. Thus, a 300 KHz bandpass receiver is used in conjunction with a tunable filter to maximize the SNR.

These waveforms were made asymetric and the measurements taken only during the longer upsweep time of the waveform due to the difficulty in creating symetrical waveforms which tune the laser identically during both the upsweep and the downsweep. Combined with the fact that the tuning linearity breaks down near the turnaround points, the usable fraction of the waveform is only ~50% of the total waveform.

Figure 6 shows the SNR for three different Hitachi HL8314 diodes as a function of optical path length difference measured in a 300 KHz bandpass. The effective range of these devices with the current receiver is in the 4.5 - 6.0 meter area.

3.3 Back Reflected Light

The effect of back reflected light on a GaAlAs laser diode's modal structure is well documented [7-10]. Depending upon the intensity and phase of the back scattered light, the laser's linewidth can be narrowed or broadened, noise properties can change

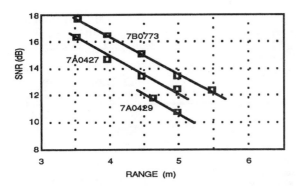

FIGURE 6. LASER RADAR SIGNAL TO NOISE RATIO FOR THREE DIFFERENT SOURCE LASERS

dramatically, and multimode operation may occur. These effects are detrimental to the operation of the coherent laser radar and, as such, optical isolators are employed to prevent them.

The tuning characteristics of a diode laser are especially sensitive to back scattered light. A total of ~90 dB isolation is needed to prevent reflection induced laser tuning nonlinearities from corrupting the measurement signal.

4.0 OVERCOMING LIMITATIONS

4.1 Optical Isolation

A diode laser is so sensitive to back reflected light that most commercial faraday isolators reflect sufficient light to corrupt the laser they are trying to protect. Any isolator used in the CLR must have a large aperture, use a crystal with very high optical transmission, and be housed with a material which has high absorption characteristics. The needed ~90 dB total isolation can include space loss and target reflectivity.

4.2 Waveform Linearization

In order to extend the linear region of the drive waveform, an adaptive measurment loop was created. The CLR diode was supplied with an approximately linear drive waveform. Then by allowing it to sweep, measuring the sweep linearity errors, and adjusting the waveform iteratively, maximum linearity is found automatically. A computer performs statistical analysis of the receiver frequency bins following each sweep waveform perturbance in order to determine which parts of the waveform cause deviation from sweep linearity.

Drive waveforms developed with this technique allow both a longer usable tuning range and a greater linear fraction of the total waveform. The percentage increase in both of these factors proprotionally improves the CLR system time-precision product.

Additionally, such a waveform linearization technique can be used to provide a symmetric waveform which sweeps the laser frequency identically in both directions. The advantages of such a waveform are twofold. First, the higher frequency components of the waveform retrace would be eliminated allowing a greater laser frequency excursion per sweep thus improving system accuracy and measurement time. Second, range errors due to the Doppler shift caused by any relative motion between the system and the target can be corrected since the Doppler shift will add to the measurement frequency in one sweep direction and subtract from it in the other direction. This Doppler shift can even be extracted to provide velocity information as well as range information.

4.3 Electronic Linewidth Narrowing

While superior receiver electronics will allow some improvement in the operating range of the CLR by permitting operation below the current 12 dB SNR limit, source devices with narrower linewidths (greater coherence lengths) can greatly extend this limit. Until such devices become commercially available, overcoming this limitation can be achieved by artificially enhancing the laser's coherence length.

Ohtsu and Kotajima [11] have reported electronic linewidth narrowing of a diode laser in a static (non-tuning) mode. We have achieved electronic linewidth narrowing using a rate-locking configuration which allows the laser linewidth to be reduced without impeding the FM tuning of the laser. The configuration used (Figure 7) incorporates a Bragg cell (Acousto-Optic Modulator) to upshift one path of the locking interferometer by 80 MHz. The laser was offset locked via an RF Oscillator to provide a radar signal of ~2 MHz/meter.

The laser linewidth was estimated from the SNR measurements. Figure 8 is a graph of the SNR versus Optical Path Length Difference (OPLD) for the locked and unlocked cases of an Hitachi HL8314 laser diode. The unlocked laser's coherence length is ~8 m. The locked laser, however, is seen to have a coherence length of 21 m or a factor of 2.6 improvement over the unlocked case. Conversely, the laser linewidth is also narrowed by a factor of 2.6 which

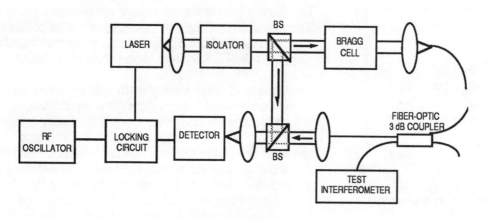

**FIGURE 7
LINEWIDTH REDUCTION TEST SET-UP**

is in reasonable agreement with a factor of 3 achieved in a previous static narrowing case.

5.0 FUTURE LASER RADAR TECHNOLOGY

The major obstacle to increasing the range capability of the CLR is the coherence length of the laser diode source. As devices exhibiting a narrower natural linewidth become available, a proportional extension in the range capability will occur. With such devices, electronic linewidth narrowing becomes less difficult to achieve due to the smaller locking circuit bandwidth involved. Thus, it is conceivable that a CLR system employing an artificially linewidth narrowed device can achieve measurement ranges beyond 100 meters.

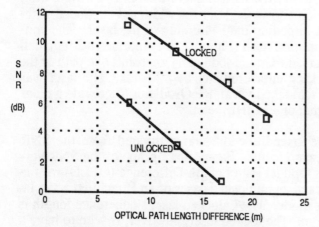

FIGURE 8. COMPARISON OF LOCKED AND UNLOCKED RADAR SIGNAL TO NOISE

Another important constraint to the CLR system performance is the laser tuning range and tuning rate currently available. The present CLR measurement systems are limited to tuning rates on the order of 24 GHz/µsec due to laser modal instability and thermal time constant. However, electronically tunable devices incorporating a phase shifting section in the laser structure have been reported to tune over 50Å [12, 13]. Since they are not limited by the thermal time constant of the laser, the frequency deviation response of these lasers remains constant for all modulation frequencies. Simpler drive waveforms can be used to tune these lasers over a wider range at greater speeds. Tuning 50 Å at the present rates will provide a time/precision improvement of ~100 for the metrology system (25 µm in 1 msec).

6.0 CONCLUSIONS

A coherent laser radar (CLR) utilizing a frequency modulated (FM) GaAlAs laser diode as an optical source has been described. Both metrology and vision measurement systems have been developed.

The coherence lengths of commercially available laser diodes limits the range of these systems to ~5 meters, and the modal and tuning properties of these lasers limit the accuracy to 4 mm (0.157") in a 3.8 µsec measurement time for the vision system and 0.025 mm (0.001") in a 0.1 sec measurement time for the metrology system.

A electronic linewidth narrowing technique was described which increased the effective laser coherence length by a factor of 2.6 thus allowing longer range systems.

Finally, it was shown that, as electronically tunable lasers become available, the time/precision tradeoff for these systems will improve by more than an order of magnitude.

7.0 ACKNOWLEDGMENTS

The authors are grateful to Bonnie Rogers and Mark Edwards for their help in the production of this paper.

8.0 REFERENCES

[1] Besl, P. J., "Active Optical Range Imaging Sensors," *Machine Vision and Applications*, Vol. 1, pp. 127-152, 1988.

[2] Binnger, N. and Harris, S. J., "Applications of Laser Radar Technology," *Sensors*, Vol. 4, pp. 42-44, 1987.

[3] Goodwin, F.E., "Coherent Laser Radar 3-D Vision Sensor," *Proceedings Sensors '85 Conference*, 1985.

[4] Hersman, M., Goodwin, F., Kenyon, S., and Slotwinski, A., "Coherent Laser Application to 3-D Vision," *Proceedings Vision '87 Conference*, pp. 3-1 thru 3-12, 1987.

[5] Clark, George L., Heflinger, Lee O., and Roychoudhuri, Chandrasekhar, "Dynamic Wavelength Tuning of Single-Mode GaAlAs Lasers," *IEEE Journal of Quantum Electronics*, Vol. QE-18, No. 2, February 1982, pp. 199-204, 1982.

[6] Welford, David, and Alexander, Stephen B., "Magnitude and Phase Characteristics of Frequency Modulation in Directly Modulated GaAlAs Semiconductor Diode Lasers," *Journal of Lightwave Technology*, Vol. LT-3, pp. 1092-1099, 1982.

[7] Lang, R. and Kobayashi, K., "External Optical Feedback Effects on Semiconductor Injection Laser Properties," *IEEE Journal of Quantum Eletctronics*, Vol. QE-16, pp. 347-355, 1980.

[8] Golberg, L., Taylor, H.F., Dandridge, A., Weller, J.F., and Miles, R.O., "Spectral Characteristics of Semiconductor Lasers with Optical Feedback," *IEEE Journal of Quantum Electronics*, Vol QE-18, pp. 555-563, 1982.

[9] Lenstra, D., Verbeek, B.V., and denBoef, A.J., "Coherence Collapse in Single-mode Semiconductors Lasers due to Optical Feedback," *IEEE Journal of Quantum Electronics*, Vol QE-21, June 1985.

[10] Henry, C.H., and Kazarinov, R.F., "Instability of Semiconductor Lasers due to Optical Feedback from Distant Reflectors," *IEEE Journal of Quantum Electronics*, Vol. QE-22, pp.294-301, 1986.

[11] Ohtsu, M., and Kotajima, S., "Linewidth Reduction of a Semiconductior Laser by Electrical Feedback," *IEEE Journal of Quantum Electronics*, Vol. QE-21, pp. 1905-1912, 1985.

[12] Westbrook, L.D., Nelson, A.W.,Fiddyment, P.J., and Collins, J.B., "Monolithic 1.5 µm Hybrid DFB/DBR Laser with 5 nm Tuning Range," *Electronic Letters*, Vol. 20, pp. 957-959, Nov. 1984.

[13] Kobayashi, K., and Mito, I., "Single Frequency and Tunable Laser Diodes," *Journal of Lighwave Tech.*, Vol 6, pp. 1623-1633, 1988.

Invited Paper

Novel Device Functions and Applications of
Two-Electrode Distributed Feedback Lasers

K.-Y. Liou

AT&T Bell Laboratories
Crawford Hill Laboratory
Holmdel, New Jersey 07733

ABSTRACT

By splitting the electrical contact of a conventional distributed feedback (DFB) laser into two sections, the frequency tuning characteristics of the DFB laser are modified and the DFB two-mode degeneracy becomes electrically controllable. As a result, novel device functions can be achieved. Several applications of two-electrode DFB lasers are described: (1) active single-mode stablization, (2) control of spectral reliability and wavelength chirp under amplitude modulation, (3) logic gate operations utilizing the DFB two-mode degeneracy for switching, routing, and optical computing, and (4) frequency modulation of the DFB laser for FSK coherent communication systems and optical sensing.

1. INTRODUCTION

Distributed feedback (DFB) injection lasers are promising single-wavelength (frequency) sources for long-haul or high-bit-rate optical fiber transmission systems, where the effect of fiber dispersion should be suppressed. The lasers are also proposed for use as narrow-linewidth sources in coherent communication systems employing heterodyne detection methods. These applications require that the laser oscillate with a single longitudinal mode. Hence the main effort in the development of practical DFB lasers has been centered around single-mode stabilization.

One problem that degrades the single-mode stability of DFB lasers is the tendency to simultaneous oscillation at two degenerate DFB modes that have equal threshold currents. This two-mode degeneracy [1] is an intrinsic property of an axially symmetric DFB laser without facet reflections from both ends. In the general case when there are facet reflections, two-mode oscillations in DFB lasers occur with a statistic determined by the probability distribution of the positions of randomly cleaved facets relative to the grating corrugation [2].

By splitting the electrical contact on top of a DFB laser into two sections with separate currents applied to them, we have demonstrated that the two-mode degeneracy becomes electrically controllable [3]. The DFB laser can then be actively stabilized either as a single-wavelength source for conventional use or as a two-wavelength laser for new applications. Furthermore, the two wavelengths can be switched at speeds higher than 1 GHz for optical switching and logic gating [4]. Similar two-electrode operation can also increase the frequency modulation (FM) response of DFB lasers, which has been proposed for use in FSK coherent communication systems [5,6] and for heterodyne distance sensing. This paper discusses the various applications of two-electrode DFB lasers.

2. TWO-MODE DEGENERACY AND ELECTRICAL CONTROL WITH TWO-ELECTRODE DFB LASERS

The two-mode degeneracy of the DFB laser can be derived from the coupled-wave theory [1] of a periodic waveguide resonator. The optical feedback required for the lasing action in a DFB laser arises from the distributed Bragg scattering from the corrugated grating. Such a grating waveguide has a "stop band" centered at the Bragg wavelength, within which wave propagation is inhibited. The grating can be considered as a periodic structure that is conceptually analogous to a one-dimensional crystal, and the stop band of a DFB laser here corresponds exactly to the well known energy band gap of a crystalline solid [7]. Using the coupled-wave approach, the electric field of light propagating along the laser axis in z direction can be written as

$$E(z) = E_f\exp(i\beta z) + E_b\exp(-i\beta z)$$

where E_f and E_b are amplitudes of the forward and backward waves and β is the propagation constant. The corresponding coupled-wave equations are given by

$$\frac{dE_f}{dz} = ikE_b \exp(-2i\Delta\beta z)$$

$$\frac{dE_b}{dz} = -ikE_f \exp(2i\Delta\beta z)$$

where $\Delta\beta = \beta - \beta_{Bragg}$ and k is the coupling constant of the DFB grating. The solution leads to the dispersion relation

$$u = \pm[(\Delta\beta)^2 - k^2]^{1/2}$$

that determines the possible wave number u in the DFB resonator. We note that u is pure imaginary if $-k < \Delta\beta < k$, for which wave propagation is prohibited. Therefore the width of the stop band equals $2k$. In this symmetrical case, the lowest order resonances are located one on each side of the stop band and have equal lasing threshold [1].

Since k is determined from the periodic index variation of the DFB grating and is independent of the length of the laser, the width of the stop band can be preselected by controlling the grating profile and the waveguide layers. The effect of facet reflections can be suppressed by applying anti-reflection coatings.

Figure 1 shows a longitudinal mode spectrum recorded for a DFB laser operating below threshold. The spectrum clearly shows a stop band of 20Å width and the two degenerate DFB modes, λ_{-1} and λ_{+1}, separated by the stop band. Equal intensities of these two modes in the figure indicate that the two modes have the same mode gain. Above threshold, the λ_{-1} and λ_{+1} modes oscillate simultaneously.

Two-electrode control of the DFB laser is relatively simple. Figure 2a shows a schematic diagram of the two-electrode DFB laser. The separate electrodes are produced by conventional photolithography and the conducting p layers between the two contacts are partially etched away to produce an electrical isolation of about 100 Ohms. The separation between the two contacts is about 25 μm. The two-electrode lasers discussed here are of the SIPBH (semi-insulating planar buried heterostructure) type with a first-order grating, which we have reported previously [3,4]. Non-uniform excitations in the two sections by varying the two injection currents, I_1 and I_2, introduces asymmetry into the laser and removes the two-mode degeneracy [3]. Figure 2b shows the CW lasing spectra of a two-electrode laser when the two currents, I_1 and I_2, are adjusted. The laser can be controlled to oscillate at either the λ_{-1} mode or the λ_{+1} mode, or both together. The power distribution between the two modes changes continuously from λ_{-1} to λ_{+1}, without hysteresis, when either I_1 or I_2 is varied. The current changes, in either I_1 or I_2, required for complete mode switching are typically less than 10 mA. This method can be applied to lasers with randomly cleared facets, and the length ratio L_1/L_2 is not critical.

3. ACTIVE SINGLE-MODE STABILIZATION AND CHIRP CONTROL UNDER AMPLITUDE MODULATION

Single mode control in two-electrode DFB lasers requires relatively non-critical adjustment of the two applied currents. Also, we will see that the effect of temperature change is insignificant because the DFB two-mode degeneracy is a temperature independent property. Thus the two-electrode laser may provide a viable alternative to the 1/4-wavelength shifted DFB laser [8] or the asymmetric facet reflectivity DFB structure [2] for single DFB mode operation. Wavelength chirp under amplitude modulation has also been measured, and we show that chirp can be reduced by using a filtered wavelength modulation method.

Figure 3 shows the spectral property of the laser of Fig. 2b characterized on a I_1/I_2 map. The measured threshold curve and the mode switching boundary, where the λ_{-1} and λ_{+1} mode have equal intensities, are plotted. The changes in I_1 or I_2 required for complete mode switching are shown by the horizontal and vertical bars at two data points in the figure. Outside of this mode switching band, the laser oscillates with a single mode with side mode suppression greater than 30 dB.

Figure 4 shows the I_1/I_2 characteristics for another laser measured at 15 °C, 23 °C, and 40 °C. The lasing threshold increases with temperature as usual, but the two-mode operation line remains nearly unchanged. In an ideal symmetrical DFB laser, two-mode oscillation occurs along the $I_1 = I_2$ line (or more precisely, $I_1/L_1 = I_2/L_2$) where the laser is uniformly pumped. Mode switching occurs when the two sections are unequally pumped (most effectively, along the $I_1 + I_2 =$ constant line). This characteristic is true at all temperatures.

With cleaved facets, however, the I_1/I_2 maps are different for different lasers. This is simply due to reflections from the randomly cleaved facets that shift the mode switching boundary away from the $I_1 = I_2$ line by the grating/facet phase effect. Material non-uniformity can also vary the I_1/I_2 map among lasers. With these complications, however, large single-mode regimes on the I_1/I_2 plane are still observed, and nearly all two-electrode DFB lasers can be controlled to operate with a single mode.

The I_1/I_2 maps can be used for DFB laser screening. Two-electrode DFB lasers with a large single-mode regime on the I_1/I_2 map can be selected and set to operate at a distance from the two-mode boundary to assure long-term single-mode operation with margin for laser degradation. On the contrary, a conventional single-electrode DFB laser can operate only along the $I_1/L_1 = I_2/L_2$ line without active control.

Wavelength chirp under amplitude modulation (AM) is dependent on the current modulation path on the I_1/I_2 plane. Figure 5 shows the chirp width at 20 dB down from the peak measured for a two-electrode DFB laser under pseudorandom pulsed operation. The laser was pulsed from near threshold to 5 mW output by splitting the applied current at different I_1/I_2 ratios. Chirp is minimum when the laser is pulsed along $I_1 = I_2$. It increases when I_1/I_2 deviates from unity. The increased chirp in the latter case is related to an increased FM modulation efficiency, which is discussed in section 5 for FM applications. The results in Fig. 5 show that the chirp width is less than 3 Å for modulation up to 5 Gbit/s.

Chirp can be reduced significantly by using a different modulation method, in which the laser output is switched between the λ_{-1} and λ_{+1} mode and a wavelength filter that passes only one mode is used to convert the wavelength modulation to amplitude modulation. This method is similar to that used previously for a cleaved coupled cavity laser [9]. Since a small modulation current (only a few mA) is necessary for switching between the two DFB modes, the measured chirp due to current modulation was reduced to less than 1 Å at 3 Gbit/s using this method. This result is attractive when the DFB laser is used as a single-mode AM source for direct-detection optical fiber transmission systems.

4. OPTICAL SWITCHING AND LOGIC GATING

The unique two-mode DFB laser degeneracy can be used for optical switching, routing, wavelength division multiplexing, and logic gating. The two wavelengths are switched by electrical signals applied to the two electrodes, and light pulses containing the two wavelengths can be multiplexed or demultiplexed into different fiber lines. We describe here the general case of a complete set of AND, OR, NAND, NOR, and INVERT logic gate operations that we have demonstrated for information processing [4].

The schematic diagram in Fig. 6 illustrates how electro-optical logic operations can be performed. The solid line is the mode switching boundary on the I_1/I_2 plane. The laser is dc biased at the (00) point. The vectors, (10) and (01), represent the current signals applied to I_1 and I_2, respectively. When the output light powers of the two modes are separated by a wavelength filter and a photodiode is used to detect either the λ_{-1} or the λ_{+1} mode, logic operations shown in Fig. 6 can be obtained.

The oscillograms in Fig. 7a show the applied signals and the operations of AND and OR gate with a two-electrode DFB laser by detecting the λ_{-1} mode as illustrated in Fig. 6. Figure 7b shows, similarly, the operations of NOR, NAND, and inverted $I_1 \cdot I_2$ gates by detecting the λ_{+1} mode. The inverted $I_1 \cdot I_2$ gate was done by setting the (00) bias point below threshold and pulsing the laser with logical signals such that only the (01) point is in the λ_{+1} mode. The laser with the I_1/I_2 map in Fig. 3 was used for this demonstration, and a diffraction grating was conveniently used as a filter to separate the two wavelengths. A switching time of 400 psec, limited by the speed of the electrical signal, was demonstrated [4].

5. FM CHARACTERISTICS AND APPLICATIONS TO COHERENT SYSTEMS AND OPTICAL SENSING

The two-electrode DFB laser is attractive for use as a tunable local oscillator or as an FM transmitter for coherent detection systems. Here the DFB laser is used as a single-mode source, but the frequency (wavelength) tuning efficiency is increased by unequal carrier injections into the two sections.

Frequency shift results from refractive index change due to carrier injection by the plasma effect [10]. Carrier injection also increases the gain coefficient, which again varies the refractive index through the Kramers-Kronig relation [10]. The FM efficiency can be increased by using one of the two laser sections as a modulator, which is kept at a low injection level to avoid carrier or gain saturation due to stimulated emission.

Continuous wavelength tuning over 20Å has been reported by Yoshikuni et al for a two-electrode DFB laser [11]. Typically, we can obtain a tuning range of only about 5 Å. This is in agreement with theoretical modeling by Kuznetsov [12]. A broader tuning range may be possible if the Bragg wavelength is detuned to the longer wavelength side of the gain peak to obtain a large linewidth enhancement factor [13,14].

Figure 8 shows the measured FM response of a typical two-electrode SIPBH DFB laser, whose I_1/I_2 characteristic is shown in Fig. 4. The laser is biased at $I_1 = 60$ mA and $I_2 = 18$ mA at 20°C with a 6 mW output from the I_1 side. The FM modulation current was added to I_2, which resulted in negligible AM of the output from the I_1 side. A flat FM response of 3 GHz/mA was obtained, with comparatively negligible temperature modulation at low frequency ($\lesssim 1$ MHz). The high frequency roll off is due to the injected carrier life time.

The observed FM behavior is typical of a composite-cavity laser with two optically coupled active sections [15-17]. It can be analyzed using coupled rate equations for the optical fields and carrier densities in the two sections. The modulation condition of Fig. 8 is optimized for FM applications. If the modulator bias $I_2 \simeq 0$, it becomes an absorber and may introduce bistability. If $I_2 \simeq I_1$, the laser is uniformly pumped and the FM response reduces to that of a standard single-contact DFB laser.

The two-electrode SIPBH DFB lasers have been used as an FM source in FSK coherent lightwave systems [18]. Other than as a broadband FM source, the flat FM response at low frequency can be particularly interesting for heterodyne distance sensing [19]. For this application, the optical frequency of the laser is swept by current modulation at a known frequency, and the returning light reflected from a distant object is heterodyned with the immediate laser output. The heterodyned beat frequency and the source FM frequency then determine the distance of the object.

6. CONCLUSIONS

The properties of the two-electrode DFB laser we have reviewed here illustrate the potential of the DFB laser for various applications as a conventional single-mode source or as a two-wavelength laser. The DFB two-mode degeneracy, which has always been considered as a problem for single-mode operation, is resolved using the two-electrode control method. Furthermore, while this active control can be used simply to stablize the laser output in a single mode, it can also be used to switch rapidly between the two DFB degenerate modes. The single-mode stabilization, chirp control, wavelength division multiplexing, optical routing, logic gate operations, heterodyne FSK communication, and optical sensing that we have discussed, can all be realized by simply splitting the electrode of a conventional uniform-grating DFB laser into two contacts.

REFERENCES

1. H. Kogelnik and C. V. Shank, J. Appl. Phys. 43, 2327 (1972).
2. W. Streifer, R. D. Burnham, and D. R. Scifres, IEEE J. Quantum Electron. QE-11, 154 (1975).
3. K.-Y. Liou, C. A. Burrus, U. Koren and T. L. Koch, Appl. Phys. Lett. 51, 634, (1987).
4. K.-Y. Liou, C. A. Burrus, U. Koren and T. L. Koch, Appl. Phys. Lett. 51, 1777 (1987).
5. Y. Yoshikuni and G. Motosugi, page 32, Proc. 9th Conf. Optical Fiber Communication, Atlanta, GA. 1986.
6. Y. Yoshikuni and G. Motosugi, J. Lightwave Technol. LT-5, 516 (1987).
7. S. Wang, IEEE J. Quantum Electron. QE-10, 413 (1974).
8. K. Utaka, S. Akiba, K. Sakai, and Y. Matsushima, IEEE J. Quantum Electron. QE-22, 1042 (1986).
9. W. T. Tsang, N. A. Olsson, R. A. Logan and R. A. Linke, Electron. Lett., 19, 341 (1983).
10. G. H. B. Thomson, "Physics of Semiconductor Laser Devices", John Wiley & Son, 1980, p. 535.
11. Y. Yoshikuni, K. Oe, G. Motosugi, and T. Matsuoka, Electron. Lett. 22, 1153 (1986).
12. M. Kuznetsov, IEEE J. Quantum Electron. QE-24, 1837 (1988).
13. C. H. Henry, IEEE J. Quantum Electron. QE-18, 259 (1982).
14. K.-Y. Liou, E. C. Burrows, and N. K. Dutta, page 218, Technical Digest, Conf. Lasers and Electro-Optics, Baltimore, 1987.
15. S. Yamazaki, K. Emura, M. Shikada, M. Yamaguchi, and I. Mito, Electron. Lett. 21, 283 (1985).
16. S. Yamazaki, K. Emura, M. Shikada, M. Yamaguchi, I. Mito, and K. Minemura, Electron. Lett. 22, 5 (1986).
17. C. Y. Kuo and N. K. Dutta, Electron. Lett. 24, 947 (1988).
18. L. J. Cimini, I. M. I. Habbab, S. Yang, A. J. Rustako, K.-Y. Liou, and C. A. Burrus, Electron. Lett. 24, 358 (1988)
19. L. A. Coldren, private communication.

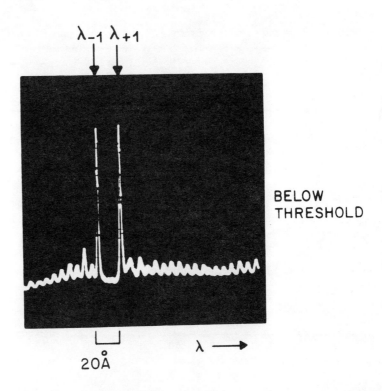

Fig. 1. Spontaneous emission spectrum of a 1.3 µm DFB laser showing the DFB stop band and two-mode degeneracy.

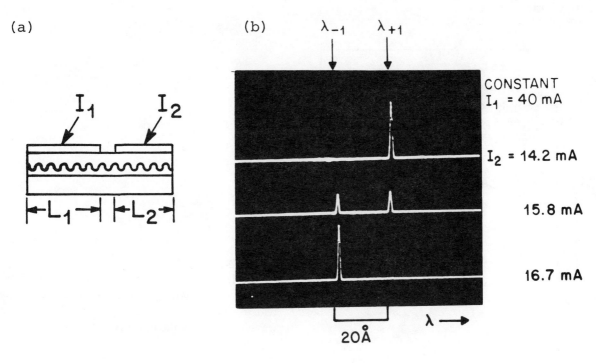

Fig. 2. (a) Schematic diagram of a two-electrode DFB laser. (b) Lasing spectra showing electrical control of the two modes, λ_{-1} = 12960Å and λ_{+1} = 12980Å.

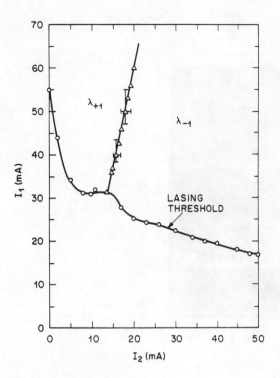

Fig. 3. I_1/I_2 Characteristic of the laser of Fig. 2 ($L_1 = 178\ \mu m$, $L_2 = 133\ \mu m$). Required current changes in I_1 and I_2 for complete mode switching are shown by the vertical and horizontal bars.

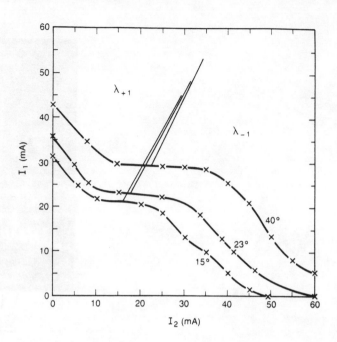

Fig. 4. I_1/I_2 maps for a two-electrode DFB laser ($L_1 = 210\ \mu m$, $L_2 = 200\ \mu m$) showing negligible temperature effect on mode switching boundary.

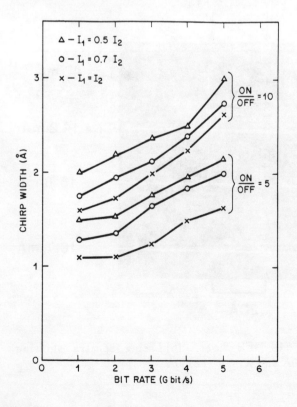

Fig. 5. Measured chirp width for a two-electrode DFB laser ($L_1/L_2 = 1.1$) under direct current modulation with different I_1/I_2 ratios. Chirp reduced to $\lesssim 1$ Å using the filtered wavelength-modulation method.

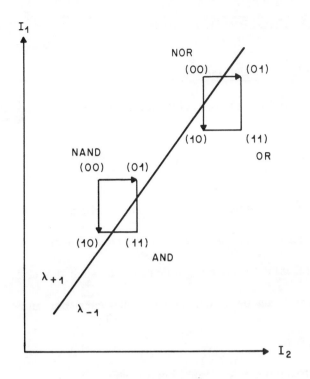

Fig. 6. Schematic diagram illustrating logic operation using two-electrode DFB laser.

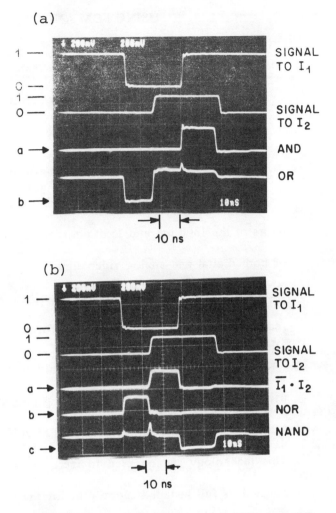

Fig. 7. Oscillograms showing (a) AND and OR gate operations, and (b) NOR, NAND, and inverted $I_1 \cdot I_2$ operations.

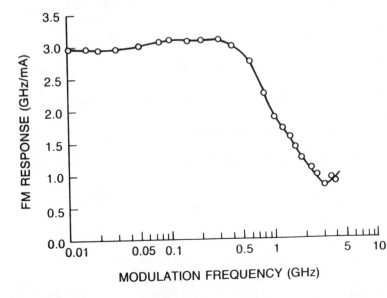

Fig. 8. Frequency modulation response of a two-electrode DFB laser.

SEMICONDUCTOR LASER-BASED MULTI-CHANNEL ANALOG VIDEO TRANSMISSION USING FDM AND WDM OVER SINGLE MODE FIBER

P.S. Natarajan, P.S. Venkatesan, C.W. Lundgren and Chinlon Lin *

BELLCORE, Red Bank, New Jersey 07701 and *Morristown, New Jersey 07960.

Improved, yet cost-effective laser-based analog video transmitters are required for single mode fiber for video distribution to subscribers. Both Fabry-Perot and DFB lasers in the 1300 nm and 1550 nm regions are commercially available which facilitate transmission of both digital and analog video signals. Three representative system applications of such devices explored recently by Bellcore are described with emphasis on desirable laser characteristics and requirements which govern overall performance.

First, an FM electrically multiplexed multichannel television fiber overbuild technology using Wavelength Division Multiplexing (WDM) for the simultaneous transmission of a digital 405 Mbps channel at 1300 nm and several FM video channels at 1550 nm on the same fiber is discussed. This technology can be used to increase the bandwidth utilization of the optical fiber that has reached its full installed capacity or for the overbuild of analog services on a fiber presently used for digital transmission and vice-versa. Inexpensive fusion-type WDM couplers, injection lasers and DFB lasers are used in this application. It was found that for a three video channel overbuild, using Pulse Frequency Modulation (PFM) for transmitting video, an injection laser performed satisfactorily over a 20 km standard single mode fiber in spite of the high dispersion at 1550 nm. When large numbers of channels had to be transmitted, (eight in this case), Frequency Modulation (FM) was used to transmit the video signals (the wide-spectrum square-wave shape of the PFM signal limited its use to a few channels; multiplexing several heavily-filtered PFM channels results in a degradation of PFM performance to that of FM). In this case a narrow-spectrum DFB laser had to be used to overcome the large dispersion at 1550 nm in a fiber optimized for zero dispersion at 1300 nm, to obtain "entertainment" quality multichannel video over distances of approximately 25 km.

The second representative application involves electrical FDM of a baseband digital data channel and a PFM video signal on the same laser (same wavelength) for transmission on one single mode fiber. This is a variation of typical FDM, where-in two or more electrical signals separated in frequency are combined resistively for transmission over a common medium. In this case, a fixed bandwidth allocated in the low-end of the electrical spectrum is reserved for the digital baseband signal, which is band-limited (by passing the baseband signal through a low-pass filter network before the FDM process). The modulated analog video signal on a higher-frequency carrier is then electrically multiplexed with the filtered digital baseband signal for transmission over one fiber. Bellcore Technical Advisory, TA-TSY-000 758,"Customer Controlled DS3/PFM Video with Audio Bridging", outlines Bellcore's view on the preliminary technical requirements on transmitting a baseband DS3-rate video signal, a PFM video signal, and a Quadrature Amplitude Modulated DS1-rate data channel over a single mode fiber. The principal requirements on the laser transmitter for such applications are (1) sufficient linearity is required over the modulation bandwidth and (2) the laser transmitter should have a good low-frequency response to transmit the baseband digital signal. The same concepts can be extended to include higher baseband digital data rates and upgraded television channels such as HDTV.

The third application describes the use of WDM to multiplex closely spaced wavelengths for the analog transmission of full-bandwidth High Definition Television (HDTV) on one single mode fiber. In this application, highly selective WDM devices and lasers exhibiting long term stability are crucial to acceptable performance, suggesting temperature sensitivity pre-screening of devices and thermally controlled transmitters. Such requirements are imposed by the need to maintain alignments between each optical signal, eg., three fabry-perot lasers with Thermo-electric Coolers (TEC) and a spectral width of 2.5 nm (FWHM) operating at 1270, 1300 and 1330 nm, and the corresponding narrow optical pass-band of the four-port grating-type demultiplexer.

Combinations of electrical and optical multiplexing using a variety of long-wavelength semiconductor lasers and WDM components can be used to accomplish hybrid single-fiber transport of baseband digital and multiple channels of both standard television and HDTV as well as two way transmission of broadband information on the same fiber. While it is clear that digital video transmission is the desired method, transitory technologies such as PFM may be used to transmit video until a digital standard is adopted by the various standards organizations.

High stability frequency and timing distribution using
semiconductor lasers and fiber optic links

George Lutes

Jet Propulsion Laboratory
California Institute of Technology
Pasadena, California

1. INTRODUCTION

Modern frequency standards, such as hydrogen masers, generate very stable frequency references for various applications in communications and metric tracking systems. The frequency stability of some standards currently exceeds 1×10^{-15} for 1000 second averaging times.[1] For various reasons of redundancy and cost efficiency there is a need to distribute stable reference signals to remote users without significantly degrading their frequency stability. However, distribution systems generally degrade the frequency stability of transmitted signals by degrading the Signal-to-Noise-Ratio (SNR) of the signal and causing group delay variations in the signal path with respect to time. Thus achieving the required frequency stability in frequency distribution systems has become a difficult technical challenge.

The ability to distribute precise frequency references over distances of tens of kilometers will result in considerable cost savings, improved performance and better reliability in the NASA/JPL Deep Space Network (DSN). This ability, for instance, will enable the use of a centralized frequency and timing facility and therefore reduce the number of expensive frequency standards needed in a Deep Space Communications Complex (DSCC). To this end, fiber optic frequency reference distribution system development is an ongoing task at JPL. The present goal is to achieve a transmission stability of 1×10^{-18} for 1000 seconds averaging times over a distance of 29 kilometers.

This paper will describe the mechanisms in a distribution system that cause degradation of frequency stability of a transmitted signal. In particular instabilities that result from the use of a semiconductor laser transmitter will be discussed. Finally, it will describe the fiber optic frequency reference distribution systems developed at the Jet Propulsion Laboratory, and now in use at the Goldstone DSCC.

2. DEGRADATION OF FREQUENCY STABILITY

For short averaging times on the order of a few 10s of seconds and less, the frequency stability of a frequency reference signal is set by its SNR. In this range the plot of the frequency stability (σ) with respect to averaging time (τ) has a $1/\tau$ slope. Frequency variations due to environmental effects and aging occur too slowly to predominate in this range. A typical frequency stability value for a hydrogen maser frequency standard in this range is 3×10^{-13} for 1 second averaging time. The level of the frequency stability changes as $S_\phi(f)^{1/2}$ where $S_\phi(f)$ is the spectral density of phase noise of the signal. Therefore, if the SNR of the transmitted signal is reduced by the distribution system the frequency stability of the signal will be degraded.

Since the bandwidth of the signal generated by the frequency standard is reduced within the standard to a very narrow value (typically < 100 Hz) the bandwidth of the signal at the output of the fiber optic link must also be reduced. This is necessary to preserve the SNR of the transmitted signal. A Phase Locked Loop (PLL) filter is usually used for this purpose.

At longer averaging times frequency drift due to environmental effects and aging predominates. The frequency stability of a hydrogen maser, for instance, is best at around 1000 second averaging times where it reaches a level of about 1×10^{-15}. As the averaging time increases beyond 1000 seconds the frequency stability degrades due to long term drift caused by sensitivity to various environmental effects.[2,3] Group delay variations in a distribution system, caused primarily by thermal effects, result in degradation of the frequency stability of a transmitted signal for averaging times greater than a few tens of seconds.

The dependence of frequency stability caused by group delay may be obtained in the following way. The phase of the output of a distribution system relative to the phase of the input signal is

$$\theta_{out} = \theta_{in} + \theta_d = \theta_{in} + \omega_o(D_o + (dD_{(t)}/dt)t) \tag{1}$$

where θ_{in} is the radian phase of the signal at the input to the distribution system, θ_d is the radian phase delay through the distribution system, ω_o is the nominal radian frequency at the input to the distribution system, D_o is the nominal group delay through the distribution system, and $D_{(t)}$ is the group delay through the line as a function of time.

The rate of change of output phase with respect to time is, from 1,

$$d\theta_{out}/dt = \omega_o(dD_{(t)}/dt) \tag{2}$$

Dividing both sides of (2) by 2π gives the frequency offset, Δf, in Hz at the output of the distribution system,

$$\Delta f = (1/2\pi)(d\theta_{out}/dt) = (\omega_o/2\pi)(dD_{(t)}/dt) = f_o(dD_{(t)}/dt) \tag{3}$$

The actual frequency at the output of the distribution system is

$$f_{out} = f_o + \Delta f = f_o + f_o(dD_{(t)}/dt) \tag{4}$$

The change in output frequency with respect to time caused by group delay variations in the distribution system is given by

$$df_{out}/dt = f_o(d^2D_{(t)}/dt^2) \tag{5}$$

The absolute frequency at the output of a distribution system at any moment in time is given by (4) and the frequency stability of the signal at any moment in time is given by (5). It can be seen from (4) and (5) that if the group delay with respect to time, $D_{(t)}$, is linear, the offset frequency, Δf, will be constant and the frequency instability added to the signal will be zero. However, if the group delay through the distribution system with respect to time is not linear, as is usually the case, an additional frequency instability is added to the transmitted signal.

Frequency stability is usually measured in time domain in terms of Alan deviation σ which is given by

$$(\sigma_{\Delta f/f}(2,T,\tau)) = 1/f_o \sqrt{(1/2N) \sum_{i=1}^{N} (f_i - f_{(i-1)})^2} \tag{6}$$

Here $f_i - f_{(i-1)}$ are individual successive measurements of the frequency being measured, N is the number of measurements, f_o is the nominal mean frequency, T is the time between measurements, and τ is the averaging time of each frequency measurement.[4]

3. SEMICONDUCTOR LASER CONTRIBUTION TO STABILITY DEGRADATION

Semiconductor laser transmitters are used almost exclusively in frequency reference distribution systems. These are the only devices that can provide adequate optical power in a single-mode fiber optic system to transmit high SNR analog signals over the required distance. However, semiconductor lasers are also one of the major sources of degradation to the frequency stability of a transmitted signal.

The maximum SNR that can be achieved with a typical single-mode fiber optic link using a semiconductor laser is about 120 dB/Hz when used to transmit analog signals.[5] The SNR of short links with less than about 20 dB optical loss is relatively constant at this level because laser noise predominates. This level of SNR is more than adequate for today's distribution systems since the SNR of a typical frequency standard in use today is < 100 dB/Hz. However, the SNR of future frequency standards is expected to be much higher resulting in better short term frequency stability. This will require a fiber optic system with better performance. Since the noise of short (<30 km) fiber optic links is due primarily to the semiconductor laser, the RIN and linearity of the lasers must be improved. It is gratifying that substantial improvements in these parameters have been made recently to satisfy the needs of the cable television industry.

Changes in reflection from the fiber back into the laser diode cause delay variations across the laser which may be as great as 100 ps.[6] These changes in reflection result from vibration or flexure of the fiber optic cable. Optical isolation of the laser on the order of 60 dB can reduce such changes to less than 0.03 ps. Commercial optical isolators typically have 35 to 40 dB isolation and less than 2 dB loss in the forward direction. This level of isolation is not great enough for frequency reference distribution applications.

JPL has developed a suitable optical isolator assembly for use with single-mode optical fiber.[7] This assembly provides greater than 60 dB isolation with only 1.3 dB loss in the forward direction. The assembly uses a commercial bulk optical isolator unit and high quality expanded beam connectors. The expanded beam connectors expand the light from the 10 micrometer diameter core of the single-mode fiber to 1.5 millimeters and collimate it. The narrow acceptance angle of the connectors provides the additional isolation in the isolator. Light scattered in the isolator no longer has the proper polarization to be rejected by the output polarizer which it passes through. This decreases the isolation of the isolator. However, most of this scattered light is also not parallel to the axis of the isolator and falls outside of the acceptance angle of the connector. Since the scattered light is not accepted by the collecting connector the isolation of the isolator assembly is greatly improved.

An isolator that is external to the semiconductor laser package, however, presents some problems. If a fiber is used between the laser and the isolator assembly the laser can be very sensitive to movement or vibration of that fiber. Ideally there should be no discrete reflections between the laser diode and the isolator. At least reflected light should not be permitted to reenter the laser diode.

Delay variations across a laser diode have been measured which are apparently due to the reflection from the near end of the fiber pigtail. Because of the thermal coefficient of expansion in a fiber optic transmitter assembly the spacing between the fiber end and the laser changes with temperature, changing the phase of the reflected signal and resulting in delay variations across the laser diode. Figure 1 shows the measured change in delay due to this effect for one laser transmitter that has been tested.

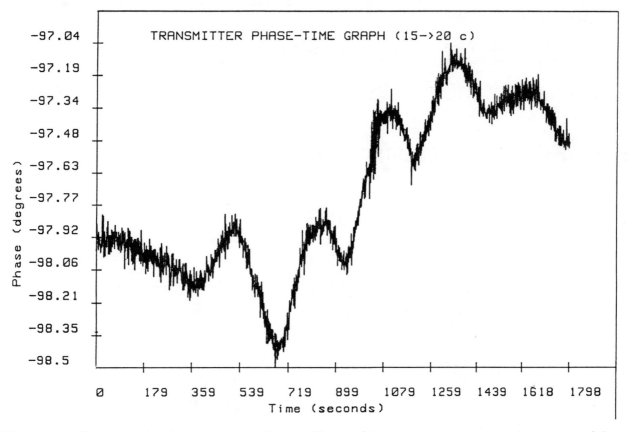

Figure 1. Phase variations across a laser diode with respect to temperature caused by changes in the distance between the laser diode and the near end of the fiber pigtail.

Other possible sources of degradation to a transmitted signals frequency stability are being examined. For instance the magnitude of instabilities due to the lasers linewidth and its interaction with fiber dispersion can impact the stability of a reference signal transmitted as the modulation of the laser light in the fiber. Low frequency noise modulation due to laser nonlinearities are also being examined.

4. PERFORMANCE OF PRESENT SYSTEMS

Figure 2 shows a block diagram of a long distance frequency reference distribution link. A reference signal to be transmitted is applied to the modulation input of the semiconductor laser transmitter. The modulated optical carrier passes through a high isolation optical isolator having greater than 60 dB isolation. After passage through the fiber optic cable a receiver detects and amplifies the 100 MHz modulation signal. The output of the receiver is filtered by a phase locked loop filter to limit the noise bandwidth of the signal.

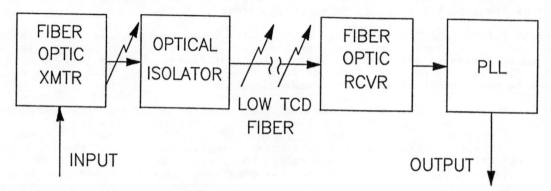

Figure 2. A block diagram of a long distance fiber optic frequency reference distribution link.

Figure 3 is a block diagram of the measurement system used to measure the stability of this link. A 100 MHz reference signal was transmitted round trip over a cable 29 kms long for a total distance of 58 km. A receiver transmitter pair at the far end of the link was used as a repeater. A network analyzer was used to measure changes in phase across the link by comparing the phase of the input signal to the phase of the return signal as shown. The total measurement time was 5 days.

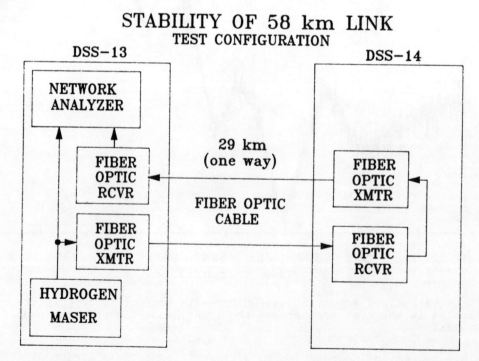

Figure 3. A block diagram of the measurement system used to measure the stability of the 58-km fiber optic link.

Figure 4 shows the measured phase across the link which is about +/- 1° of phase at 100 MHz over a 24-hour period. The data from this test was used to calculate the Alan deviation which is shown in Fig. 5. The degradation to the stability of the transmitted hydrogen maser frequency reference was quite small.

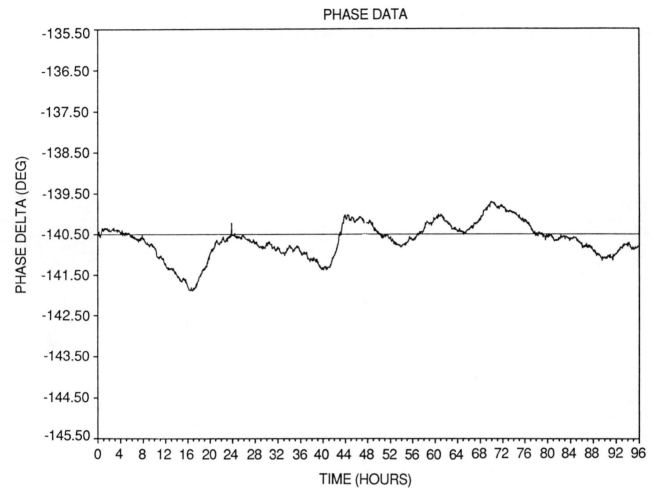

Figure 4. A plot of the phase measurement across the 58-km fiber optic link with respect to time.

Another experiment was performed on a fiber optic system to be used to transmit frequency references through an antenna wrap-up where the fiber optic cable is flexed. The phase across the link was measured using the test configuration shown in Fig. 6. Measurements were made with and without an optical isolator to isolate the laser diode from external reflections. Figure 7 shows the measured phase without the isolator and Fig. 8 shows the measured phase with the isolator. Without the isolator, phase jumps are seen when the antenna is moved. These phase jumps are eliminated when the isolator is used. The effect of phase jumps on the Alan variance is shown in Fig. 9. Elimination of the phase jumps results in a substantial improvement of the Alan variance and performance that surpasses today's requirements.

The stability of present links is adequate for today's frequency standards. However, frequency standards now in development are expected to achieve frequency stabilities on the order of 1×10^{-17} for 1000 second averaging times. In order not to excessively degrade the frequency stability of the transmitted signal the frequency stability of the distribution link should be at least 10 times better than the frequency stability of the signal. Therefore, in the future the distribution link frequency stability will have to improve accordingly to about 1×10^{-18} for 1000 second averaging times.

Passive means to improve the stability of fiber optic distribution links, such as burying the cable, have been exhausted in the present systems. Active systems using optical and electronic feedback are currently being developed at JPL to meet the improved long term stability performance required in the future. Improvements in short term

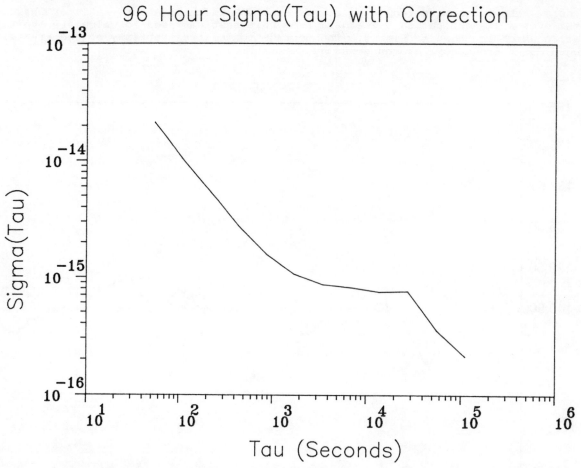

Figure 5. The frequency stability (Alan deviation) calculated from the measured phase data for the 58-km fiber optic link.

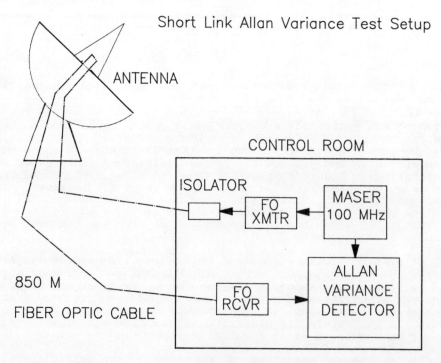

Figure 6. A block diagram of the measurement system used to measure the frequency stability and phase of a reference signal transmitted through the wrap-up of an antenna. The fiber optic cable was flexed when the antenna was moved.

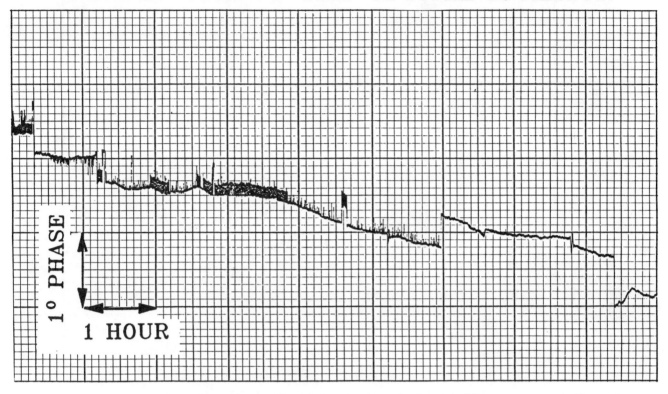

Figure 7. The measured phase of a signal transmitted through the wrap-up of the antenna when no optical isolator was used.

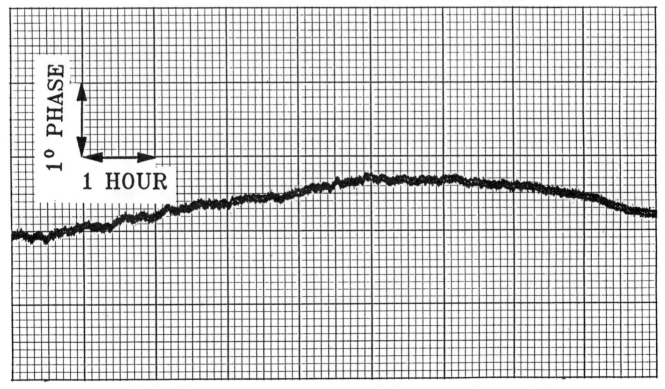

Figure 8. The measured phase of a signal transmitted through the wrap-up of the antenna when the optical isolator was used.

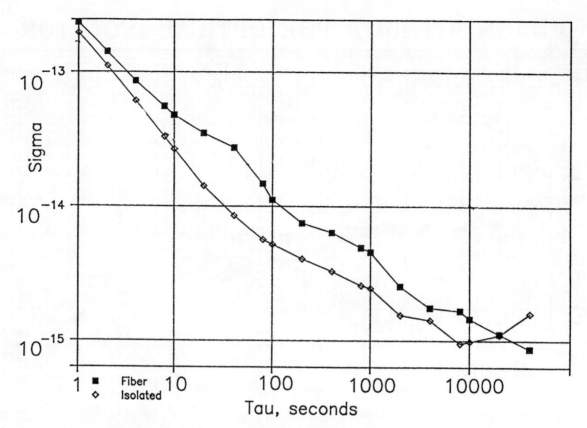

Figure 9. The measured Alan deviation of the signal transmitted through the antenna wrap-up with and without the optical isolator.

frequency stability of a transmitted signal must come from improvements in semiconductor laser diodes which permit better SNR performance.

5. CONCLUSION

Because of optical fiber's low loss, wide bandwidth, superior thermal stability and immunity to RFI and EMI it is the medium of choice for transmitting precise frequency references. Fiber optic frequency reference distribution links have been demonstrated at JPL and are in limited use in the JPL/NASA DSN. These systems can meet the stability requirements for transmitting signals generated by today's frequency standards. More stable links being developed at JPL will meet the stability requirements for transmitting signals generated by the frequency standards of the future. Improved semiconductor lasers which are less affected by outside influences and can provide better SNR are needed to meet the requirements of future distribution systems.

6. ACKNOWLEDGMENTS

This work represents the results of one phase of research carried out at the Jet Propulsion Laboratory, California Institute of Technology, under contract with the National Aeronautics and Space Administration.

The author thanks L. Maleki and L. Primas for their help and support in writing this paper.

7. REFERENCES

1. A. Kirk, P. Kuhnle, and R. Sydnor, "Evaluation of modern hydrogen masers," Proc. 14th Ann. Precise Time and Time Interval (PTTI) Applications and Planning Meeting, pp. 359-392, NASA Conference Publication 2265, Nov./Dec. 1982.
2. J. A. Barnes, A. R. Chi, L. S. Cutler, D. J. Healey, D. B. Leeson, T. E. McGunigal, J. A. Mullen, W. L. Smith, R. Sydnor, R. F. C. Vessot, and G. M. R. Winkler, "Characterization of frequency stability," Technical Note 394, National Bureau of Standards, Oct. 1970.
3. L. S. Cutler and C. L. Searle, "Some aspects of the theory and measurement of

frequency fluctuations in frequency standards," Proc. IEEE, special issue on Frequency Stability, Vol. 54, p.136, Feb. 1966.

4. D. W. Alan, "Statistics of Atomic Frequency Standards," Proc. IEEE, vol. 54, pp. 221-230, February 1966.

5. K. Lau, "Signal-to-noise calculations for fiber optics links," The Telecommunications and Data Acquisition Progress Report 42-58, pp. 41-48, Jet Propulsion Laboratory, May-June 1980.

6. K. Y. Lau, "Microwave phase stability of directly modulated semiconductor injection lasers," Applied Physics Letters 52(17), pp. 1377-1378, 25 April 1988.

7. G. Lutes, "Optical isolator system for fiber-optic uses," Applied Optics, Vol. 27, No. 7, pp. 1326-1328, 1 April 1988.

LASER DIODE TECHNOLOGY AND APPLICATIONS

Volume 1043

SESSION 6

Novel Semiconductor Laser Applications II

Chair
David L. Begley
Ball Aerospace Systems Group

Invited Paper

Applications and requirements of laser diodes for free-space laser communications

David L. Begley

Ball Aerospace Systems Group
P.O. Box 1062, Boulder, CO 80306

1. INTRODUCTION

Communications in space utilizing lasers has been considered since their realization in 1960. It was soon recognized that, though the laser had the potential for the transfer of data at extremely high rates, much work was required in system and component development, particularly for space-qualified hardware. Advances in system architecture, data formatting, and component technology over the past quarter century have now made laser communications in space a viable and attractive approach to space based communications. In particular, semiconductor laser diodes offer important advantages over other laser sources, in size, weight, volume, efficiency, and data rate. There are however, performance restrictions which impact the system design and the direct application of laser diodes for communications in space. This paper presents an overview of space-borne laser communication systems and key laser diode parameters which affect their application.

2. LASER COMMUNICATION SYSTEMS

The high data rate and large information throughput available are many times greater than in r.f. systems. The small aperture size requires only a small increase in the weight and volume of the host platform. With telescope diameters typically less than 12 inches the smaller apertures create less momentum disturbance to any sensitive platform sensors or other position sensitive subsystems. The narrow beam divergence affords private or secure communications and interference free operation. Laser communications security can be illustrated in Figure 1; clearly a very small area (in comparison with r.f.) exists where interception of transmitted data is possible. For extremely long range applications, out-of-orbit, and planetary missions the beam sizes are on the order of one-earth diameter (three orders of magnitude less than conventional r.f. systems). The narrow beam divergence places stringent requirements on the pointing and tracking subsystems, (narrow beams must be pointed with much greater precision and stability).

A block diagram of a typical terminal is illustrated in Figure 2. Information is input to the transmit data electronics circuitry that modulates the laser source and thereby impose the data signal on the output beam.. The laser source output (with encoded information) passes through an optical system (transfer optics and telescope) into the free-space channel. The receiver beam comes in through the optics system and is directed to detectors and signal processing. The control electronics must control the gimbals, servos, and other steering mechanisms required to perform acquisition and tracking subsystem functions. Acquisition and tracking may be performed by the same laser source as the communication function, however, in most applications separate lasers are employed because of the different performance requirements.

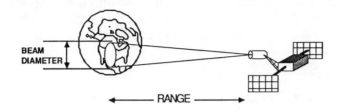

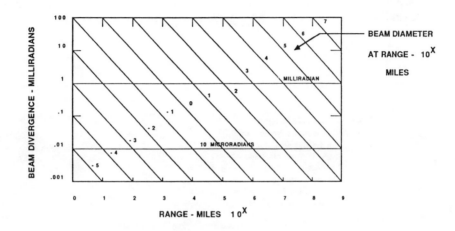

Figure 1. Beam divergence and diameter versus range.

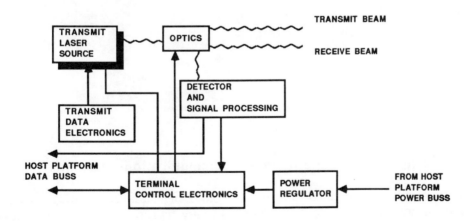

Figure 2. Functional block diagram of a laser communications terminal

Of the three acquisition is generally considered to be the most difficult. Communications depends on bandwidth or data rate, but is generally less demanding than acquisition unless very high data rates are required. Acquisition is the most difficult because laser beams are smaller than the area of uncertainty. All objects move with some uncertainty, placing restrictions on the length of time available to perform acquisition prior to the loss of the reference. A lower pulse rate is required for acquisition than for tracking or communications. It is possible therefore to operate specific lasers at high peak power and low duty cycle. A high brightness, short duration, optical pulse serves as a beacon signal to make the acquisition process less demanding. High energy pulses more easily overcome the receiver set threshold (keeping the false alarm rate low). Use of a continuous source for acquisition becomes more feasible as the uncertainty area decreases.

A conceptual drawing of a generic laser communications terminal is shown in Figure 3 with basic components and subsystem elements. In this design the electronic subsystems (power conditioning, communication, processor, servo and laser drive) are modularized and integrated in the upper half of the terminal. All optical/electro-optical components are attached to an optical platform comprising the lower section of the terminal. The telescope and gimbal are the physically dominate subassemblies in this terminal design.

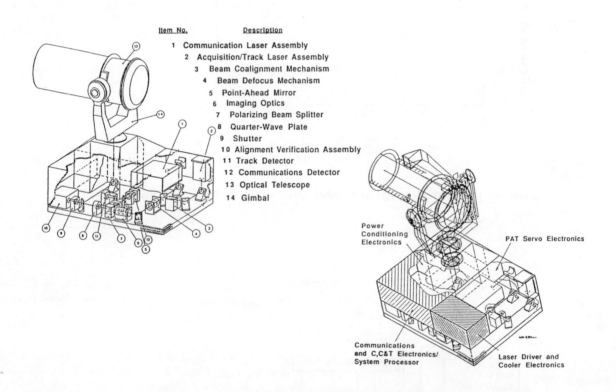

Figure 3. Generic laser communications terminal

To achieve the potential diffraction-limited beamwidth from a high quality telescope, a single-mode, high beam quality laser source is required, together with very high quality optical components throughout the transmitting optical system. The output beam quality in the free-space channel cannot be better than the worst element in the optical chain. Because of the requirement for both high efficiency and high beam quality, many lasers which are suitable in other applications are unsuitable for long-distance free-space communications. In order to communicate, adequate power must be available at the detector surface to distinguish signal from noise. Optical noise (in this portion of the electromagnetic spectrum quantum noise is dominate) can greatly affect the laser communication system performance. For orbital platform applications the main background noise source is the sun.

The earth, moon, atmospheric scattered sunlight, clouds, and the planets exhibit similar radiances and are as much as eight orders of magnitude below the sun. The optical noise introduced by background sources can be reduced by making the receiver field of view and spectral bandpass as narrow as possible.

The link equation presented in Figure 4 is utilized to establish hardware requirements and evaluate system design concepts. Laser power, transmitter optical system losses, pointing system errors, transmitter and receiver antenna gains, receiver losses and receiver tracking losses, are all factors that go into establishing the required receiver power. Transmitter output power has been identified as a key subsystem parameter governing the total link performance. System size, weight, efficiency, and complexity can all be reduced, given adequate source power. This can be graphically demonstrated by Figure 5, where aperture size and data rate are presented as a function of laser power. The size of the primary aperture is directly related to system weight and information transmission rate. Data rate, detector sensitivity, modulation formats, noise and detection methods are key parameters in system performance and are governed in part by the specific mission.

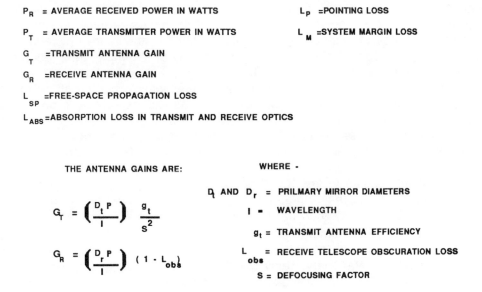

Figure 4. Link equation for received optical power

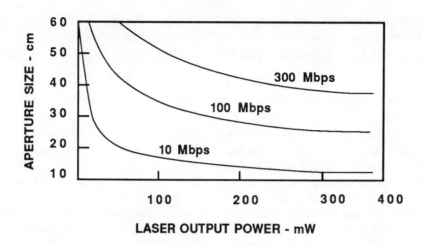

Figure 5. Telescope aperture diameter as a function of data rate and laser power

3. APPLICATIONS AND HOST SPACECRAFT MISSIONS

The form of a laser communication system and its impact on the host platform are highly dependent upon mission constraints and technology limits. Different scenarios require, in general, different system configurations (choice of laser, detector, optics, etc.) for maximum efficiency in performance. The host platform also has a significant role on the system. As an example, integration of a lasercom terminal with a platform for geosynchronous orbit involves more coordination than a sole use platform (high cost of geosynchronous launch may dictate laser communication system shared with other mission payloads). Power and weight allowances will also be limited as well as access to on board telemetry and control facilities. The lack of recovery demands the system be fully redundant with ground control of essential terminal functions. Placement of the terminal and telescope assembly will depend on other facility integration and required total field of view given platform orbit and orientation.

Table 1 presents a listing of some of the applications for space-borne laser communications existing in both the commercial and defense areas. In Japan efforts have been directed at an intersatellite communication system to be integrated on the Engineering Test Satellite-VI scheduled for launch in 1992 [2]. The National Space Development Agency of Japan (NASDA) initiated a study of intersatellite laser links in 1985 for the application of communication between a low earth orbit satellite and a space station via high earth orbit (geostationary) relay satellites. Semiconductors laser diode technology is planned for the acquisition (0.8 micron wavelength at high powers) and communication (1.3 micron wavelength for internal fiber optic data bus and free-space propagation).

In Europe the European Space Agency plans an on-orbit demonstration of laser communication capability. Their mission scenario consists of two geostationary spacecrafts and a low earth orbiting satellite [3]. The French SPOT 4 earth observation spacecraft is scheduled to be the first platform to carry a laser communication terminal with launch in 1992. Although the present experiment will be performed with 0.8 micron semiconductor lasers there has been some consideration to solid state laser integration in following programs.

A team at the Jet Propulsion Laboratory has considered the system and component technologies required for laser communications to improve data transmission during future deep-space missions [4]. These missions, beyond earth orbit, have data rates not easily satisfied by r.f. technology. The Cassini spacecraft offers the first planetary mission opportunity for laser communications demonstration. A data rate 1,000 times that utilized on previous missions is possible during the crafts journey past

Mars and Saturn. Integration of a terminal on the Mariner Mark II spacecraft, to be launched in 1996 for a voyage to Saturn, and other planned missions are also under consideration. JPL has concentrated

SPACE BORNE LASER COMMUNICATION APPLICATIONS IN COMMERCIAL AND DEFENSE AREAS	LASER TECHNOLOGY PREFERED/BACKUP
SPACE-TO-SPACE	
NASA TDAS (TRACKING AND DATA ACQUISITION SYSTEM)	LASER DIODE
NASA SPACE STATION TO CO-ORBITING PLATFORMS	LASER DIODE
SDI	---
DOD	---
INTELSAT	LASER DIODE
JPL INTERPLANETARY MISSIONS	DIODE PUMPED SOLID STATE
JAPAN ETS (ENGINEERING TEST SATELLITE)	LASER DIODE
ESA DRS (EUROPEAN SPACE AGENCY DATA RELAY SATELLITE)	LASER DIODE
SPACE-TO-AIRCRAFT	
DOD	...
SDI	...
SPACE-TO-GROUND	
NASA ACTS (ADVANCED COMMUNICATION TECHNOLOGY SATELLITE)	LASER DIODE
NAVY SLC-SAT (SUBMARINE LASER COMMUNICATION SATELLITE)	RAMAN SHIFTED XeCl/DIODE PUMPED SOLID STATE
SDI	...
DOD	...

Table 1. Space-borne laser communications applications

its transmitter development efforts on solid state lasers that produce very high-quality, diffraction-limited beams, during high peak pulse power operation [5].

NASA (Goddhard Space Flight Center) has been investigating the utility of laser communications on the Space Station for video, voice, and data transmission between the Station, co-orbiting platforms, and extra vehicular units (astronauts is free flying vehicles). It is anticipated that laser communications will provide relief from the projected r.f. congestion and interference on the space station during its growth phase.

The Navy SLC-SAT program will provide one-way communication via satellite to submarines [6]. A space-borne laser emitting in the blue-green portion of the spectrum will transmit data to receivers on submarines that may be operating at depths several hundreds of feet below the ocean surface. Although a Raman shifted XeCl laser has received the most development, solid state laser concepts have been and are presently under investigation.

A study of the application of laser communications to the TDAS satellite data transmission requirements was funded by NASA-GSFC. Although the feasibility of a laser intersatellite crosslink capable of 2 Gbps data transfer was validated, the implementation of flight hardware required technology advancements; specifically in high power semiconductor lasers and high speed processing electronics.

The NASA ACTS satellite represented the earliest introduction of laser communications in space. Originally planned to accommodate two experimental packages; a direct detection and a coherent terminal, with a common optical subsystem, the funding was greatly reduced in early 1988. The direct detection transmitter utilized an incoherent beam combiner approach for multiple semiconductor laser diodes. The coherent transmitter consisted of a highly controlled single frequency laser diode to produce the stable emission required for heterodyne detection.

4. REQUIREMENTS FOR LASER DIODES

As illustrated in Table 1 and the discussion above semiconductor laser diodes have been selected as a key technology component for the success of major space communication missions. Recent advances in semiconductor laser diodes have direct application to space-borne systems[7,8]. There are however critical performance characteristics which must be addressed before application is possible as either an optical pump or direct source. Table 2 presents the general requirements of laser diode performance for diode pumping of solid state lasers [9,10] and as sources for direct and coherent (heterodyne) detection systems.

CHARACTERISTIC	DIODE PUMPING	DIRECT	COHERENT
OUTPUT POWER-mW	50 TO 1,0000	50 TO 1,000	50 TO 200
BEAM PROFILE	20 X 70 DEG. NOT CRITICAL	DIFFRACTION LIMITED	DIFFRACTION LIMITED
SPECTRAL DIST.	± 3 nm	SINGLE FREQ. < 10 GHz	SINGLE FREQ. <5 MHz
THERMAL CONTROL	± 5 C	± 0.1 C	$\pm 10^{-4}$ C
OUTPUT COMBINATION	STRAIGHT FOWARD	ACHIEVABLE	VERY DIFFICULT
RELIABILITY	DEGRADATION AFFECTS NOT MAJOR CONCERN	DEGRADATION AFFECTS OF SOME CONCERN	DEGRADTION AFFECTS CRITICAL

Table 2. General laser diode requirements

The employment of semiconductor lasers as optical pumps requires the least stringent performance of the three applications. Figure 6 illustrates the three conventional approaches to diode pumping. The end pumping configuration produces the highest total efficiency. The optical mode from the pump laser can be matched to the lasing mode of the solid-state material, thus maximizing the coupling efficiency between pump and laser. The output power from this approach is, in general limited by the power obtainable from a single (or very few) diode emitter. Pumping of a crystalline rod along the longitudinal axis can provide a versitle approach to achieving higher powers in a compact laser. Since the pump radiation must propagte through the periphery of the rod, fundamental mode operation utilizes a region of the rod extending less than half of the diameter, resulting in lower efficiency compared to end pumping. Another physical configuration which is of considerable interest is the slab laser. Slab lasers are pumped at a geometrical surface generating a laser mode which propagates through the material by total internal reflection. The greater effective length of the active material and large surface pump area affords high peak powers.

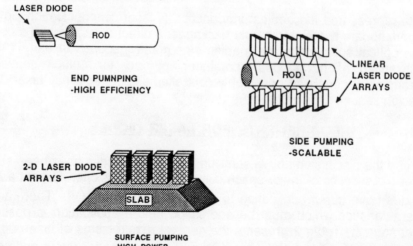

Figure 6. Diode pumped solid state laser configurations.

In most applications high available output power is an advantage, however the 50 mW value represents a lower bound below which the size of the pump array becomes to large or to costly (for stacked discrete devices). The 1 watt upper limit represents a reasonable value for a single emitter device with acceptable reliability (the reliability issue will be addressed later in this paper). The beam profile is not critical since the pump device (or array) can be positioned close to the surface of the laser crystal or coupled to beam forming optics. The spectral distribution must be within the 6 nanometer spread to insure efficient absorption (here the 808 nanometer pump band of Nd:YAG is used as an example). Because one in general will be working with a distributed active medium pump surface area (except for end pumping) output combining is straight forward. Reliability can be addressed in a conventional manner in that devices can be screened and burned-in individually prior to assembly into the pump array whether composed of discrete emitters or stacks of monolithic linear arrays. The early failure of any single device (or multiple devices) will degrade the performance of the laser by only the contribution of that element. Graceful degradation is there inherent in diode pumping. End pumping presents a somewhat greater challenge particularly when reliability issues are addressed.

For application in direct detection systems perhaps the most critical characteristics are the beam profile and output power. There are short range communication missions requiring low output powers of approximately 50 mW, however, most requirements are placed at the 500 to 1000 mW level. As mentioned previously a greater output power affords a smaller telescope aperture and simpler terminal design. A diffraction limited beam is required to insure optical system throughput efficiency. A wide output beam or a beam with multiple farfield lobes can not efficiently be accommodated by transfer and beam shaping optics. A graphical comparison of laser diode performance availability versus the system need or requirement is shown in Figure 7. Clearly the 1000 mW output power level is a challenge to the technical community. A varity of concepts have been investigated over the years with limited success. All monolithic approaches have failed to control the output beam form to a diffraction limit at any significant power levels. Discrete emitter beam combiners have been physically large and complex, althouth they have a built-in reliability advantage similar to the pump array discussed above.

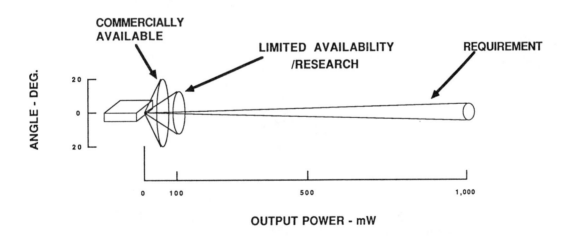

Figure 7. Laser diode performance availability versus need.

Typical space missions demand a system lifetime from three to ten years or more. These missions lifetimes places stringent requirements on the reliability of laster diodes and the steps involved in their processing and fabrication. Devices and fabrication processed must be designed to reduce or eliminate degradation mechanism effects. Burn-in and screening criteria applied must be applied to device populations to eliminate infant mortalities and select potentially long life lasers. Figure 8 presents a typical output power performance history for a laser diode. Early degradation is seen to occur in the first few hundred hours of operation. Once stabilized, very gradual reduction in optical power may occur over the lifetime of the device. Failure of the laser diode occurs when the output power reaches fifty percent of the beginning of life value. This point may occur a varied operating times depending on the type of degradation mechanism (or the number of mechanism) present in the device. The burn-in and screening criteria are determined for the particular device under qualification with these procedures providing the framework for reliable device selection. Tests performed on a number of devices will produce a distribution of failure times , assumed to be Gaussian in Figure 8. The distribution of failures about the median lifetime must be considered to insure that the laser diode lifetime exceeds the system requirements i.e. the three sigma point should be close to the system requirement.

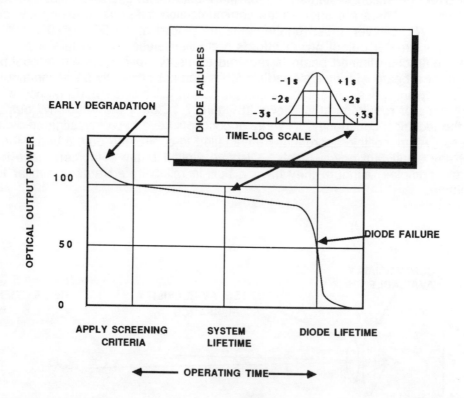

Figure 8 Laser diode output power performance history

The growing requirements for efficient, secure, high data rate communication has led to growing interest in the operational deployment of laser communication systems for a wide range of space missions. Through the history of free-space optical communications, programs have been initiated and terminated[11]. The system and component technology necessary for successful flight operation exist today.and operational systems are being developed. Following the first successful space-borne demonstration, providing validation of the technology maturity a rapid growth and expansion in this area of optical communications is anticipated. Further advances in laser diode performance will have a critical role in bringing these expectations to a reality.

REFERENCES

1. R.D. Nelson, T.H. Ebben, and R.G. Marshalek "Experimental verification of the pointing error distribution of an optical-intersatellite link". Free-Space Laser communication Technologies, Proc. SPIE 885, p. 132-142, 1988.

2. Y. Furuhama, K. Yasukawa, K. Kashiki, and Y. Hirata "Present status of optical isl studies in japan", Optical Systems for Space Application, SPIE Proc. 810, p. 141-149, 1987.

3. L. Frecon, J.C. Boutemy, E. Sein, "The use of optical intersatellite links for the european relay system", Optical Technologies for Communication Satellite Applications, SPIE Proc. 616, p.49-68, 1986.

4. M.D. Rayman and J.R. Lesh (1988) Optical communications for future deep-space missions. AIAA Space Programs and Technology Conference, Houston TX. AIAA-88-3507, June 1988.

5. Lesh, J.R. and M.D. Rayman "Deep-space missions look to laser communications", Laser Focus/Electro-Optics. October, p. 81-86, 1988.

6. G.W. Goodman, "Laser communications eyed by navy and air force for key 1990s applications", Armed Forces Journal International, p 86-89,1988.

7. D.L. Begley, D.K. Wagner, D.S. Hill, "Advanced laser diode structures for space communication systems", Optical Technologies for Space Communication Systems, Proc. SPIE 756, 19-24, 1987.

8. D. Botez "High-power diode lasers for space communications: a review", Free-Space Laser Communication Technologies, Proc. SPIE 885, 100-110, 1988.

9. D.L. Begley, D.J. Krebs, and M. Ross, "Diode pumped Nd:YAG lasers and their unique features", Lasers in Medicine, Proc. SPIE 712, 42-47, 1986.

10. D.J. Krebs, "Solid state lasers for space communication", Free-Space Laser Communication Technologies, Proc. SPIE 885, 191-194, 1988.

11. M. Ross, "The history of space laser communications", Free-Space Laser Communication Technologies, Proc. SPIE 885, 2-9, 1988.

AN ALL FIBRE LASER LOW COST "RANGEFINDER" FOR SMALL VIBRATION MEASUREMENTS.

Y.N. Ning+, B.T. Meggitt*, K.T.V. Grattan+, A.W. Palmer+

+Measurement and Instrumentation Centre
Department of Electrical, Electronic
and Information Engineering,
City University, Northampton Square,
London, EC1V 0HB, England.

*Department of Electronic and Electrical Engineering
Kings College London, Strand,
London WC2R 2LS, England.

ABSTRACT

An all fibre interferometer device is presented which allows the measurement of speed to be made using an electronic processing system and is contrasted with the measurement of velocity through an optical processing technique which, however, is more complex and expensive to implement. The overall simplicity of the electronic technique, the low cost of components and the use of an all-fibre arrangement make this a convenient system to implement.

INTRODUCTION

There is an increasing interest in the use of optical fibre interferometer based sensors for the measurement of a range of parameters such as temperature, pressure and chemical variables such as the presence of dangerous gases. In these cases, the parameter itself is usually converted to a change of displacement of a component of the interferometer which yields a change in the optical path length of one of the 'arms' of the device. The details of their operation are discussed elsewhere (1) and the current at a photodetector where the outputs of the two 'arms' combine has a factor dependent upon the time - dependent phase difference between the two optical signals in the 'arms'. This phase difference, $\phi(t)$ is proportional to $/x_1(t) - x_2/$ where x_1 and x_2 are the distances the light travels in arm one (which is displaced) and arm two respectively. It is possible to detect very small changes of phase and thus displacement with the device and Moss et al(2) have determined periodic displacement amplitudes of 10^{-14}m, with the detection limit set by the photodetector.

The alignment problems in the use of conventional interferometers for sensing purposes have largely been overcome by the use of fibre optic systems, allowing the development of a range of sensor devices based on displacement monitoring.

In general, the relationship between the interferometer intensity modulation and the displacement of the reflective body at the end of arm one of the device, ΔL, is given by:

$$I = \varepsilon \left(1 + K \cos \frac{4\pi n \Delta L}{\lambda}\right) \qquad (1)$$

where I is the output of the photodetector, ε and K are constants under constant illumination and λ and n are the wavelength of the light used and the refractive index of the material respectively.

It is not trival to demodulate this signal directly and various optical schemes have been devised to accomplish this (3,4,5). One commercial method (Polytech) described in reference 4 operates by incorporating the interogating fibre into one arm of a laser based interferometer (Mach-Zehnder and/or Michelson) and incorporating a Bragg frequency shifter in the other arm of the interferometer. The signals from the two arms are allowed to interfere and this results in an R.F. carrier which is frequency modulated by the Doppler shift of light returned from the vibrating body. The fibre version of the above scheme is not inherently "down lead" insensitive although acoustic screening of the fibre has been achieved. This is a major disadvantage when considering measurement of displacement in engine and other similiar industrial environments. In addition, these types of systems require external bulk optic interferometers which are inconvenient to align and operate.

Herein we propose a method of demodulating the characteristic vibration and displacement pattern of the body encoded as in equation (1) which does not require any such bulk external optical components and has the distinct advantage in being "down lead" insensitive. The scheme has not been discussed previously and relies for its operation on a wide band electronic phase shifter to achieve electronic demodulation. It is compared with a familiar all optical demodulation scheme. The use of all optical schemes is not new and reports of earlier and unsophisticated methods are seen in the literature. For example, the feasibility of the technique was reported by Cookson et al (6) and Ueha et al (7). The work of Parmigiani (8) showed the use of a fibre optic probe to couple the light from a conventional interferometer, in spite of a decrease in fringe visibility with the use of 600 μm step index fibre. A simple, bulk optical heterodyne technique with basic signal processing was reported by Sheng et al (9) recently.

THEORETICAL BACKGROUND

The displacement characteristic is determined by analysis of the optical signal returned from the device illuminated. This arises from a direct reflection from the end of the fibre combined with a reflection from the displacement of the vibrating body. This is shown schematically in Figure 1. The light reflected from the fibre

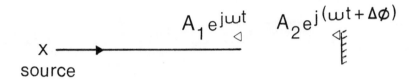

Figure 1: Schematic reflections from fibre end and vibrating body

end is given by $A_1 e^{j\omega t}$ and from the vibrating body is $A_2 e^{(j\omega t + \Delta\phi)}$, where A_1 and A_2 are constants. $\Delta\phi$ is given as

$$\Delta\phi = 2\pi/\lambda \ [L_o + L_s \sin\omega_s t] \qquad (2)$$

where $\Delta\phi$ is a phase difference factor, L_o is the cavity length at zero displacement, L_s is the maximum magnitude of the displacement on either side of L_o and ω_s is the frequency of vibration, for a light source of wavelength λ. The two returning light beams from the reflective surfaces add and their sum has a dependence on $\Delta\phi$ of the form:

$$k[1 + \cos(\pm\Delta\phi)] \qquad (3)$$

where this is the form of signal detected (this assumes $A_1 = A_2$), the + or - term being dependent on the direction of motion, where k is a constant. Demodulation of this expression is a means of obtaining the displacement information and various optical schemes have been developed (3,4,5).

OPTICAL DEMODULATION SCHEME

An optical method which has been used to demodulate this relies upon achieving a $90°$ optical phase shift in the Doppler shifted optical frequency (where the Doppler shift is induced by the movement of the object under study) giving an expression of the form:

$$k [1 + \cos(\pm \Delta\phi + 90°)] \qquad (4)$$

for the optical beam.

This expression can be rearranged to give:

$$k [1 \pm \sin(\Delta\phi)] \qquad (5)$$

The two signals in equations (3) and (5) are multiplied by a carrier frequency and a carrier quadrature introduced as a modulation of the original optical signal at a frequency ω_c. Thus the form of the two output signals multiplied by the appropriate carrier, is as shown below, when they are added to give:

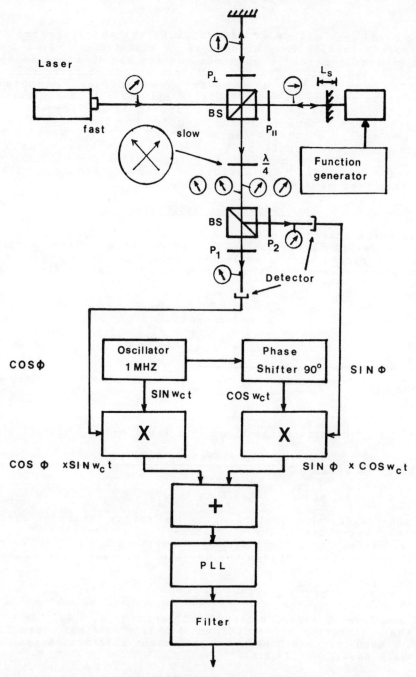

Figure 2: Schematic optical demodulation technique

```
        P    -    Polarizer
       BS    -    Beam splitter
      λ/4    -    Quarter wave plate
      PLL    -    Phase Lock Loop
        X    -    Multiplier
   Filter    -    Electronic Filter
```

$$A'\{[\cos(\pm\Delta\phi)][\sin\omega_c t] + [\sin\mp(\Delta\phi)][\cos\omega_c t]\} \quad (6)$$

where A' is a constant. This can be reduced to:

$$A'\{[\cos(\Delta\phi)\sin\omega_c t + \sin(\mp\Delta\phi)\cos\omega_c t]\} \quad (7)$$

which may further be simplified to:

$$A'\sin(\omega_c t \mp \Delta\phi) \quad (8)$$

This signal can now be demodulated relatively simply using an electronic phase locked loop (PLL) to give a demodulation of the original signal with the sense of direction of the motion preserved due to the $\mp\Delta\phi$ term in equation (8) causing a decrease and increase of the carrier frequency ω_c, as a result of vibration to be measured in the interferometer.

ELECTRONIC DEMODULATION SCHEME

However, by comparison, a simple system can be developed where the direct modulation of the optical signal is replaced by an **electronic** modulation of the appropriate signals. The main advantage of such an arrangement is the simplification of the optical scheme which is now almost entirely fibre optic based in contrast to the previous scheme which uses bulk optics. However, the disadvantage that ensues is that the direction of motion is lost, as will be shown, but nevertheless the fundamental frequency of the movement may be monitored, thereby enabling the **magnitude** of the displacement of be determined.

RESULTS OF THIS WORK

(a) Optical Demodulation Scheme

Figure 2 illustrates the optical demodulation scheme, in a simple block diagram approach. The technique is as follows. Light from a laser source (~ few mW of radiation from either a He-Ne gas laser or other coherent laser sources) is launched into an interferometer, as shown. This arrangement was configured using bulk optics, in contrast to the electronic demodulation system which used an 'all-fibre' approach. The vibration to be measured is simulated by the movement of the mirror over a distance L_s, as shown in the diagram. To achieve this under laboratory conditions, a function generator, operated at a known frequency drives a piezo-electric transducer (PZT) which induces the vibration. The polarization directions of the light are as shown in the diagram. The displacement characteristic is then determined using the analysis shown in the section discussing the theoretical background. Figure 3A shows the unmodulated signal described by equation (3) and Figure 3B a 90° phase shifted version. This shift has been achieved by optical means and its significance was shown in equation (5). Figure 4 illustrates the Lissagous figure obtained by applying the signals representing equations (3) and (5) to the x and y plates of an oscilloscope. As expected, a well defined circle is obtained. This indicates that the optical scheme does indeed provide a 90° phase shift between these two signals.

(b) Electronic Demodulation Scheme

Figure 5 illustrates the simplified 'all-fibre' electronic demodulation scheme. Again light from the laser source is launched into an interferometer, this time a fibre optic system. Light only emerges from the fibre to interrogate the vibrating body, which is again simulated in this laboratory study through the use of a PZT-driven mirror, with a function generator providing the oscillation over a distance L_s, at a fixed frequency. The light leaves the fibre interferometer to fall on the optical p-i-n diode.

This single detector is used, which gives a signal output as shown in equation (3). In the signal received, as $\cos(+\Delta\phi) = \cos(-\Delta\phi)$ the directional information is now lost as the magnitude only of the signal is preserved. The details of the electronic demodulation scheme are as shown in Figure 5. A wide band phase shifting circuit operating from 10Hz to 30kHz gives the phase quadrature of the function shown in equation (3), i.e. the detected signal to within a small angular error.

Similar traces to those of Figures 3 and 4 cannot be obtained in this electronic system as these two systems are not strictly comparable at this stage. For example, all the harmonics of the detected signal of the form of equation (3) are shifted by 90°.

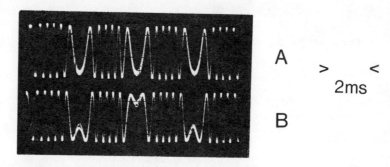

Figure 3: A -   Original signal
          B - 90° phase shifted signal
          (Vertical scale - arbitrary units)

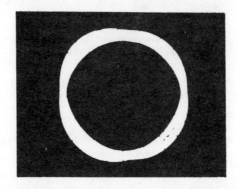

Figure 4: Lissagous Figure obtained by applying signals represented by
           equations (3) and (5) to the x and y plates of the oscilloscope.

(c) Comparison and contrast of the two systems

Figure 6A trace illustrates the demodulated output of the optical scheme, showing the velocity change of the vibrator. For comparison, the trace B is the signal applied by the function generator to the mirror. The signal frequency is 100 Hz.

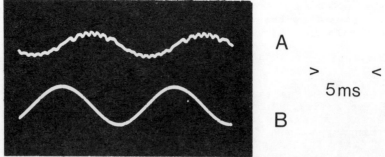

Figure 6: A - Demodulated output of the optical scheme
           B - Signal applied to function generator
           (vertical scale - arbitrary units)

By way of comparison Figure 7, trace A shows the demodulated output of the electronic system under the same conditions, with trace 7B again being the function signal at the same frequency. It may be noted from these results that rectification of the signal has occurred and thus the distinction between positive and negative directions of motion as discussed in the earlier text, is lost. However, the fundamental velocity **magnitude** i.e. speed can be deduced from the frequency, and of course, the displacement of the mirror may be obtained by integration.

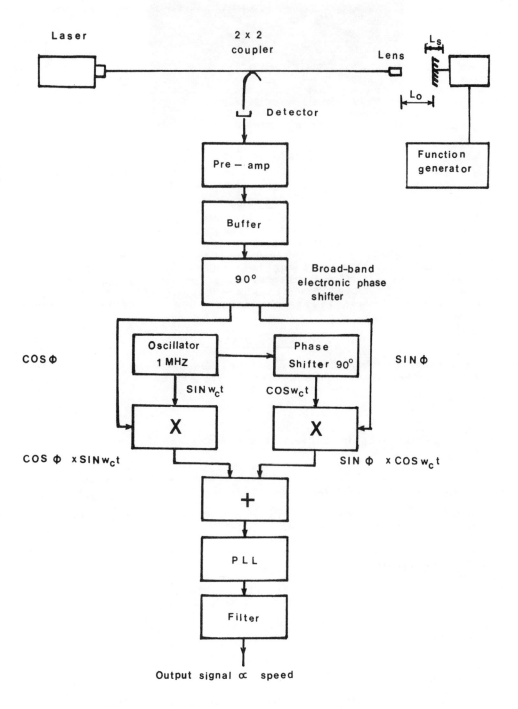

Figure 5: Schematic electronic demodulation technique

X - Multiplier
PLL - Phase Lock Loop
Filter - Electronic Filter

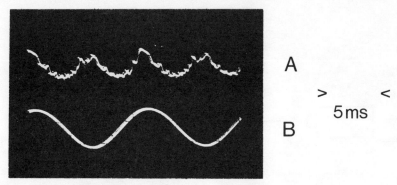

Figure 7: A - Demodulated output of the electronic scheme
B - Signal applied to function generator
(Vertical scale - arbitrary units)

DISCUSSION

Two schemes have been illustrated and shown to provide information on the velocity/speed of the mirror motion studied. The objective of this feasibility study has been the demonstration of the **principle** of the use of the electronic technique, rather than a detailed study of the range of velocity/speed which can be measured. The electronic system, although providing less information, is extremely simple in concept by virtue of the all fibre interferometer and direct electronic processing and is an attractive proposition for use where this limited information only is required. Further work is continuing to study the use of these interferometric techniques for such measurement.

ACKNOWLEDGEMENTS

Two of the authors (AWP and BTM) acknowledge support from the Royal Society/SERC by their tenure of Industrial Fellowships which have allowed this cooperative work to proceed.

REFERENCES

1. D.A. Jackson 'Monomode optical fibre interferometers for precision measurement' J.Phys. E. 18, 981-1001, 1985.

2. G.E. Moss, L.R. Miller, R.L. Forward 'Photon-noise-limited laser transducer for gravitational antenna' Appl. Opt. 10, 2495-7, 1971.

3. N.A. Halliwell 'Laser Doppler measurement of vibrating surfaces: a portable instrument' J. Sound. Vibration, 62, 312-15, 1979.

4. P. Bushave 'Laser Doppler vibration measurements using variable frequency shift' DISA Inf. 18, 15-29, 1975.

5. N. Fox 'A Prototype Non-Contacting Velocity Sensor' MSc Thesis, City University, London, 1987.

6. R.A. Cookson, P.Bandyopadhyay 'Mechanical vibration measurements using a fibre-optic Laser Doppler Probe' Opt. Laser Tech 10, 33-36, 1978.

7. S. Ueha, N. Shibata, J. Tsujivchi 'Flexible Coherent optical probe for vibration measurements' Opt. Commun. 23, 407-09, 1977.

8. F. Parmigiani 'A high sensitivity laser vibration meter using a fibre optic probe' Opt. Quant. Electron. 10, 533-5, 1978.

9. S.Y. Sheng, Y. Yongdong 'Laser Heterodyne vibration measuring method' Opt. Laser Tech. 20, 100-2, 1988.

Radiation Pattern of a Laser Diode Collimator as a Function of Driving Current and Frequency

J. Cabrita Freitas (1), F. Carvalho Rodrigues (1), V. M. Silvestre (2), Rogério D. Prina (3), L. Cadete (4), Mateus da Silva (4)

1) LNETI - 1699 Lisboa Codex - Portugal

2) EID - Quinta dos Medronheiros, Lazarim, - 2825 Monte da Caparica - Portugal

3) INDEP - 1802 Lisboa Codex - Portugal

4) EME - Largo do Museu de Artilharia - 1196 Lisboa - Portugal

Abstract

To write messages with diode lasers they are current driven. The words correspond to different impulse packets. The size of the pulses and the repetition rate are variables which are organized to suit the needs to convey a particular phrase.

The radiation pattern of a diode laser is influenced by both current and pulse signal and repetition rate. The emitted light is structured in a way that the area where the message can be read varies strongly. This is used to make some messages reach into wider areas and some messages into more confined space.

This paper shows the results pertaining a collimator for two types of pulse sizes and two different messages. One which is aimed very precisely and the other which is meant to cover a larger portion of space.

The diagrams of spot size and its evolution through space are presented. As an example and for the best situation as regards our application the area of the narrow beam passes through a minimum along its propagation path. Also changes in the elliptical orientation of the pattern are reported.

Introduction

Semiconductor laser devices designed to convey any message at great length compared to the real size of the source are being deployed in a large number of applications.
The present paper presents a comprehensive study of the radiation pattern of a laser diode being driven at a rate of 2 KHz at distances from one meter to several hundred meters from the source. The effect of collimation on the shape of the radiation pattern along the line of propagation is demonstrated to be of great value when sending simple messages to small dimensions receptors.

The Process of Measurement

Two types of set-up were devised to visualise the shape of the radiation pattern. At close range an infra red sensitive paper card was used. The glowing portion of the sensitive paper was strong enough to be registered by a camera.
For distances in the region of the several hundred meters, an array of detectors was employed. Techniques of collimation to create large optical distances over short lengths were not employed as they always induce some alterations in the pattern which are difficult to assess. The array of photodetectors was monted on a movable X-Y table which scanned the area where the beam was detected. From the data gathered in this way radiation patterns were drawn for distances of up to 600 meters.
The semiconductor laser was driven with a current of 4 A and 4,5 A at a frequency of 2 KHz.
The laser beam was collimated by a lens of 46.5 mm focal distance and 20 mm of diameter.
The distance between the lens and the laser aperture was varied +/- .2 mm from the focal distance.

Results

At short distances typically at 2 meters the round shape (Fig. 1a) changed to a structured pattern (Fig. 1b).

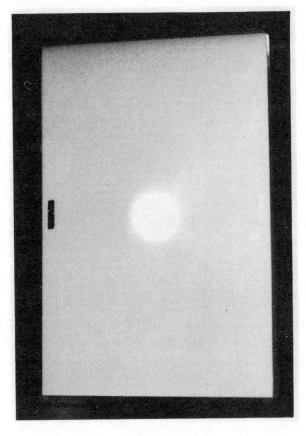 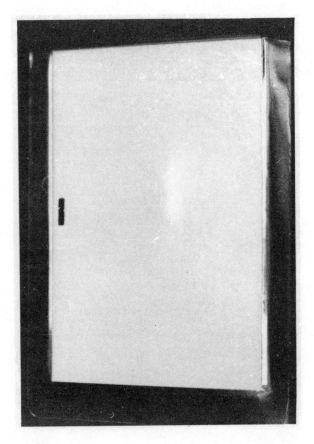

Fig. 1a   Fig 1b

As the distance from the laser collimator increased the pattern evolution along the distance is shown in Fig. 2.
The results in Fig. 2 correspond to a distance between the laser and the lens equal to the focal distance.
The evolution of the radiation pattern was very sensitive to the distance between the laser and the lens. Fig. 3 shows the shape of the radiation field when the distance between the laser and the lens changes .2 mm.
Fig. 2 and Fig. 3 pertain the laser out-put for a drive current of 4A for one message and 4.5 A for the other. Fig. 4 represent the data when the current is changed from threshold current to a higher value, i.e., 3,5 and 6A.

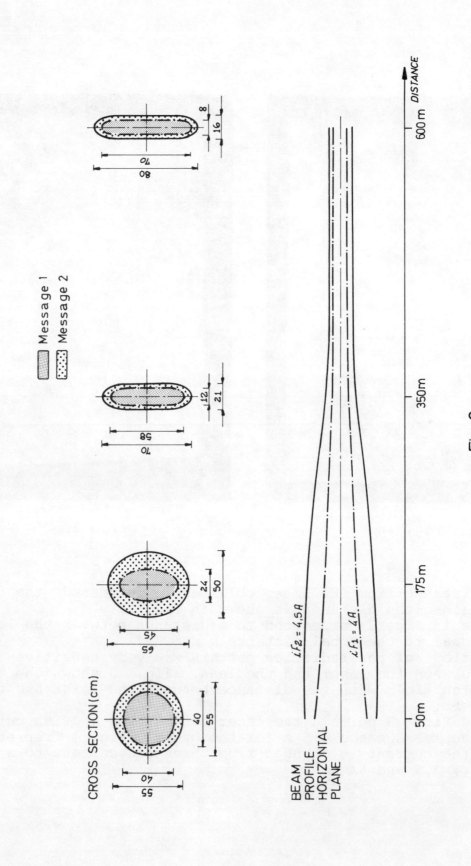

Fig. 2

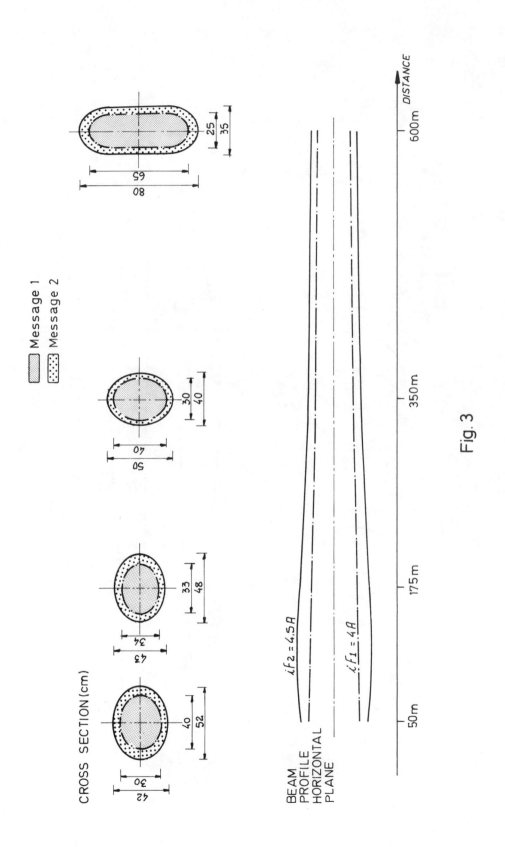

Fig. 3

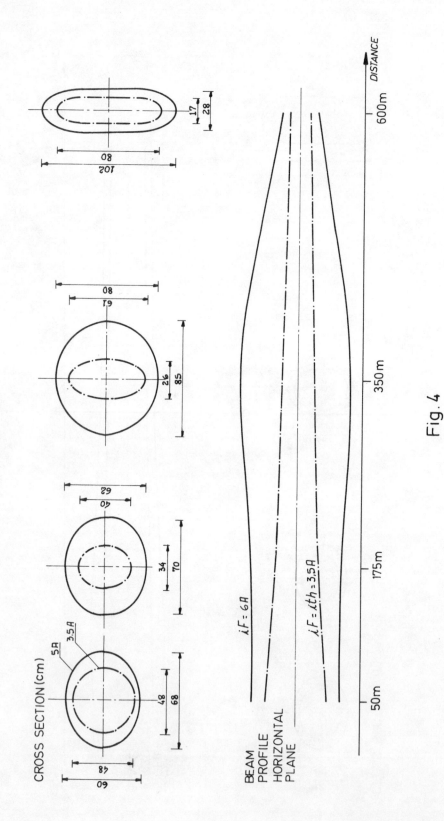

Fig. 4

Conclusions

The far field patter of collimated semiconductor laser beam is highly sensitive to the distance between the collimating lens and the laser. The present data also shows that, in regard to a specific application, the exact knowledge of the shape and extension of the radiation pattern must be known. It's dependence on the laser driving current it is also an important factor when deciding what region is to be reached by a particular message. Due to the nature of the source the radiation pattern is highly structured.

LASER DIODE TECHNOLOGY AND APPLICATIONS

Volume 1043

SESSION 7

Semiconductor Laser Optoelectronics Packaging and Reliability

Chair
Randy Randall
Tektronix, Inc.

Invited Paper

High Frequency Characteristics of 1.3 μm Lasers

D. Renner, W. H. Cheng, J. Pooladdej, and A. Appelbaum
Rockwell International Corporation
Network Transmission Systems Division
Dallas, Texas 75356-8842

K. L. Hess and S. W. Zehr
Rockwell International Corporation
Science Center,
Thousand Oaks, California 91360

ABSTRACT

A review of high frequency InGaAsP/InP laser structures is presented. The performance of these devices is analyzed based on a rate equations model. The effects of packaging and device parasitics on high speed modulation are also considered through a circuit configuration. The model is used to compare the relative advantages of the main high frequency laser structures in order to maximize the obtainable modulation bandwidth. The characteristics of buried crescent lasers with semi-insulating current-blocking layers are highlighted. A 3-dB direct modulation bandwidth of 11 GHz together with 42-mW output power has been achieved with this device.

1. INTRODUCTION

Requirements in both digital and analog lightwave communication systems have created a strong interest in developing reliable high frequency InGaAsP semiconductor lasers. Buried crescent lasers with semi-insulating InP blocking layers have demonstrated the capability for achieving both wide modulation bandwidth and high reliability.

High-frequency modulation characteristics of 1.3-μm InGaAsP lasers with semi-insulating layers have been reported.[1-7] Although lasers with semi-insulating blocking layers can achieve high-power operation, the 3-dB modulation bandwidth of these lasers has been found to be very sensitive to the linearity of the light-current characteristics. A slight increase in leakage current drastically reduces the modulation bandwidth and is likely caused by a drastic increase in the parasitic capacitance. In our previous work we have reported a significant improvement[8] in the modulation bandwidth of 1.3-μm semi-insulating buried crescent (SIBC) lasers by using a thick semi-insulating (SI) layer and by forming a double-channel structure. In this paper we extend our work by modeling the laser intrinsic response together with the parasitic responses from the semi-insulating layer and packaging. The model is fitted with the measurement data, and then used to predict the maximum obtainable bandwidth. The measured relative intensity noise of the semi-insulating buried crescent laser is also presented.

2. STRUCTURE AND FABRICATION

The laser structure and the fabrication steps are shown schematically in Fig. 1. The structure is realized in two epitaxial steps: a planar low-pressure metalorganic chemical vapor deposition (LPMOCVD)[9] growth for the Fe-doped InP SI current blocking layer, followed by a liquid phase[6] epitaxy (LPE) for the buffer, active, cladding, and contact layers. After the first MOCVD growth, arrowhead-shaped channels are etched down to the n-InP layer. Then an LPE regrowth is executed to form an n-ZnP buffer layer in the channel, a 0.15-μm thick crescent-shaped active region, a P-InP cladding layer, and a P+ InGaAs contact layer. Two channels are now etched with 20-μm spacing and a depth of 8 μm. The channel helps reduce the parasitic capacitance. Si_3N_4 is then deposited on the mesa structure wafer and an 8-μm wide contact window is opened. The wafer is, finally, processed to form p- and n-contact metallizations.

3. STATIC PERFORMANCE

The cw light-current (L-I) characteristics of a SIBC laser at 23°C is shown in Fig. 2. The laser is mounted p-side up and has a cavity length of 275-μm width with as-cleaved facets. It has a threshold current of 10 mA and a total differential quantum efficiency of 60% from threshold to 8-mW optical power. The maximum cw power output is 42 mW/facet. This high-power operation indicates that the SI blocking layer is effective for dc current blocking.

The far-field patterns at various light output powers have been measured (Fig. 2). The single-lobed emission at 10 mW has a full width at half-maximum (FWHM) of 20° and 26° in the direction parallel and perpendicular to the junction plane, respectively. The device operates in a stable single transverse mode over the full output power range.

The temperature dependence of the cw L-I characteristics for an SIBC laser is shown in Fig. 3. The laser exhibits a characteristic temperature To of 63 K between 25° and 70°C, and cw operation up to 100°C with optical power of 9 mW.

4. DYNAMIC PERFORMANCE

The small-signal frequency response of a 1.3-μm SIBC laser measured at various output power levels is shown in Fig. 4. A 3-dB bandwidth of 11 GHz was obtained at 28-mW optical power. The wide bandwidth achieved indicates that the laser structure is suitable for application as a source in high-speed fiber optic transmission systems.

A plot of the 3-dB modulation bandwidth as a function of the square root of optical power for the SIBC laser of Fig. 4 is shown in Fig. 5. The 3-dB bandwidth is linear at the lower bias power and is saturated at higher bias power. This can be understood by the effect of nonlinear gain suppression, which will be described in detail in the next section.

5. DEVICE MODELS

Three models are used to describe the intrinsic laser modulation, SI layer dynamic behavior, and packaging circuit response, respectively. These models are then, combined together to predict the packaged device response, to compare with experiment, and to predict the maximum obtainable bandwidth.

5.1 Intrinsic laser model

The rate equations of a laser with nonlinear gain can be expressed as[10,11]

$$\frac{dN}{dt} = -\frac{g_o(N - N_t)S}{1 + \epsilon S} + \frac{I}{qV} - \frac{N}{\tau_n} \tag{1a}$$

$$\frac{dS}{dt} = \frac{\Gamma g_o(N - N_t)S}{1 + \epsilon S} - \frac{S}{\tau_p} + \frac{\beta \Gamma N}{\tau_n} \tag{1b}$$

where N and S are the electron and photon densities, respectively, g_o is the differential gain, N_t is the carrier density for transparency, ϵ is the parameter for nonlinear gain suppression, Γ is the optical confinement factor, I is the current through active layer, V is the volume of the active region, is the electron charge, τ_n and τ_p are the electron and photon lifetimes, respectively, β is the fraction of spontaneous emission coupled into the lasing mode. The rate equations can be solved by using the standard small-signal analysis $S = S_o + se^{j\omega t}$, $N = N_o + ne^{j\omega t}$, and $I = I_o + ie^{j\omega t}$. The static photon density S_o can be obtained by solving the third-order polynomial equation,

$$A S_o^3 + B S_o^2 + C S_o + D = 0 \tag{2}$$

where $A = \frac{\epsilon}{\tau_p}(g_o + \frac{\epsilon}{\tau_n})$

$$B = (g_o + \frac{\epsilon}{\tau_n})(\Gamma g_o N_t + \frac{1}{\tau_p}) + \frac{\epsilon}{\tau_n \tau_p} - (g_o N_t + \frac{\epsilon I_o}{qV})(\Gamma g_o + \frac{\beta \Gamma \epsilon}{\tau_n})$$

$$C = \frac{1}{\tau_n}(\Gamma g_o N_t + \frac{1}{\tau_p}) - \frac{\beta \Gamma}{\tau_n}(g_o N_t + \frac{\epsilon I_o}{qV}) - \frac{I_o}{qV}(\Gamma g_o + \frac{\beta \Gamma \epsilon}{\tau_n})$$

$$D = -\frac{I_o}{qV}\frac{\beta \Gamma}{\tau_n}$$

The static electron density N_o is related to S_o by

$$N_o = \frac{(\Gamma g_o N_t + \frac{1}{\tau_p}) S_o + \frac{\varepsilon}{\tau_p} S_o^2}{(\Gamma g_o + \frac{\beta \Gamma \varepsilon}{\tau_n}) S_o + \frac{\beta \Gamma}{\tau_n}} \qquad (3)$$

The normalized intensity modulation response is

$$\frac{S(\omega)}{S(o)} = \frac{\omega_o^2}{\omega_o^2 - \omega^2 + j\omega \Gamma_d} \qquad (4)$$

where

$$\Gamma_d = \frac{g_o S_o}{1 + \varepsilon S_o} + \frac{1}{\tau_n} - \frac{\Gamma g_o (N_o - N_t)}{(1 + \varepsilon S_o)^2} + \frac{1}{\tau_p}$$

$$\omega_o^2 = \frac{\Gamma g_o (N_o - N_t)}{(1 + \varepsilon S_o)^2} (\frac{g_o S_o}{1 + \varepsilon S_o} + \frac{\beta}{\tau_n}) - (\frac{\Gamma g_o (N_o - N_t)}{(1 + \varepsilon S_o)^2} - \frac{1}{\tau_p})(\frac{g_o S_o}{1 + \varepsilon S_o} + \frac{1}{\tau_n})$$

The transfer function, shown in equation (4), has a peak (or resonance) response at the frequency,

$$\omega_r = (\omega_o^2 - \frac{\Gamma_d^2}{2})^{1/2} \qquad (5)$$

The output optical power P is related to the photon density S by

$$P = \frac{S V h\nu \alpha_m}{2\Gamma \tau_p (\alpha_m + \alpha_i)} \qquad (6)$$

where $h\nu$ is the photon density, α_m is the mirror loss, and α_i is the internal loss.

5.2 SI layer circuit model

The circuit model of SI layer can be represented by[8] Fig. 6, where C_1 is the capacitance due to displacement current through the SI layer, C_2 is the capacitance due to finite carrier life time of the electron and iron acceptor recombination process, and R is the resistance of the SI layer.

The Fe-doped InP SI layer can be characterized with two different regimes[12,13] from its current-voltage (I-V) curve. Below a critical voltage, the I-V characteristic is ohmic with high resistivity. Above the critical voltage, the leakage current increases superlinearly due to the space-charge-limited (SCL) effect. The critical voltage is dependent on the thickness of the SI layer. For a typical thickness of 5 μm, the breakdown voltage is about 10 V, which is much higher than the operating voltage of a laser diode. Table 1 lists the typical parameter values of SI layer in ohmic regime.

5.3 Packaged device model

The laser chip is mounted at the end of microstrip line, which is connected to K Launcher[14] through a glass bead. The overall packaged device can be represented by the circuit model of Fig. 7. An impedance-matched resister is serially connected to the laser diode to reduce the microwave reflection.

Table 1. Typical Parameter Values for SI Layer in Ohmic Regime

Element	Symbol	Unit	Value
SI resistivity	ρ	Ohm-cm	3×10^8
SI thickness	d	μm	5
Bond-pad area	A_1	cm^2	3.6×10^{-4}
Mesa area	A_2	cm^2	5.5×10^{-5}
SI carrier lifetime	τ	s	2.8×10^{-7}
Bond-pad capacitance	C_1	pF	1
Mesa capacitance	C_2	fF	0.9

5.4 Comparison between model analysis and measurement data

Since intrinsic laser diode can be regarded as a short circuit[15] at all frequencies for the laser biased above the threshold, the analysis can ben separated into two parts: intrinsic laser modulation response, R_I and parasitic modulation response, R_p. Thus, the total response, including the detector's response, R_D, is expressed as

$$R_T = R_I \times R_P \times R_D \qquad (7)$$

or

$$R_T (dB) = R_I (dB) + R_P (dB) + R_D (dB)$$

To compare with experiment, first the parameters for the intrinsic laser are chosen such that the theoretical calculation of L-I curve based on equations (2), (3), and (6) is fitted with experimental L-I curve. Fig. 8 shows this comparison and Table 2 lists the values of the parameters used for the calculation.

Table 2. Parameters Used in Calculation for SIBC Lasers

Element	Symbol	Unit	Value
Photon energy	hν	eV	0.95
Active thickness	t	μm	0.15
Active width	w	μm	2.0
Cavity length	l	μm	275
Group refractive index	μ_g	—	3.9
Confinement factor	Γ	—	0.34
Facet reflectivity	R_f	—	0.31
Internal loss	α_i	cm^{-1}	25
Differential gain	g_o	m^3/s	1.8×10^{-12}
Gain suppression	ϵ	m^3	1.7×10^{-23}
Electron lifetime	τ_n	ns	1.65
Carrier density for transparency	N_t	m^{-3}	1×10^{24}
Spontaneous emission coupling	β	—	10^{-4}

Second, from the experimental relation between the resonance frequency and the square root of optical power, the nonlinear gain of 1.7×10^{-23} m^3 is used to calculate the theoretical relation based on equations (5) and (6), which is shown in Fig. 9. Then, the intrinsic laser modulation response is obtained by equation (4) and is shown in Fig. 10(a). Third, using Super-Compact[16] software, the parasitic modulation response is analyzed based on the circuit model of Fig. 7. The result is shown in Fig. 10(b), and Table 3 lists the values of the parasitic elements. The bondwire inductance is 1.0 nH, measured from

S_{11} data of the Smith chart at 2 GHz. The chip parasitic capacitance is approximately 2 pF, which includes the bond-pad capacitance, the mesa capacitance, and the channel capacitance. Finally, the intrinsic laser response, the parasitic response and the detector response are added together, according to equation (7), to get the total response. The slight difference between the theoretical calculation and the measured frequency response could be attributed to the variation of the nonlinear gain with modulation frequency and driving current. From Fig. 9, this variation is estimated from 1.5×10^{-23} m^3 to 2.0×10^{-23} m^3.

Table 3. Parameter Values for Parasitic Elements

Element	Symbol	Unit	Value
Source impendance	R_{so}	Ohm	50
Coaxial Cable:			
Characteristic impedance	Z	Ohm	50
Physical length	P	Inch	12
Glass bead capacitance	C_g	pF	0.015
Microstrip Line:			
Substrate thickness	H	mil	10
Conductor width	W	mil	10
Conductor thickness	T	mil	0.1
Conductor length	L	Inch	0.15
Impedance-matched resistor	R_m	Ohm	46
Bondwire inductance	L_b	nH	1.0
Chip parasitic capacitance	C_p	pF	2.0
Chip contact resistance	R_c	Ohm	5.0

5.5 Maximum obtainable bandwidth

From Fig. 9, it can be seen that the experimental resonance frequency saturates around 8.5 GHz. This seems to be the major limitation of the device. To understand how this restriction can be removed under reasonable fabrication change, two parameters are changed: One is the active layer width changed from 2 to 1 μm; one is the differential gain changed from 1.8×10^{-12} m^3/s to 2.7×10^{-12} m^3/s. The channel width could be made smaller by using a smaller opening line or by reactive ion etching to reduce undercut. The differential gain could be improved[17] by slightly raising the active doping level without degrading the carrier lifetime and the internal absorption of the laser diode. Fig. 11 shows the intrinsic laser response with these new changes. It can be seen that a 3-dB bandwidth of 20 GHz can be obtained at 80-mA driving current.

Improving laser intrinsic response alone is not enough for the total response to achieve a 20-GHz bandwidth. The bondwire inductance needs to be reduced to less than 0.1 nH and the chip parasitic capacitance needs to be reduced to less than 1 pF. The bondwire inductance can be improved by using the beam-lead to connect the laser chip to the microstrip line and by flip-chip bonding of impedance matching resistor. The chip parasitic capacitance can be reduced by coating a thick polyimide layer under the bonding pad. Fig. 12 shows the Super-Compact simulation of parasitic response under these new changes.

6. RELATIVE INTENSITY NOISE

The relative intensity noise (RIN) is an important parameter to evaluate the suitability of an injection laser diode to be used in high quality analog fiber optic systems.[18,19] RIN is defined as[20]

$$RIN = \frac{\langle \Delta P \rangle^2}{\langle P \rangle^2} \frac{1}{\Delta f}$$

where $<P>$ is the average laser light intensity, $<\Delta P>$ is the root-mean-square light intensity fluctuation, and $<\Delta F>$ is the frequency range of measurement.

The RIN spectrum of SIBC lasers was measured by using an HP 71400A lightwave signal analyzer, and is shown in Fig. 13 for bias currents of 50 and 102 mA, respectively. Since there is no optical isolator used in this experiment, the measured RIN should include the intrinsic relative intensity noise, RIN_i, and the relative intensity noise induced by the reflection from single-mode optical fiber, RIN_r. The laser coupled optical power, C, reflected back from the far end of the single-mode fiber is estimated about -40 dB. The noise spectrum clearly shows that the maximum noise happens at the resonance frequency, and the noise is substantially decreased with higher bias current.

7. CONCLUSIONS

We have developed a high-speed and high-power 1.3-μm InGaAsP laser with a semi-insulating current blocking layer. The lasers have a 3-dB bandwidth of 11 GHz and high-power output of 42 mW/facet. In addition, the lasers have CW threshold current as low as 10 mA at room temperature, total differential quantum efficiency of 60%, and high-temperature operation up to 100°C. Packaged device models are developed which include the intrinsic laser response and the parasitic modulation response. The experimental results are compared to the model analysis with reasonable agreement. The model is also used to predict maximum obtainable bandwidth of 20 GHz with proper changes in the fabrication process. Finally, the measured relative intensity noise of SIBC Laser was also presented.

8. ACKNOWLEDGEMENTS

The authors wish to thank C. B. Su of Texas A&M University for stimulating discussions, D. Wolf, K. D. Buehring, and B. DeFoe for their contribution to this work, and L. Wicker for typing the manuscript.

9. REFERENCES

1. K. Tanaka, M. Hoshino, K. Wakao, J. Komeno, H. Ishikawa, S. Yamakoshi, and H. Imai, "Semi-insulator-embedded InGaAsP/InP flat-surface buried heterostructure laser", Appl. Phys. Lett. 47, 1127-1129 (1985).

2. N. K. Dutta, J. L. Zilko, T. Cella, D. A. Ackerman, T. M. Shen, and S. G. Napholtz, "InGaAsP laser with semi-insulating current confining layers", Appl. Phys. Lett. 48, 1572-1573 (1986).

3. D. P. Wilt, J. Long, W. C. Dautremont-Smith, M. W. Focht, T. M. Shen, R. L. Hartman, "Channelled-substrate buried-hetrostructure InGaAsP/InP laser with semi-insulating OMVPE base structure and LPE regrowth", Electron. Lett. 22, 869-870 (1986).

4. S. Sugou, Y. Kato, H. Nishimoto, K. Kasahara, "Planar surface buried-heterostructure InGaAsP/InP lasers with hydrid VPE-grown Fe-doped highly resistive current-blocking layers", Electron. Lett. 22, 1213-1215 (1986).

5. C. Z. Zah, J. S. Osinski, S. G. Menocal, N. Tabatabaie, T. P. Lee, "Wide-bandwidth and high-power 1.3-μm InGaAsP buried crescent lasers with semi-insulating Fe-doped InP current blocking layers", Electron. Lett. 23, 52-53 (1987).

6. K. Wakao, K. Nakai, T. Sanada, M. Kuno, T. Odagawa, and S. Yamakoshi, "InGaAsP/InP Planar buried heterostructure lasers with semi-insulating InP current blocking layers grown by MOCVD", IEEE J. Quantum Electron., QE-23, 943-947 (1987).

7. W. H. Cheng, C. B. Su, K. D. Buehring, J. W. Ure, D. Perrachione, D. Renner, K. L. Hess and S. W. Zehr, "Low threshold and wide-bandwidth 1.3-μm InGaAsP buried crescent injection lasers with semi-insulating current confinement layers", Appl. Phys. Lett. 51, 155-157 (1987).

8. W. H. Cheng, C. B. Su, K. D. Buehring, S. Y. Huang, J. Pooladdej, D. Wolf, D. Perrachione, D. Renner, K. L. Hess and S. W. Zehr, "High-speed and high-power 1.3-μm InGaAsP buried crescent injection lasers with semi-insulating current blocking layers", Appl. Phys. Lett. 51, 1783-1785 (1987).

9. K. L. Hess, S. W. Zehr, W. H. Cheng, and D. Perrachione, "Semi-insulating InP grown by low pressure MOCVD", J. Electron. Mater. 16, 127-131 (1987).

10. J. E. Bowers, B. R. Hemenway, A. H. Grauck, and D. P. Wilt, "High-speed InGaAsP constricted-mesa lasers", IEEE J. Quantum Electron. QE-22, 833-844 (1986).

11. J. E. Bowers, "High-speed semiconductor laser design and performance", Solid-state Electron. 30, 1-11 (1987).

12. J. Cheng, S. R. Forrest, B. Tell, D. Wilt, B. Schwartz, and P. D. Wright, "Semi-insulating properties of Fe-implanted InP. I. Current-limiting properties of $n\pm$ semi-insulating $-n+$ structures", Journal of Appl. Phys. 58, 1780-1786 (1985).

13. A. T. Macrander, J. A. Long, V. G. Riggs, A. F. Bloemeke, and W. D. Johnston, Jr., "Electrical characteristics of Fe-doped semi-insulating InP grown by Metalorganic Chemical Vapor Deposition", Appl. Phys. Lett. 45, 1297-1298 (1984)."

14. Wiltron Company, K connector

15. K. Y. Lau, and A. Yariv, "Ultra-high speed semiconductor lasers", IEEE J. Quantum Electron. QE-21, 121-138 (1985).

16. Compact Software, Inc. Super-compact revision 1.91.

17. C. B. Su, and V. Lanzisera, "Effect of doping level on the gain constant and modulation bandwidth of InGaAsP semiconductor lasers", Appl. Phys. Lett. 45, 1302-1304 (1984).

18. H. B. Kim, R. Maciejko, and J. Conradi, "Effect of laser noise on analogue fiber optic systems", Electron. Lett. 16, 919-920 (1980).

19. K. I. Sato, "Intensity noise of semiconductor laser diodes in fiber optic analog video transmission", IEEE J. Quantum Electron. QE-19, 1380-1391 (1983).

20. H. Jackel and H. Melchior, "Fundamental limits of the light intensity fluctuations of semiconductor lasers with dielectric transverse mode confinement", Proc. 5th Euro. Conf. Opt. Commun. Amsterdam, The Netherlands, Sept. 17-19, 2.5 (1979).

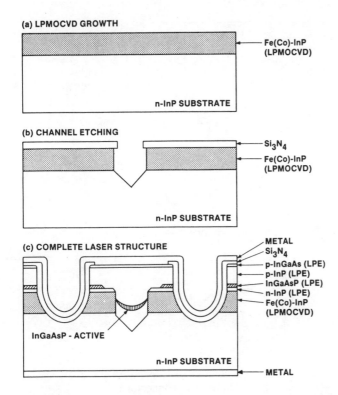

Figure 1. Schematic diagram of SIBC laser structure
a) After LPMOCVD growth
b) After channel etching
c) Complete laser structure

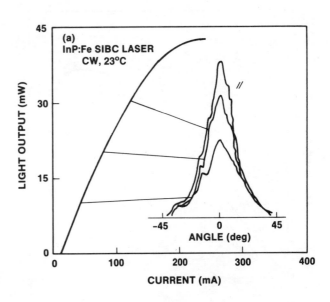

Figure 2. CW L-I characteristics of SIBC laser at 23°C and far-field patterns parallel to the junction plane at various light output powers

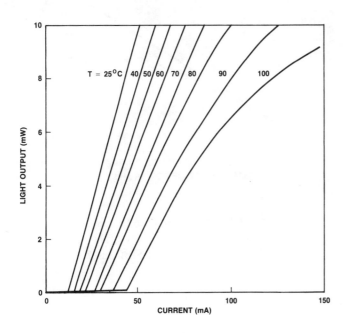

Figure 3. CW L-I characteristics of an SIBC laser at various temperatures

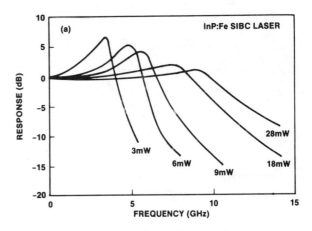

Figure 4. Small-signal modulation responses of an SIBC laser at various optical power levels

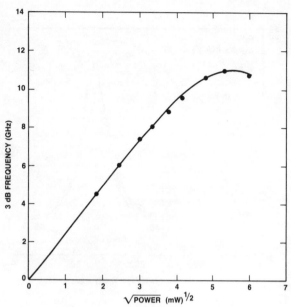

Figure 5. 3-dB modulation bandwidth as a function of the square root of optical power

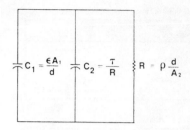

Figure 6. A simple circuit model for SI layer

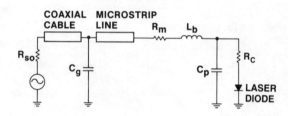

Figure 7. A packaged device model for the SIBC laser mounted on a K connector

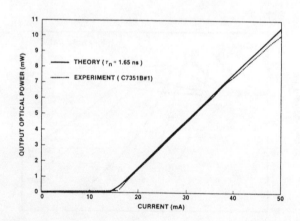

Figure 8. Comparison of L-I curves between experiment and theoretical calculation

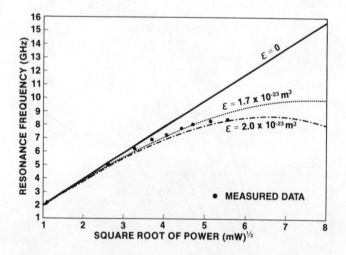

Figure 9. Dependence of resonance frequency on the square root of optical power. The data points are measurements on a SIBC laser

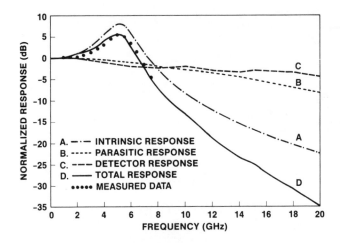

Figure 10. Small-signal modulation response of a SIBC laser at a bias current of 40 mA
  a) Intrinsic laser response
  b) Parasitic roll-off
  c) Detector response
  d) Total response
  e) Data points of measurement

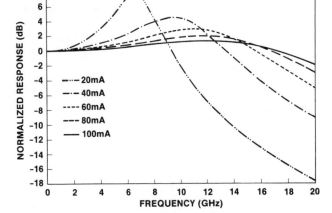

Figure 11. Intrinsic laser modulation response for an active-layer of 1-μm, a differential gain of 2.7×10^{-12} m^3/s, and a nonlinear gain suppression of 2.0×10^{-23} m^3

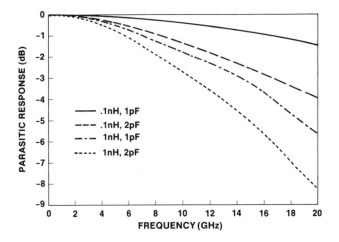

Figure 12. Parasitic modulation response for different values of capacitance and inductance

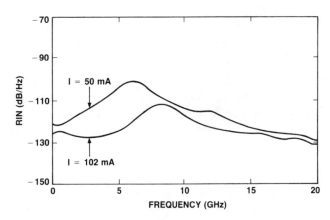

Figure 13. RIN spectra of a SIBC laser

Invited Paper

THE INFLUENCE OF In ON THE PERFORMANCE OF (Al)GaAs
SINGLE QUANTUM WELL LASERS

R. G. Waters, C. M. Harding and B. A. Soltz

McDonnell Douglas Astronautics Co.
350 Executive Boulevard
Elmsford, NY 10523

P. K. York, J. N. Baillargeon and J. J. Coleman

Dept. of Electrical and Computer Engineering
University of Illinois at Urbana-Champaign
Urbana, IL 61801

S. E. Fischer, D. Fekete and J. M. Ballantyne

School of Electrical Engineering and Field of Applied Physics
Cornell University
Ithaca, NY 14853

ABSTRACT

Strained-layer $In_x Ga_{1-x} As$ quantum well lasers have attracted considerable attention of late due to the materials configurations made possible. Interest in the semiconductor laser community stems in part from the prospect of accessing the spectral window near 1 um for pumping new solid state hosts and in part for space communications if an advantage can be demonstrated. Technologists in these areas have fostered the hope that strain accommodation[1] and perhaps lattice hardening[2-4] by In can enable viable long-lived devices. Steady progress in the development of high-performance $In_x Ga_{1-x} As$ lasers[5-11] has been encouraging with the first cw life-test reports coming quite recently.[ivl] Among other recent advances we cite achievement of high-power, low-threshold buried heterostructure devices operating near 1.1 μm.[12] We will be presenting recent progress in performance and reliability of (In)GaAs lasers of three very different types. First we will discuss devices emitting near 1 μm with demonstrated cw lifetimes exceeding 5000 hours. Next we turn our attention to two extreme cases. The first structure utilizes low levels (2.5%) of In in the quantum well of an otherwise conventional (Al)GaAs graded-index separate confinement heterostructure single quantum well (GRINSCH-SQW) laser and thus constitutes a small perturbation on a familiar device. Finally, a step-index structure with a $In_{0.51} Ga_{0.49} As$ quantum well will be discussed.

1. DEVICES OPERATING NEAR 1 μm

The device structure, grown by low-pressure metalorganic vapor deposition, incorporates a single $In_{.37}Ga_{.63}As$ strained layer quantum well (L_z=40 Å) in a GaAs/AlGaAs graded-index separate confinement heterostructure and is shown in Fig 1. The quantum well (remainder of the structure) was grown at 650°C (750°C) and 240Å/min (1000Å/min) except for the graded region which was grown at 400Å/min. Oxide-defined, 60 μm wide stripes were formed using standard processing.[13] Facets were formed by cleaving and 600 μm long uncoated devices were mounted to a copper heat sink. (This configuration will apply throughout unless otherwise stated.) The resulting devices operated cw at 1010 nm with threshold current (density) of 128 mA (356 A/cm^2) and slope efficiency of 0.25 W/A per facet.

Life testing was carried out at 30° heat sink temperature in a constant-power mode on devices operating cw at 70 mW/facet. A total of 30 devices were placed on life test. They were not screened in any way. Device histories are shown in Fig. 2 for 15 devices. (Half of the population was removed at the 1000 hour point due to equipment needs but said devices were virtually indistinguishable from those shown.) Lasers have surpassed the 5000-hour mark with an average degradation rate of 1.8% per kh (fractional current increase). This is to be compared with degradation in GaAs quantum wells in which rates below 2% have been achieved[14,15] although in our experience 7-12% is more typical[15] at these current densities.

The apparent immunity to sudden failure is striking and, we believe, significant since our statistical base is greater than the figure would indicate. Recall that 30 devices were operated to 1000 hours. In addition, an earlier population of 8 devices were tested to current doubling ($\gtrsim$ 4000 hours in that case). In spite of the large population, we have yet to see a sudden failure. Put simply and conservatively 38 devices have shown 100% survival to 1000 hours. Such a large population may be necessary to be convincing since experience with GaAs quantum wells has taught us that the survival rate depends on handling artifacts as much as anything. Whatever the cause, total survival for GaAs devices is seen in no more than 3% of the populations. In the present case, therefore, it is unlikely that we are being deceived by a fortuitous population of damage-free lasers.

Some other devices were placed on life test at an earlier date. The results for three lasers are shown in Fig. 3. While the statistics here are meager, the data does constitute an existence proof for lifetimes exceeding 10,000 hours. In addition, five lasers operating at λ = 967 nm (from a separate growth run) were tested. Of these, two reached the current limit at 4000 and 7000 hours respectively and three continue to operate beyond 10,000 hours.

2. $In_{.025}Ga_{.975}As$

The next structure we consider incorporates a small concentration (2.5%) of In in the quantum well of an otherwise conventional graded-index separate confinement heterostructure (GRINSCH) laser and is schematized in Fig. 4. The purpose of this experiment was to determine whether small amounts of In afforded a performance advantage. "Small" in this context implies a small wavelength change so that the devices may be considered as replacements for binary (GaAs) devices in conventional applications. A control growth was conducted and the structure is shown in Fig. 5. Structurally, it is the same in every respect except for the omission of the In. Growth-wise it is as similar as is possible with typical reactor reproducibility and the changes needed to facilitate In incorporation. These structures consist of a .25 μm GaAs buffer, 1.5 μm $Al_{.6}Ga_{.4}As$ confining lasers, .12 μm parabolically graded $Al_xGa_{1-x}As$ layers with .2 < X < .6, a 50Å (In) GaAs quantum well and a .2 μm p+ GaAs cap. Growth temperature was 800°C except for the In-bearing quantum well and its adjacent graded regions for which 625°C was used. Mg and Si were used as dopants.

Table 1 shows how the performance parameters compared to those of the control structure. Results are averages over twenty devices of each type with one growth per structure. The apparent performance enhancement for the (In)GaAs case is the subject of confirmatory studies.

TABLE I - PERFORMANCE COMPARISON

	λ	J_{th}	Slope Eff.	T_o
GaAs	829nm	375A/cm^2	0.43W/A	140K
$In_{.025}Ga_{.975}As$	838nm	308A/cm^2	0.49W/A	172K

3. $In_{.51}Ga_{.49}As$

The final structure to be discussed is shown in Fig. 6. A 30 Å quantum well of $In_{.51}Ga_{.49}As$ is incorporated into a step-index AlGaAs structure to achieve a lasing wavelength of 1102 nm. Similar material with a similar wavelength has been used to produce buried heterostructure lasers with thresholds of 7 mA.[12] This separate confinement structure has $Al_{.2}Ga_{.8}As$ confining layers, .1 μm GaAs to either side of the quantum well, and a step-graded quantum well region. The buffer and confining layers were grown at 720°C and the temperature was lowered (raised) to 625°C (720°C) at the beginning (end) of the .1 μm GaAs layer.

Threshold current (densities) were measured to be 90mA (250A/cm^2) and the slope efficiencies were .26W/A. This efficiency in conjunction with a characteristic temperature of 90K causes the cw output to be thermally limited to 240 mW per facet. Laser parameters for this and the other structures previously described are given in Table II.

TABLE II - LASER PARAMETERS

Structure	λ (nm)	J_{th} (A/cm^2)	Slope Eff(W/A)	T_0	Max. Power (mW)
GaAs	829	375	0.43	140	**
$In_{.025}Ga_{.975}As$	838	308	0.49	172	**
$In_{.37}Ga_{.63}As$	1010	356	0.25	147	350-400
$In_{.51}Ga_{.49}As$	1102	250	0.26	90	240-260

* All cw, L=600 μm, W=60 μm, oxide-defined, uncoated
** Not thermally limited

4. ACKNOWLEDGEMENTS

The authors are grateful to Y. Chen, K. Bystrom, S. Yellen, R. Soltz, S. Schultz and T. Guido for valuable technical assistance.

5. REFERENCES

1. R. M. Kolbas, N. G. Anderson, W. D. Laidig, Y. Sin, Y. C. Lo, K. Y. Hsieh and Y. J. Yang, IEEE J. Quantum Electron. 24, 1605 (1988)

2. P. A. Kirby, IEEE J. Quantum Electron. QE-11, 562 (1975)

3. M. Ettenberg and C. J. Nuese, J. Appl. Phys. 46, 2137 (1975)

4. G. H. B. Thompson, "Physics of Semiconductor Laser Devices" (John Wiley and Sons, New York, 1980)

5. W. D. Laidig, P. J. Caldwell, Y. F. Lin, and C. K. Peng, Appl. Phys. Lett. 44, 653 (1984)

6. W. D. Laidig, Y. F. Lin and P. J. Caldwell, J. Appl. Phys. 57, 33 (1985)

7. D. Fekete, K. T. Chan, J. M. Ballantyne and L. F. Eastman, Appl. Phys. Lett. 49, 1659 (1986)

8. Y. J. Yang. K. Y. Hsieh and R. M. Kolbas, Appl. Phys. Lett. 51, 215 (1987)

9. J. N. Baillargeon, P. K. York, C. A. Zmudzinski, G. E. Fernandez, D. J. Beernink, and J. J. Coleman, Appl. Phys Lett. 53, 457 (1988)

10. S. E. Fischer, D. Fekete, G. B. Feak and J. M. Ballantyne, Appl. Phys. Lett. 50, 714 (1987)

11. P. Gavrilovic, K. Meehan, W. Stutius, J. E. Williams and J. H. Zarrabi, 11th IEEE International Semiconductor Laser Conference, Boston, MA, Aug. 1988, paper L-5

12. P. K. York, K. J. Beernink, G. E. Fernandez and J. J. Coleman, Appl. Phys. Lett. (in press)

13. D. K. Wagner, R. G. Waters, P. L. Tihanyi, D. S. Hill, A. J. Roza, H. J. Vollmer and M. M. Leopold, IEEE J. Quantum Electron. 24, 1258 (1988)

14. G. L. Harnagel, T. L. Paoli, R. L. Thornton, R. D. Burnham and D. L. Smith, Appl. Phys. Lett. 46, 118 (1985)

15. R. G. Waters and R. K. Bertaska, Appl. Phys. Lett. 52, 179 (1988)

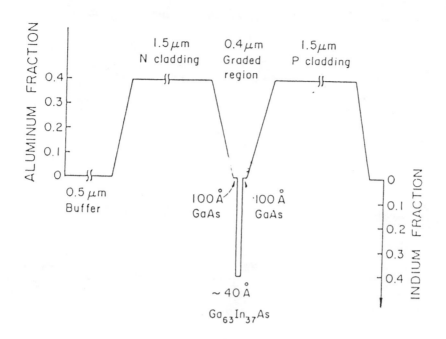

Fig. 1 In$_{.37}$Ga$_{.63}$As strained-layer structure for lasers emitting near 1 μm

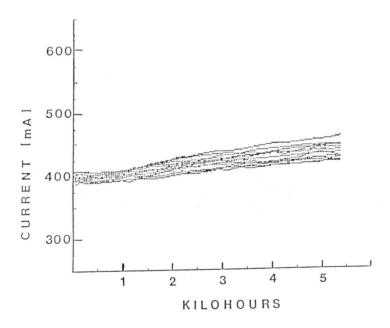

Fig. 2 Histories for In$_{.37}$Ga$_{.63}$As lasers operating cw at 70 mW per facet and at 30°C. Results for fifteen devices are shown

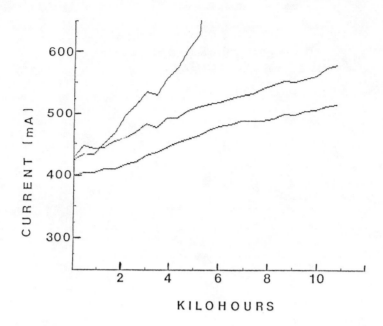

Fig. 3 Histories for three lasers. These are nominally the same as in Fig. 2 except that a different wafer section was used and testing was started earlier. Two devices continue to operate

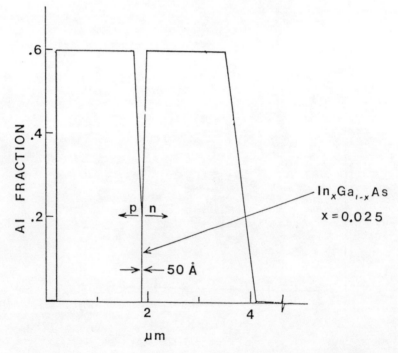

Fig. 4 GRINSCH structure with 2.5% In incorporated into the quantum well.

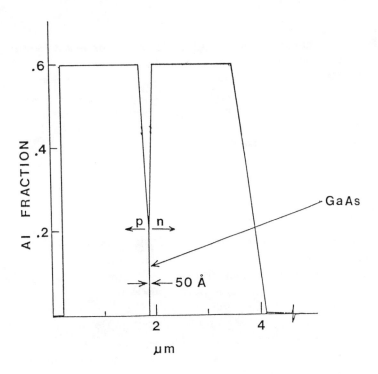

Fig. 5 GRINSCH structures with no In in the quantum well.

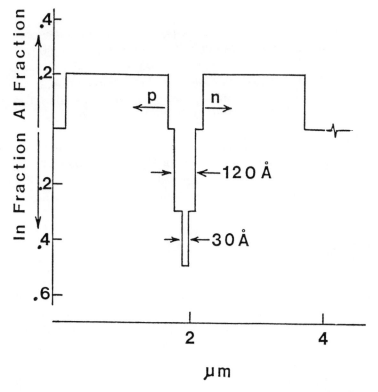

Fig. 6 Step-index In$_{.51}$Ga$_{.49}$As/AlGaAs structure.

Reliability of single-element diode lasers for high-performance optical data storage applications

M. K. Benedict, IBM Corporation, General Products Division, Tucson, Arizona 85744
C. B. Morrison, IBM Corporation, General Technology Division, East Fishkill, New York 12533
A. J. Tzou, IBM Corporation, General Products Division, Tucson, Arizona 85744
A. D. Gleckler, Kaman Aerospace, Tucson, Arizona 85711
D. W. Fried, IBM Corporation, General Products Division, Tucson, Arizona 85744
K. J. Giewont, IBM Corporation, General Technology Division, East Fishkill, New York 12533

ABSTRACT

For high-performance optical data storage applications, AlGaAs/GaAs diode lasers were stressed at various power levels, temperatures, and operating conditions. The devices tested were V-channeled structures mounted with the junction side down. These lasers came from a single production run to eliminate the statistical variances associated with multilot tests.

Cumulative failure plots for cells at 30 mW stressed at 65°C and 40 mW stressed at 55 and 65°C show that two failure mechanisms are present, which we designated as intrinsic and wear-out failure regions. Using the data from the wear-out region and assuming an Arrhenius model for the temperature dependence of the reliability function, we found that the activation energy for this lot of lasers is 0.37 eV. From this evaluation, we project a median lifetime of 3.4 khrs for 40 mW operation at 35°C, and a median lifetime of 36.7 khrs at 30 mW and 35°C, which is an order of magnitude greater. For a power model where the median lifetime is proportional to power raised to the -n, we calculated that n is 4.3 for powers between 30 and 40 mW.

Other data to be discussed was accumulated from low-power continuous-wave and pulsed stress cells. In addition, failure analysis results correlated with the various failure regions will be presented. All the devices were fully characterized prior to stressing, and throughout the stress period they were periodically characterized for changes in operating current at 7 mW and 30 mW, for parallel and perpendicular far-field distributions, and for astigmatic length. To our knowledge, this is the first experimental data that tracks these optical properties over the life of a laser diode.

With the exception of the drive current to maintain a given optical power, all other electro-optic properties exhibit stability throughout the diode lasers' lifetime. The data also shows that there is no precursor to failure. Our results show that acceptable reliability targets can be met for high-performance optical storage applications as long as the operating temperature is maintained below 35°C and the optical power is limited to 30 mW.

1. INTRODUCTION

Optical data storage products require high-power, single-element diode lasers with specialized optical and electrical characteristics. There are also requirements for defraction limited beams with a very short depth of focus. To attain these requirements, it is necessary to have a coherent energy source with beam characteristics capable of producing a reliable spot on the optical recording disk surface.[1]

The diode laser characteristics (which include spatial mode distributions, wavelength, astigmatic length, and continuous wave optical power) limit the choices of diode lasers used in the optical data storage application. In addition, these properties must be stable throughout the life of the data storage product. To our knowledge, a complete study of the stability during the lifetime of these optical properties has been never published.

This report is a study of the changes in the operating characteristics of the diode laser as it ages. Along with the characteristic changes, key failure mechanisms are identified and related to the effects on optical data storage products. Based upon this study, recommendations to the laser and the product developer are made.

2. COMPONENT DESCRIPTION

The diode laser used for this study has a maximum CW rating of 40 mW and a nominal 830 nm wavelength spectral emission. The device is packaged with a back-facet photodetector in a 3-pin, TO-5 type can. The diode laser itself is a conventional, 4-layer double heterostructure grown by liquid phase epitaxy (LPE) over an etched v-channel in a p-type GaAs substrate. An n-type epitaxial layer is used to form a p-n-p-n transistor to provide for current confinement. The device is mounted junction-side down. The electrical connections are made by ball-bonded using gold wires. There are high and low reflectivity coatings on the back and front facets, respectively.

All diode lasers were screened by a preliminary burn-in process before the start of this experiment. All diode lasers came from a single production run to remove the lot-to-lot variations in the experimental results.

3. HANDLING AND STRESS-TEST CAPABILITIES

When lasers were mounted on any of the testers, special electrostatic (ESD) discharge precautions were followed, such as the use of wrist straps, shorting bars on laser packages, grounded heatsinks and grounding mats. The two stress systems used for this experiment are as follows:

1. <u>Low power life tester</u>. The driver module monitors the laser's internal photodiode current and adjusts the drive current to maintain a constant optical power from the rear facet.
2. <u>Modulation and composite waveform tester</u>. The composite portion of this tester was used to stress 25 lasers in a simulated product environment. One cycle or period is composed of three parts: (a) optical power at 7 mW for 1 msec, (b) optical power at 25 mW for 20 msec, and (c) 40 mW 50% duty cycle pulse at a frequency of 12.5 MHz for 20 msec.

Because of the complexity of the tester, the current sources did not servo on any optical power but were fixed current sources. Solar cells were used, however, to detect the front-facet optical-output power, and the tester monitored each of the three power levels.

The modulation portion of this tester was used to stress 20 lasers in a 200 MHz, 7 mW average power level. The tester monitored the average output power, internal photodiode output, and the temperature of the lasers.

The stress systems are housed in an environmentally controlled class 10,000 room. The input power is regulated by a power conditioning system to remove powerline surges and transients.

4. ELECTRICAL AND OPTICAL PROPERTIES

At time zero, that is before any stress testing has commenced, all diode lasers were fully characterized for their electrical and optical properties. These characterizations included I-V, P-I, far-field distributions, astigmatism, spectrum, feedback noise, and near-field distributions. Where appropriate, characterizations were done at two different power levels (5 and 30 mW) with two different temperatures (25 and 50 $\pm$ 0.2°C).

A data base was generated containing results from more than 300 diode lasers. From this data, parametric changes in temperature and power can be evaluated. This same data base is used to track the parametric changes in time for this experiment. The parametric characteristics tracked in time for this experiment included threshold current, power at threshold, differential quantum efficiency, current to maintain power at 5 and 30 mW, linearity, peak wavelength, laser noise caused by optical feedback, far-field ripple, wavelength shifts, far-field full-width half-maximums (FWHMs), aspect ratio, beam pointing directions, and astigmatic length.

5. ACCELERATED STRESS TEST MATRIX

In order to understand failure mechanisms, manufacturing defects, and application specific aging mechanisms, a limited amount of stress testing is necessary. Considering application needs and the desire to know or verify certain diode laser parameters, such as the high power activation energy and the power model for mean time to failure, we devised the following test matrix:

cell (1) 40 mW, 65°C, n=16
cell (2) 40 mW, 55°C, n=16
cell (3) 30 mW, 65°C, n=16
cell (4) 7 mW, 50°C, n=25
cell (5) 7 mW, 90°C, n=25
cell (6) Composite waveform (one period includes 7 mW for 1 sec; 25 mW for 20 msec;
    40 mW peak, 50% duty cycle for 20 msec, 50°C, n=25
cell (7) Modulation stress test, 200 MHz, 7 mW avg. power, 50°C, n=20

The composite waveform stress test was devised to simulate, in some fashion, the actual usage of the diode in the application, a relatively long period at low power CW operation, a small amount of time at medium power CW operation, and a similar small time at high power pulsed operation. Data was compared between this cell and the CW cell for increase in aging rate for multi-operational points when the medium and high-power operation is a small fraction (less than 10%) of the total power on hours (POH).

One technique for reducing the effects of optical feedback (operating point shift and increased intensity noise) at lower power is to modulate the laser drive current with a high-frequency current. By comparing the results from the modulation cell to that of a similar CW cell, it is possible to determine if modulation has a detrimental effect upon the diode lasers.

By comparing the results between the various test cells, conclusions are sought to the following issues:

1. Is there a significant failure rate difference when the operating point is a low power CW or when modulated to the same average value? This comparison should detect failure mechanisms associated with peak optical powers, peak currents, or rapid thermal cycling of the facets.
2. What is the high power activation energy?
3. Can we develop a power vs. reliability model that spans the entire proposed operating range?
4. Is there any application oriented failure problems?
5. What are the various failure mechanisms and power level for which they are dominant?
6. What is the parametric stability of the diode laser during its useful life in a product?

The end-of-life definition for this experiment was defined as either a 30% change in current to maintain a given power level or a 10 mA change in drive current over a 24-hour period. This later condition was imposed to prevent the gross overpowering of the laser and destroying the original failure mechanism.

Figures 1 and 2 are plots of the cumulative diode laser failures vs. time. We can see that the tests appear to repeat at 2 temperatures at the 40 mW operation. There appears to be two failure rates present; the early failures can represent the intrinsic failure rate of these devices while the second region represents the end-of-life or wear-out region.

Assuming an Arrhenius model for the temperature dependence of the wear-out region, an estimate of the activation energy is as follows:

$$F_r = F_o \left[\exp\left(\frac{E_a}{kT}\right) \right] \qquad (1)$$

For two temperatures, the ratio of Eq.(1) can be solved for E_a:

$$E_a = \frac{k}{\frac{1}{T1} - \frac{1}{T2}} \ln R$$

where: E_a is the activation energy
k is the Boltzman's constant
R is the ratio of the median times to failure
F_r is the failure rate

The calculated activation energy of 0.37 eV for the power range of 30 to 40 mW CW is substantially less than 0.8 eV for a similar structure at a low power (5 mW) operation.[2] By contrast, a value 0.52 eV is reported for low-power operation of broad area diode lasers packaged similar to diode lasers used in this study.[3,4] In addition, 0.37 eV is very close to the value of 0.39 eV for a similar structure operated at pulsed high power.[5] We speculate the lower activation energy is associated with high-power facet aging while the higher activation energy can be associated with crystalline or carrier density induced defect growth.

Using the power model for the failure rate[6]

$$F_r \propto \left(\frac{1}{P}\right)^n$$

where: P is the power
n is an experimentally determined exponent

an estimation of the exponent n can be made from the wear-out region data. This estimation is n=4.3 which is close to the value of 4.0 for a similar structure operating at 780 nM.[6]

In addition, periodically, during all of these stress tests, the lasers were removed and characterization tests were performed. This was done to track the parametric stability of the optical characteristics.

Figure 3 is a plot of the current necessary to maintain 30 mW of optical power as a function of time for the stress cells operating at 50°C. The following are conclusions from Fig.3:

1. For optical data storage operations where the low power operating point is the dominate operation, there is no significant increase in the aging rate of the laser. The aging rate is 0.75 mA/khr for the 7 mW operation and 0.76 mA/khr for the composite operation.
2. When considering the question of average power vs. CW power, the modulation cell had a significant increase in aging rate to 1.4 mA/khr. This is because the peak powers for this modulation test reached about 17 mW, therefore, if modulation is used to reduce the noise, the product should be design to turn the modulation off when not needed.

Figures 4, 5, and 6 show the tracking of the optical properties of the laser diode in time. As we expected, these properties are independent of time and stress conditions. All the variations are within the measurement error of the characterization system.

During the characterization process, it was observed the pointing direction perpendicular to the junction changes by about 0.02°/mW while the parallel direction does not change. We speculate that this power dependency is caused by the difference in carrier densities in the two cladding layers. This difference causes the mode to shift slightly away from the substrate.

The overriding conclusion reached is that the only characteristic that changes dramatically during the aging of diode lasers on stress test is the drive current necessary to maintain a certain power level. To our knowledge, this is the first time that data has been collected on a wide variety of diode laser characteristics during stress testing, thus substantiating what previously has only been held industry-wide as an unstated assumption.

6. FAILURE ANALYSIS RESULTS

The ability to perform failure analysis is a vital part of any experiment for diode lasers. Because diode lasers are composed of a complex structure of epitaxial layers and are not surface devices, such as integrated circuits, examination of the entire laser structure for defects is extremely difficult. The structures involved are very small (for example, 3 um wide channels, and 0.1 um thick active layers), rendering all analysis techniques difficult.

Because GaAs damages easily during cross-sectioning, experience is required to differentiate polishing defects from actual device defects. Furthermore, cross-sectioning results have been very poor because of the minuteness of the structures, the delicacy of the single crystal material, and the extensive time required.

However, the weakest part of properly fabricated AlGaAs/GaAs double heterostructure diode laser is the facets. This facet is the location of high optical power density, heating effects caused by photon absorption by surface states, electrical leakage current, and poor heat sinking. Fortunately for failure analysis, the front facet is readily observed. Unfortunately, the front facet ages very quickly, always leaving some sign of degradation regardless of the actual failure mechanism.

In addition, the front facet is very susceptible to ESD damage,[7] even after the diode laser has failed. Thus, a diode laser that has been mishandled after failure might show facet damage, which is not the true cause of failure.

Manufacturing defects account for all of the early-life failures of the diodes, as shown in Figs. 1 and 2. Examination of one early-life failure revealed voids in the bonding solder material, and excessive chip overhang. Because of the resulting poor thermal dissipation, there is excessive heating at the facet.

Two devices showed a curved active region. This relates to the epitaxial crystal growth,[8] and causes the lasing spot to self-focus, reducing its size on the facet. Thus, the power limit to reach catastrophic optical damage is reduced. Another failed laser shows cracks caused by excessive pressure in the ball bonding operation.

Junction down mounting for better thermal dissipation reduces the distance the solder material must either grow whisker or diffuse through the material before it shorts the junction. This process is enhanced near the facet by the high local temperature of the region,[9] therefore, careful selection of the bonding solder is very important.[10]

Finally, in relation to manufacturing problems, the cap windows of several of the stress-tested lasers had cracks. There is some debate as to whether this is a problem with the package or with the method used for mounting the packaged lasers in stress-test fixtures (brass blocks).

Regarding intrinsic failure mechanisms, the facet is the weakest part of the diode laser. It can reach 200-300°C above the average chip temperature in normal operation. The following items have been observed at the facet:

1. <u>Football-shaped region</u>. This white football-shaped region on the facet where the light exits the facet shows up white under an optical microscope, as shown in Fig.7, and is often accompanied by a smaller black spot. Auger analysis indicates that this is in the aluminum oxide coating and it is either a photo-chemical reaction, a diffusion process whereby the Ga and As atoms physically move into the coating, or the facet coating has been eroded. The feature disappears as the facet is removed. This degradation mechanism is caused and enhanced by heating at the facet, a type of thermal run-away mechanism.
2. <u>Dark-line defects</u>. Electroluminescence studies have shown that some lasers aged for 2000 hours have dark areas which run parallel to the channel, as shown in Fig.8. These defects are caused by the high strain at the edge of the channel and the high temperatures at the facet allow the crystal defects to migrate to these points.[11]
3. <u>Catastrophic failure</u>. This mechanism is typified by one or more black spots on the facet. This is usually a melted region (the melting point of GaAs is 1500°C) and can be caused by overpowering the laser, surge currents, ESD, or continued high power usage when the facet is somewhat degraded. Additionally, the near field tends to be bimodal because of large losses at the center of the channel which results in a two spot near field, as shown in Fig.9.
4. <u>Leakage currents</u>. If the current blocking layers break down or if some leakage path is formed then the laser can suffer dramatic changes in threshold and efficiency. Electrically active blocking layers appear to be indicative of leakage paths and have been found in many failed devices during this experiment, which is EBIC image taken from the front facet, as shown in Fig.10.
5. <u>Bulk crystal defects</u>.[2] These are very difficult to find, but by using polarized infrared microscopy, we found that there is significant nonuniform stress in the cap layer of several devices. Stress is one of the major contributing factors to bulk defects. These stresses appear to be associated with the bonding process. Electron beam induced current (EBIC) studies have shown bulk defects in several devices. These defects show up as dark lines, but do not travel parallel to the junction.

7. RESULTS

The following summary was made based on the results (see Tables 1 and 2):

- Optical characteristics are stable up to the end of life.
- Modulation stress testing is more stressful than equivalent CW testing, and results in an increase of drive current of 1mA/khr at 7 mW avg. power, 200 MHz, 50°C.

The key failure mechanisms found are as follows:

1. High-power failure mechanisms
    a. Front facet damage
    b. Electrical breakdown of current blocking layer
    c. Asymmetrical current blocking layers
    d. Curved active layer
    e. Dark region and dark line defects
2. Manufacturing defects
    a. Cracked package window
    b. Poor die bonding
    c. Poor wire bonding
    d. Indium solder filamenting
    e. ESD damage
3. Low-power failure mechanisms
    a. Indium solder misdeposition
    b. Micro-cracks
    c. Bulk defect generation

The failure rate model parameter estimations are:

1. High-power activation energy of 0.37 eV.
2. High-power reliability model of n=4.3.

8. CONCLUSIONS

1. Better packaging technologies need to be developed, in particular technologies that do not require large localized pressures on the chip during the process, hard low temperature solders which are slow diffuser in GaAs, better strain relief, and thermal coefficient matching materials that unduly add to the package thermal resistance.
2. To facilitate the proper selection of laser diode for storage applications, the system architects need to determine methods of reducing the large number of power on hours where the laser is powered on but is not in use, which will improve the reliability picture for future products.
3. Applications architectures need to be constructed with the laser diode reliability in mind, that is, great care to provide a cool thermal environment for the laser is a must for reliable products. Operation near the maximum rated temperature and powers should be avoided, although package technology improvements might increase the flexibility of the thermal environment requirements.
4. Based on the results of this experiment, it appears that this laser diode technology can support optical data storage applications as long as the maximum optical power is limited to 30 mW.

9. ACKNOWLEDGEMENTS

The authors would like to express their sincere appreciation to R. Martin for failure analysis contributions.

10. REFERENCES

1. G. Bouwhuis, J. Huijser, J. Pasman, G. Van Rosmalen, and K. S. Immink, *Principles of Optical Disc Systems*, Adam Hilger Ltd., Bristol, England (1985).
2. K. Mizuishi, N. Chinone, H. Sato, and R. Ito, "Acceleration of the Gradual Degradation in (GaAl)As Double-Heterostructure Lasers as an Exponent Value of the Driving Current," J. Appl. Phys. 50(11), 6668-6674 (1979).
3. T. Hayakawa, N. Miyauchi, S. Yamamoto, H. Hayashi, S. Yano, and T. Hijikata, "Highly Reliable and Mode-Stabilized Operation in V-Channeled Substrate Inner Stripe Lasers on p-GaAs Substrate Emitting in the Visible Wavelength Region," J. Appl. Phys. 53, 7224, (1982).
4. T. Hayakawa, S. Yamamoto, S. Matsui, T. Sakurai, and T. Hijikata, "Long-lived (GaAl)As DH Lasers Bonded with In Produced by Eliminating Deterioration of In Solder," J. Appl. Phys. 21, 725, Japan (1982).
5. J. D. Barry, A. J. Einhorn, G. S. Mecherle, P. Nelson, R. A. Dye, and W. J. Archambeault, "Thermally Accelerated Life Testing of Single Mode, Double-Heterostructure, AlGaAs Laser Diodes Operated Pulsed at 50 mW Peak Power," IEEE J. Quantum Electronics 21(4), 365-375 (1985).
6. T. Hayakawa, N. Miyauchi, S. Yamamoto, S. Yano, and T Hijikata, "Highly Reliable and Mode-Stabilized Operation in V-Channeled Substrate Inner Stripe Lasers on P-GaAs Substrate Emitting in the Visible Wavelength Region," J. Appl. Phys. 53(11), 7224-7234, (1982).
7. "Hitachi Laser Diodes -- Precautions Against Surge," Document 10, Hitachi, Ltd., Japan (1986).
8. L. Figueroa and S. Wang, "Curved Junction Stabilized Filament (CJSF) Double-Heterostructure Injection Laser," Appl. Phys. Lett. 32, 55 (1978).
9. S. Todoroki, "Temperature Distribution Along the Striped Active Layer in High-Power GaAlAs Lasers," J. Appl. Phys. 58, 1124 (1985).
10. K. Mizuishi, "Some Aspects of Bonding-Solder Deterioration Observed in Long-Lived Semiconductor Laser: Solder Migration and Whisker Growth," J. Appl. Phys. 55(2), 289-296 (1984).
11. D. H. Newman and S. Ritchie, *Reliability and Degradation*, John Wiley and Sons, Ltd., New York (1981).

Table 1. Observations of failed lasers

TIME(HRS)	OHP 40mW/55C	HP2 40mW/65C	HP1 30mW/65C	LP2 7mW/90C	LP1+MOD'D 7mW/50C	COMP 7/20/40mW	FEEDBACK 40mW/50C
0– 100	(0/0)	(2/2) •Curved Act Layer •Poor Die Bond	(0/0)	(0/0)	(0/0)	(0/0)	(1/1) •Facet Def Found Sol
100–2K	(4/4) All four Facet Damage + EAB (Elec Active block layer)	(12/3) •Facet Damage •Facet Damage •Asym Block Layer on Sem	(2/2) •Cracked Window •None	(5/5) •Sol (2X) •Sol + Micro Crack (2X) •None	(2/2) •Killed/LCT •None	(3/2) •Facet Dmg + Sol •None	(3/3) •Facet+Stress •Killed 2
2K+	(6/6) •Facet Dmg 2X •Dark Zones •Killed 3	(1/0) Inconclusive	(1/0) Inconclusive	(1/0) Inconclusive	(2/2) •None •Killed 1 On LCT	(0/0)	(0/0)

Table 2. Laser failure analysis summary

33 observations on 26 lasers

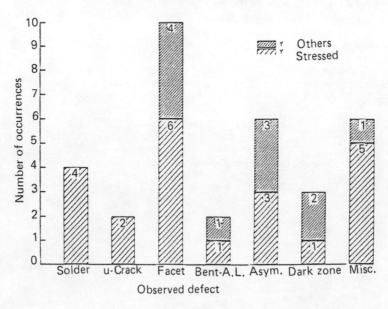

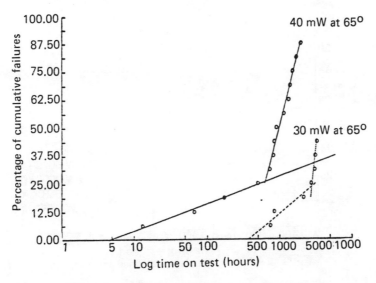

Figure 1. Reliability comparison for 30 to 40 mW

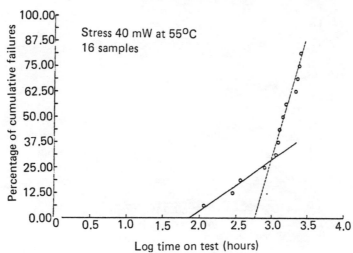

Figure 2. 40 mW data used to calculate activation energy

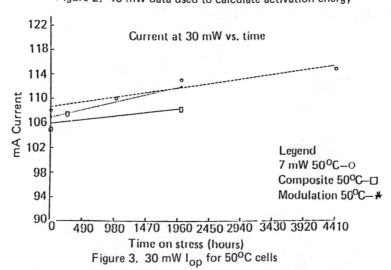

Figure 3. 30 mW I_{op} for 50°C cells

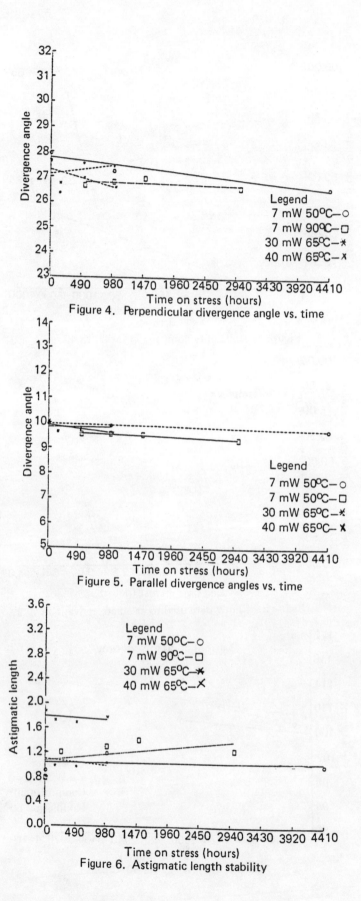

Figure 4. Perpendicular divergence angle vs. time

Figure 5. Parallel divergence angles vs. time

Figure 6. Astigmatic length stability

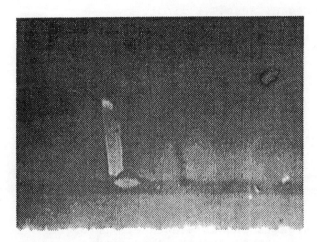

Figure 7. Optical micrograph of the front facet

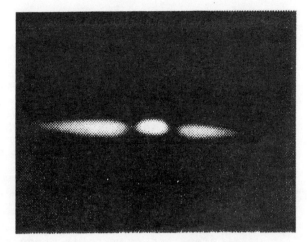

Figure 8. Near field pattern of v-groove

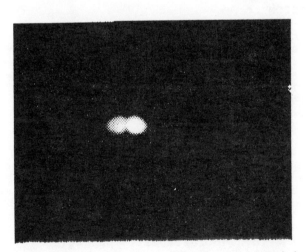

Figure 9. Near field pattern of an overpowered diode laser

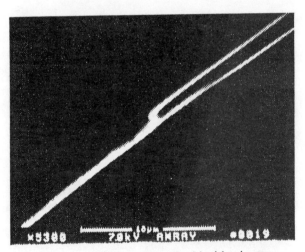

Figure 10. Electrically active blocking layer

Packaging considerations for semiconductor laser diodes

Alan.J.Perryman, James.D.Regan, Ross.T.Elliott.

STC Defence Systems, Optical Devices Division,
Brixham Road, Paignton, S.Devon, England.

ABSTRACT

The design considerations involved in the primary packaging of semiconductor laser diodes are major factors in the performance, reliability, cost and ultimate commercial success or failure of the finished device. The requirements of the package are as varied as the uses to which semiconductor laser diodes are put; they include such considerations as physical outline, ruggedness, mechanical stability, thermal efficiency, electrical characteristics, unit cost, and handlability.

The experience gained by device designers and manufacturers through development and commercial production of semiconductor laser diodes provides the data base from which design proposals are made for new products. However, performance requirements are increasing significantly beyond previous experience and both chip and packaging design engineers are having to turn to new materials and novel design methods to meet these challenges.

1. INTRODUCTION

The first commercially produced semiconductor laser diodes were designed for 'Free Space' or non fibre coupled applications, such as light sources for range finding, homing beacons, infra red illumination etc. These applications are almost entirely military and provide a large, expanding market for laser diode manufacturers. The packaging requirements for this type of device reflect the demands of operation in the military environment and standard package outlines have evolved for ease of interchangeability, ruggedness and integrity over long storage times.

The application of solid state laser diodes in the field of telecommunications has evolved through the use of glass fibre as an efficient transmission medium. Package designs evolved to provide stable chip-to-fibre alignment ensuring maximum ex-fibre outputs under the working conditions, heatpumps were incorporated to stabilise the chip output and the package outlines were designed for compatibility with DIL electronic components for circuit board mounting. These packaging techniques were developed either out of, or in parallel with high reliability packaging applications for undersea cable systems where design considerations have concentrated on very high quality materials, build standards and stable package designs to guarantee reliable operation for over 25 years.

Packages capable of handling high CW powers for Nd:YAG pumping and data storage are a growing requirement. They must be designed to maintain a constant chip operating temperature by efficient heat transfer and minimise distortion of the output beam profile by the use of non reflective components and high quality heatsink surface finishes.

1. INTRODUCTION (cont'd)

This paper will review some considerations involved in packaging GaAlAs semiconductor laser diodes designed for high speeds, narrow pulses, fibre pigtailing, beam purity and high power C.W. operation. The implementation of these features in high volume will be discussed and a number of packaging solutions offered.

2. PACKAGING FOR NARROW PULSED, FREE SPACE APPLICATIONS

A major consideration in the choice of package for narrow pulsed operation is package impedance, the most significant component of which is the inductance of the leads which carry the chip drive current. Coaxial packages are commonly used because of their small size and ruggedness. The chip is mounted on the heatsink with a suitable solder and a wire bond made to the lead out wire as shown in fig 1. The equivalent circuit of the package is shown in fig 2.

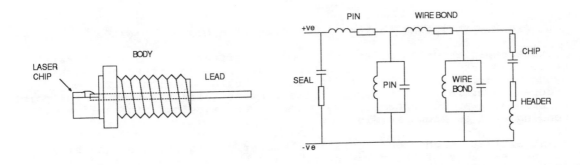

fig 1. Typical coaxial package   fig 2. Equivalent circuit

With the drive circuit connected as close to the package as possible, a total package inductance of the order of 10nH results. This, combined with the capacitive and resistive elements, restricts the minimum rise time of approximately 20ns.

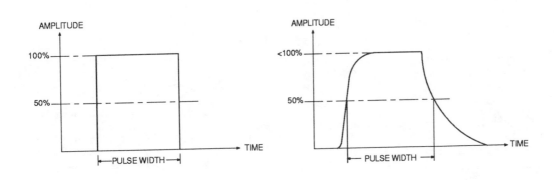

fig 3. Drive pulse   fig 4. Drive pulse when connected to laser package.

Packages designed to handle drive pulses significantly narrower than 40ns must feature lower inductive routes from drive circuit to chip; this is accomplished in two ways:-

2. PACKAGING FOR NARROW PULSE, FREE SPACE APPLICATIONS (cont'd)

a) by increasing the surface area of the current carrying lead.

b) by shortening the current carrying lead.

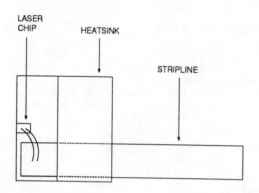

fig 5. Stripline package

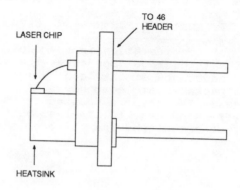

fig 6. Miniature package

Package capacitance comprises the combined effects of glass to metal seals, insulator and stray capacitance but these are often outweighed by the capacitance of the chip itself. The chip capacitance can be reduced by minimising the area of the contact surfaces, even to the point of etching away all unneccessary material to leave only the stripe and bonding area as shown in fig 7.

For ultimate high speed operation however, integration of the high current elements of the drive circuit and the laser chip, inside the package is the best solution. At present, this is accomplished with discrete charging capacitor and semiconductor switch components in chip form. The package has two isolated leads for supply and trigger inputs, the body acting as the common ground connection as shown in fig 8. Patterned substrate material has, hitherto been mainly plated BeO which has a relatively high thermal conductivity but the hazardous nature of the material has precipitated the use of AlN as a replacement.

Research is currently underway to further refine this concept by the full integration of driver and laser on a single chip but this is not commercially available at present.

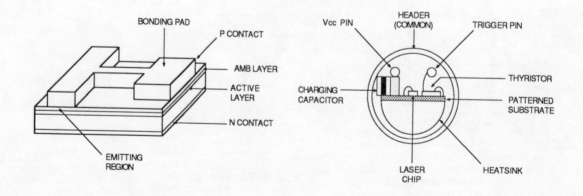

fig 7. Low capacitance chip

fig 8. Hybrid design

3. THE ATTACHMENT OF GLASS FIBRE PIGTAILS TO LASER PACKAGES

3.1 The need for fibre pigtailed laser diodes

The wide bandwidth waveguiding properties of glass fibre has revolutionised the field of data transmission to the extent that fibre coupled systems are rapidly displacing copper wire systems at all levels of telecommunications. Fibre coupled devices offer a high degree of mechanical stability and at the same time, a flexible, environment proof, direct and secure means of data transmission. Fibre pigtailed devices are offered with glass fibres of various core sizes, this allows the user to select the mode (single or multimode) of light transmission to best match the system requirements.

3.2 Considerations in fibre pigtail manufacture

The choice of fibre used for pigtailing should be carefully considered as the fibre is required to withstand not only the rigours of manufacture but also the mechanical stresses of handling when fitted to the input or output of the system. Fibre coatings must be easy to strip, must not shrink from the core during processing, be able to withstand the maximum processing temperatures and have low moisture and gas contents. The fibre-to-package interface is critical especially with respect to the choice of fibre end profile (either lensed or flat) and the method of attachment to the package. Flat fibre ends are generally associated with large core (over $50 \mu m$) diameters and are usually formed by cleaving the fibre with a diamond scriber or polishing. Lensed ends are necessary for small diameter fibres like those used in single mode systems. The most common ways of forming a lens is by selective etching in acid or melting by means of a controlled electric arc. The chosen method of mechanical connection to the package will determine the fibre end cladding design. For hermetic seals the fibre requires to be stripped of all organic coatings and plated with material suitable to form a high integrity glass to metal seal. Gold plating is the most commonly used, the fibre being soldered into a precision tube for mechanical strength and to allow soldering to the package.

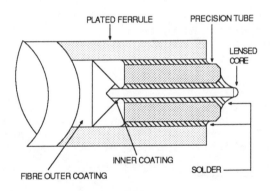

fig 9. Typical lensed fibre termination

3.3 Fibre attachment and stability

The importance of the stability of fibre to package attachments increases with reducing fibre core diameters e.g. a lens movement of $1 \mu m$ with respect to the chip can result in a 3dB power change at the output of a single mode fibre pigtail. The most important considerations are the thermally induced movements of fibre end due the expansion of the internal components of the package and the stress induced movements which are transmitted from the package walls during handling and operation.

3. THE ATTACHMENT OF FIBRE PIGTAILS TO LASER PACKAGES (cont'd)

The use of a single submount with both fibre end and chip attached reduces the respective movement of the two components to a minimum. The submount material should have a low thermal expansion coefficient and should be capable of supporting the fibre attachment method chosen.
Two popular methods of fibre attachment after active alignment are :-
1) by soft solder such as 60/40 Sn/Pb where the plated ferrule tube is locally soldered directly to the plated submount. The dissadvantage with this method of fixing is that small displacements occur as the solder cools and shrinks.
2) by laser welding of a miniature saddle to the ferrule tube and the submount, the heating effects of this type of fixing are so localised that virtually no displacement takes place, see fig 10.

The effect of stresses transmitted from the package walls to the fibre end can either be allowed for by designing a floating submount within the package so that, even if the fibre moves, the respective position of the chip is maintained, or by designing a shock absorbing mechanism to elliminate transmission of stresses through the fibre. A simple shock absorber is the unsupported fibre core itself. If the arrangement shown in fig 9. is used to terminate and attach only the end of the stripped and metalised fibre core the remaining unsupported fibre will act as an absorber, see fig 11.

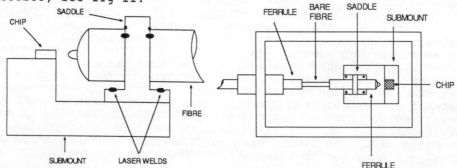

fig 10. Laser welded saddle   fig 11. Shock absorber

Large stresses are introduced into the package during device manufacture and it is important that these are completely relieved by suitable temperature soaking and cycling before final electro-optical characterisation. Typically ±1dB over an operating temperature of -20°C to +70°C and 100,000 hours life can be expected in a package designed with the above considerations.

The use of miniaturised multi-element lens systems between the chip and the fibre end is worth consideration when the methods described above are undesirable. These expanded beam optical techniques can greatly increase optical efficiencies and misalignment tolerances.

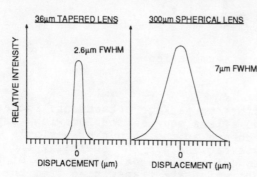
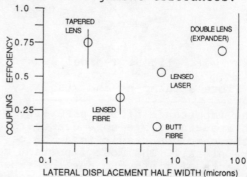

fig 12. Standard lensed fibre vs micro lens   fig 13. Effect of different coupling methods

4. CONSIDERATIONS FOR OPTIMISATION OF BEAM PROFILE

Interference phenomena result from reflections at very shallow angles from surfaces in the path of the beam. The result is far-field ripple in the plane of incidence. This is most frequently found where the chip is bonded epi-side down and often results from the chip being 'set back' or a poor edge quality to the heatsink.

Light from either the front or rear facets of the laser can couple back into the cavity if reflected off window cap or photodiode. This can lead to modal instabilities seen as optical noise or far-field ripple. The back coupling depends upon the angle of the reflecting surface, its displacement from the facet and its reflectivity. The suppression of reflections is achieved through angling, displacing or coating the surface concerned. Whereas supression of reflections from photodiodes are easily achieved by angling; for windows the choice is less obvious. Window reflections at normal incidence using Fresnel's expression for reflection becomes:-

$$r = \left(\frac{n-1}{n+1}\right)^2 \qquad (1)$$

Thus a for a typical window glass refracive index of 1.5, the reflection would be 4% at each surface i.e. approximately 8% in all. Figure 14. shows plots of farfield patterns as an uncoated window is rotated in front of the facet of a Single Spatial Mode laser. It can be seen that an angle of about 10 degrees is needed to give an acceptable far field pattern. By comparing this with a theoretical plot of power coupled back in to the cavity versus displacement for different angles (Figure 15.) it can be seen that this is equivalent to displacing the window by 500 microns or anti-reflection coating to 1% reflection.

Angling the window requires a special cap with very expensive tooling. More significantly, it inhibits the use of sophisticated coupling or collimating optics close to the chip, a problem also associated with displacing the window. The application of a dielectric coating of thickness one quarter of the wavelength of the laser ($\lambda/4$) will result in destructive interference in the backwards direction. The closest suitable material is Magnesium Fluoride with a refractive index of about 1.38. The reflectance for a material n_m with a single $\lambda/4$ coating of index n_c in a medium of index n_o is given by:-

$$r = \left(\frac{n_o \cdot n_m - n_c^2}{n_o \cdot n_m + n_c^2}\right)^2 \qquad (2)$$

from which it can be derived that a single MgF2 coating will give a total reflectivity of 3% for normal incidence. Greater reflection suppression than this is achieved through the application of multiple layers. Reflectivities lower than 1% are readily achievable with multilayer dielectric coatings which present a cost and performance effective solution.

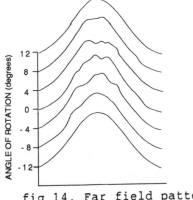

fig 14. Far field patterns

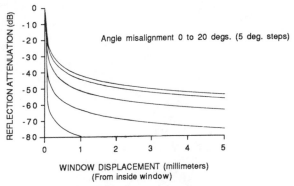

fig 15. Reflected power

4. CONSIDERATIONS FOR OPTIMISATION OF BEAM PROFILE (cont'd)

The distortion of an incident waveform by the window is determined by the surface flatness and by the presence of scattering sources. These include bulk inhomogeneities such as bubbles, and surface inclusions known as scratch and dig (MIL Spec. MIL-0-13830A). Wavefront distortion can be measured with an interferometer and consequently is specified as a fraction of the wavelength of the HeNe laser (633nm). The most common materials for windows for use at this wavelength are borosilicate glass and sapphire. Crystalline sapphire is homogeneous and highly resistant to scratch and dig. It can be polished flat then brazed into the cap. Its refractive index at about 1.75 is high and leads to initially large reflection losses but provides a good match to MgF2 coatings. These benefits however, must be balanced against the greater cost of the sapphire technology over glass, which if specified with care is sufficient for most applications.

5. PACKAGES FOR HIGH POWER C.W. DEVICES

5.1 Devices for data storage systems

The use of high power C.W. laser diodes for both read, write and erase applications in the field of digital data storage has grown out of Compact Disc and Video Disc technology. Package design considerations are largely concerned with beam profile requirements (discussed in section 4.), thermal energies, ease of manufacture and low unit cost.

Packages developed for Compact Disc (CD) applications are readily available and have been evaluated successfully at power outputs of 100mW, they are relatively cheap in quantity and are designed with high quality edge and surface finishes in the region of the chip mounting position. Two similar outlines available have 6mm or 9mm diameter heatsinks and comprise either three (fig 16.) or two part construction. For output powers over 10mW it is advised that the larger heatsink version is used and at powers over 20 mW an additional press fitted heatsink flange is fitted to further improve cooling. Coatings on window caps are selected for minimum reflection at the required operating wavelength. The wavelength may be carefully controlled during operation by the use of thermally efficient device mounting surfaces to maintain stable chip operating temperatures.

Since the active surface area of the chip is small (typically $2\mu m \times 300\mu m$), the selection of chip to heatsink bonding medium is critical to prevent mechanical instability, molecular migration and stresses in the chip. Integral Preform Contact (IPC), where the bonding medium is evaporated onto the chip contact during fabrication, has given encouraging results, the best alloy being Au/Sn which is very stable after bonding and is well suited to fluxless bonding techniques on automatic equipment.

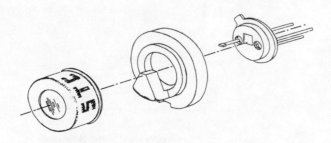

fig 16. Three part CD package

5. PACKAGES FOR HIGH POWER C.W. AND QUASI-C.W DEVICES

5.2 Devices for Nd:YAG pumping

The growing military and commercial requirement for diode pumped Nd:YAG lasers has led to increased efforts worldwide to develop high power Ga:Al:As diodes to replace far less efficient Krypton flash lamps as the pumping source. The high pumping efficiencies require precise wavelength control to match the absorption peak and operating pulse lengths between 100µs and 400µs to align with the inversion lifetime of Nd:YAG although high CW power is required for some applications.

As a result, the major package design considerations are focussed on efficient heatsinking of the chip to provide the kind of temperature control required. Chip temperature must be maintained within $\pm$ 2°C to achieve the required $\pm$ 0.5nm tolerance of output wavelength. Operating at 1 watt C.W., the chip produces 3 watts of heat, this means that a heatsink with a thermal efficiency of at least 0.67W/°C is required at this output. Changes in wavelength at different output powers are a good indicator of the thermal efficiency of a package in practice if the temperature coefficient of the chip is known.

Various heatsinking methods are being actively pursued by the industry, which range from traditional transistor package outlines, to custom designs such as large copper slabs bolted together with the chip sandwiched between. The TO3 transistor package is now established, to some extent, as a standard outline for output powers of up to 1 watt CW, incorporating either a large copper heatsink or a peltier heat pump. Where a heat pump is used, a heat spreader will be required to maximise the heat transfer from the relatively small area chip surface to the large area heat pump surface. Surface quality of the chip mounting area on the heatsink is important so that the thickness of solder under the chip is kept to a minimum as excess solder can severely increase thermal resistance. Simple copper heatsinks on TO3 headers have been shown to be capable of stable operation at up to 3.2 watts CW and 10W at 400µs pulse widths with the best designs.

6. ACKNOWLEDGEMENTS

The authors wish to thank the management of STC Defence Systems, Optical Devices Division, Paignton, England for their encouragement. Also Mark Tonkiss for preparing the illustrations.

Opto-mechanical packaging for extended temperature performance

Scott Enochs

Tektronix, Inc., P.O. Box 500, Beaverton, OR 97077

ABSTRACT

The ability of a laser diode module package to maintain precise laser-to-fiber alignment with mechanical stress or temperature change is critical for stable performance. This paper examines an optical-mechanical package configuration in which both laser and fiber are mounted on the same surface with high-temperature solder, thereby minimizing degraded package performance caused by exteraneous thermal or mechanical changes.

1. INTRODUCTION

Opto-mechanical stability—the ability of a laser diode package to maintain precise laser-to-fiber alignment during a change in temperature or application of mechanical stress—is critical if stable optical performance is to be achieved. Extending the operating or storage temperature range of a single-mode laser diode package below −40°C or above 100°C while maintaining laser-to-fiber alignment is a severe design challenge. Stability is most difficult to achieve when direct-coupled semispherically[1] or conically[2] lensed single-mode fiber is used. Thermally or mechanically induced lateral displacement of a few tenths micron between fiber and laser can cause 1 dB or greater change in fiber-coupled power.[3,4,5]

Conventional packages typically employ spot welding[3] or soldering[4,6,7] techniques to fix the fiber in alignment with the laser. These techniques generally require mechanical elements such as pedestals or substrates, tubes, and weld clips, to facilitate fiber handling and retention within the package. These mechanical elements can contribute to instability by: introducing mismatches in thermal expansion between laser and fiber supporting members; introducing mechanical strain that could cause sub-micron yielding of elements; and introducing joints that could weaken or fracture due to formation of intermetalic compounds.[8]

Environmental and mechanical stress tests such as those required by MIL-STD-833 can cause laser-fiber displacement. Such displacements limit the range of operating and storage temperatures for fiber-optic devices. Typical storage temperature range is −40°C to +100°C. Typical operating temperature range is 0°C to 50°C. Adding a temperature-stabilizing heat pump to the package typically extends the operating temperature range to −20°C to +70°C.

This paper examines a laser diode module package construction that places both the laser and fiber on the same surface, eliminating separate laser and fiber mechanical supports and creating a near-planar structure. The fiber is retained with high-temperature solder. Careful selection of materials has avoided the formation of detrimental intermetallic compounds. Opto-mechanical performance data is included for this near-planar package over an extended temperature range of −65°C to +150°C.

2. PACKAGE DESCRIPTION

2.1 Conventional packaging

Examples of conventional opto-mechanical packaging constructed with a soldering[4,7] technique and a spot welding[3] technique are depicted in Figures 1 and 2 respectively. In both figures the laser and fiber are coupled through a supporting superstructure of elements. Laser mounts, multiple solder or spot weld sites, and fiber-handling aids such as mounting substrates or mounting tubes and clips are used to fix the laser and fiber in position. These extraneous elements become integral parts of the laser-to-fiber alignment process. Any strain that eminates from or any stress that acts on these elements also acts directly on the optical coupling between fiber and laser, generally causing degraded performance.

2.2 Near-planar packaging

A near-planar package construction is illustrated in Figure 3 and shown photographically in Figure 4. Unlike conventional laser-diode packages, both laser and fiber are soldered directly to the same planar substrate surface. This construction represents a significant reduction in the number of mechanical elements and joints required to fix the laser and fiber in place and reduces the possibility of optical misalignment caused by thermal or mechanical stress. A major benefit of near-planar construction is the ability to integrate a laser diode and optical fiber directly onto a hybrid microcircuit.

A key element in near-planar package construction is the small "T-bar" shown in Figures 3 and 4. The T-bar is soldered to the fiber and provides a method to position the fiber with almost zero clearance between fiber and substrate. Mechanical rigidity of the fiber (and thus, the ability to solder it to the substrate without significant flexing) is maintained by extending the fiber only a few fiber diameters beyond the leading edge of the T-bar.

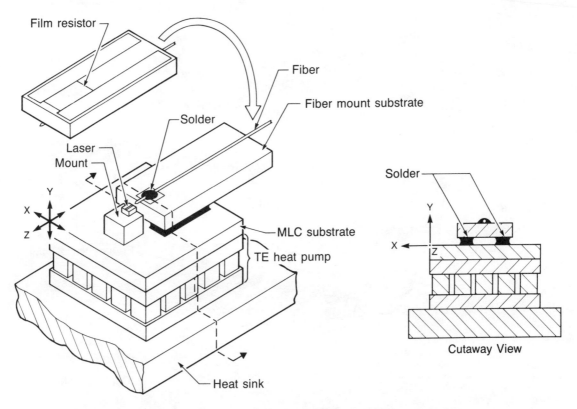

Figure 1. Package construction with a conventional soldering technique.

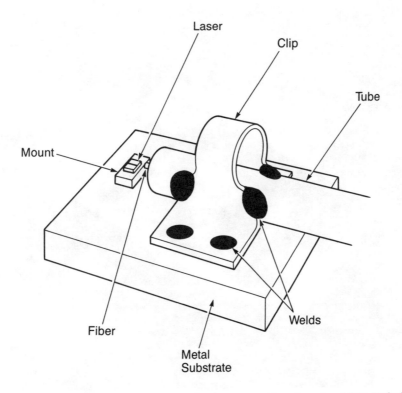

Figure 2. Package construction with the conventional spot-welding technique.

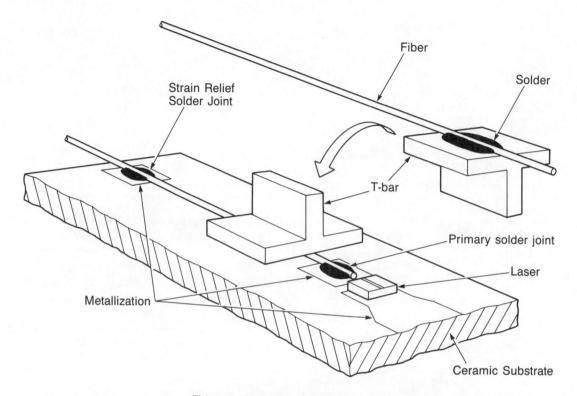

Figure 3. Near-planar package construction.

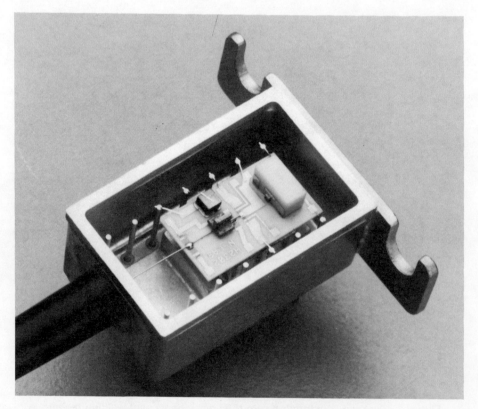

Figure 4. Near-planar laser diode module.

3. MATERIALS SELECTION

Various substrates and solders could be used for the near-planar package construction shown in Figure 3. Assuming however, that a ceramic substrate, InGaAsP laser, and fused-quartz fiber incorporate metalization schemes with gold top-metal, solder choices for reliable high-temperature-withstanding joints are, for practical purposes, limited to indium-lead[8] or gold-tin[9] compositions. Performance data included herein is for packages using 80 wt % gold, 20 wt % tin solder for the critical laser-to-substrate and primary fiber-to-substrate joints. This solder (which melts at 280 °C and is highly reliable for contacting gold films) allows a wide variety of lower-melting-temperature solders to be used for subsequent assembly operations. These include installation of the substrate into a metal package enclosure and sealing the metallized fiber into the exit tube of the package.

4. OPTO-MECHANICAL PERFORMANCE

4.1 Fiber-laser tracking

Fiber-laser tracking over the temperature range of −60°C to +70°C is shown in Figure 5 for devices assembled using the near-planar construction technique. All data is for opto-mechanical devices operated without a heat pump. Tracking performance is related to the accuracy (percent retained coupling) of the laser-to-fiber alignment. Percent retained coupling is a measurement of the fiber-coupled power after the fiber is fixed to the substrate, compared to the maximum fiber-coupled power achieved during initial alignment. Power reductions can occur due to thermal or mechanical stresses, which cause fiber-laser displacement during the fiber attachment process.

Exceptional tracking results were obtained for devices with high (95%) retained coupling. Less than 0.2 dB tracking error was demonstrated by a device with 95% retained coupling over the temperature range of −60°C to +70°C. Even those devices showing poor retained coupling (40% and 25%) met current laser-fiber-tracking standards, which vary from ±0.5 dB to ±1.0 dB for devices (without heat pumps) operating over the temperature range 0°C to 50°C.

The magnitude of laser-fiber displacement required to produce the tracking results shown in Figure 5 can be estimated from Figure 6, a plot of typical fiber-coupled power versus lateral laser-fiber displacement. Comparing the change in optical power from the tracking data with the displacement data yields an estimated ±0.25 μm maximum displacement occuring for all devices over the temperature range −60°C to +70°C, regardless of percent retained coupling. (A 0.5 μm total displacement window is indicated in Figure 6.) This displacement data suggests that laser-fiber-tracking performance can be predicted, provided that power-versus-lateral displacement characteristics and percent retained coupling power of a device are known.

Laser-Fiber tracking data for two devices fabricated with spot-welded (conventional) construction is shown in Figure 7. This data is included for reference only. It cannot be directly compared to tracking data for the near-planar devices, since these welded devices are rated for −10 dBm optical power, and thus, exhibit reduced sensitivity to lateral displacement when compared to the 0 dBm-rated near-planar devices. It is expected that the conventional devices would exhibit degraded performance if fabricated with lensed fiber equal in coupling efficiency and position sensitivity to that used in the near-planar package samples.

4.2 Temperature cycling, temperature storage

Figure 8 shows output power levels of a near-planar construction laser diode module in sequential tests: A) Temperature cycling from −65°C to +150°C; B) storage at 150°C; and C) storage at 125°C. Similar to laser-fiber tracking, performance appears to be related to the percent retained coupling of the device. Devices with good (95%) retained coupling show less than 0.5 dB change through each of these severe thermal stress tests. Stability through 168 hours of 125°C storage is excellent, regardless of percent retained coupling.

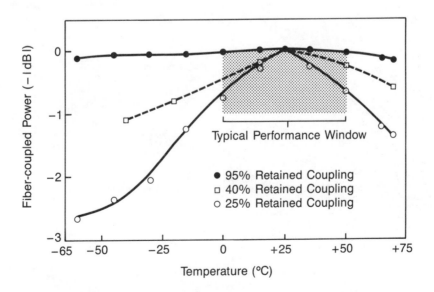

Figure 5. Fiber-laser tracking, near-planar construction.

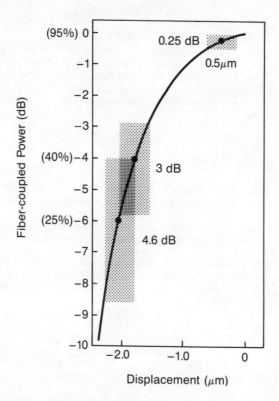

Figure 6. Fiber-coupled power versus lateral displacement for a fiber with conical lens.

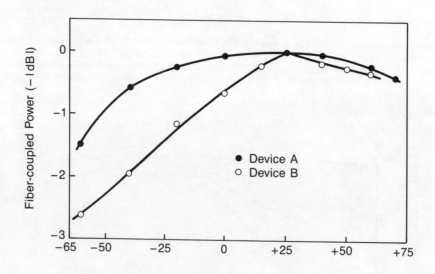

Figure 7. Fiber-laser tracking, spot-weld construction.

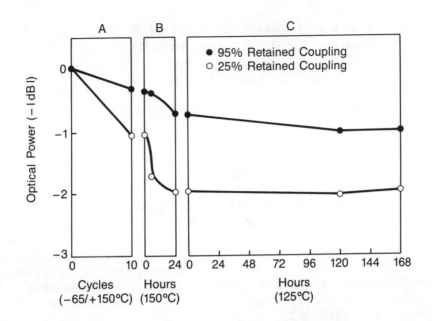

Figure 8 Temperature cycle (A) and temperature storage (B, C) performance data.

5. SUMMARY AND CONCLUSIONS

Near-planar construction and high-temperature solder has been demonstrated as a viable laser diode module packaging technique. Opto-mechanical device performance data suggests that the near-planar package is capable of withstanding non-operating storage over the extended temperature range of −65°C to +125°C, with limited exposure to 150°C. Exceptional fiber tracking capabilities enable operation of the package without a heat pump over the temperature range −60°C to +70°C. Operating temperature range can be extrapolated to 125°C, assuming a suitable heat pump is incorporated to cool the laser diode from 125°C to 70°C or less or if 125°C operating laser diode technology is established.

6. REFERENCES

1. G. Ebata, "Semispherical ended fibers and their applications," IEEE Tokyo Section, 1985, pp. 76-79, vol. 24, (1985).

2. G. Eisenstein and D. Vitello, "Chemically etched conical microlenses for coupling single-mode lasers into single-mode fibers," Applied Optics , pp. 3470–3474, vol. 21, no. 19, (Oct. 1982).

3. A. Rosiewicz, "High reliability by packaging for fiber optic sources," Proc. SPIE Reliability Considerations in Fiber Optic Applications, Cambridge, MA, pp. 63-73, vol. 717, (Sept. 1986).

4. S. Enochs, Opto-mechanical stability of a laser-diode module with soldered fiber, Proc. Seventh Annual International Electronics Packaging Conference, Boston, MA, pp. 799-804, (Nov. 1987).

5. Reith, Sumatte, and Koga, "Laser coupling to single-mode fiber using graded index lenses and compact disk 1.3 μm laser package," Electronics Letters, pp. 836–838, vol. 22, no. 16 (July 1986).

6. E. Grard and E. Duda, "A 1.3 μm module for and undersea transmission system," Proc. Optical Fiber Communication Conference, Atlanta, GA, pp. 8–9, (Feb. 1986).

7. Dodson, Enochs, and Randall, "Electro-optical transducer module," U.S. Patent No. 4,722,586, (Feb. 2, 1988).

8. F. Yost, "Soldering to gold films," Gold Bulletin, vol. 10, no. 4 (Oct. 1977).

9. Mizuishi et al., "Reliability of InGaAs P/InP buried heterostructure 1.3 μm lasers," IEEE Journal of Quantum Electronics, pp. 1294– 1301, vol. QE-19, no. 8, (Aug. 1983).

Self Consistent Heat Load Evaluation of Laser Diode
Modules for High Temperature Operation

Eric Y. Chan and C. C. Chen

Boeing Electronic High Technology Center
P. O. Box 24969, MS#7J-05
Seattle, Wa 98124.

ABSTRACT

An experimenal approach to evaluate the heat load of a laser diode module has been performed. In this experiment, stable CW light output operation up to 125° C was achieved by adding an external high capacity thermoelectric cooler to the laser diode module. By monitoring the temperature of the laser diode package, the cold side of the thermoelectric cooler, the heat sink temperature, the ambient temperature and compare these temperature data with the performance curves of the thermoelectric cooler, we have identified that the major source of heat is from the laser diode package case. Heat is originated from both the ambient and the hot side of the thermoelectric cooler. Proper thermal design of the module package is important to the optimum performance of the laser diode in an actual operating environment. These results are of considerable significance for the development of temperature stable diode laser source for military and aerospace application.

1. INTRODUCTION

Recently, there has been strong interest in laser diode module that operates from -55° C to 125° C for military and aerospace applications. Commercially available laser diode modules operate between -40° C to 70° C range. In this paper, we study the feasibility to extend the operating temperature range of a laser diode module up to 125° C by adding a high capacity thermoelectric cooler external to the laser module. We have experimented with two different size laser modules, one with a built-in thermoelectric cooler, one without a built-in thermoelectric cooler and thus much smaller in size. We found that the heat load of the smaller size module is about 7 times lower than the larger module. Therefore, the efficiency of the external thermoelectric cooler to cool the smaller module at 125° C is better than the larger module.

2. EXPERIMENTAL SET-UP

Figure 1 shows the computer controlled experimental set-up for the laser diode module heat load evaluation experiment. The laser diode module under test is put inside an environmental chamber with temperature controlled by the computer. The laser diode module was connected electrically to the driver and controller external to the environmental chamber. This avoided the controller electronics being heated during the experiment. Attached below the laser module was a thermoelectric cooler (TEC) with heat sink, all put inside the environmental chamber. The TEC was driven by a separate external power supply. Two different models of TEC were used in the experiment. The light output from the pigtail of the laser diode module was monitored by the Ge detector of the power meter. Thermocouples TC1, TC2 and TC3 monitored the ambient temperature (T_A), the laser module's case temperature (T_c) on the cold side of the TEC and the TEC hot side temperature (T_h) at the surface of the heat sink respectively. The environmental chamber was cooled by injection of liquid nitrogen into the chamber.

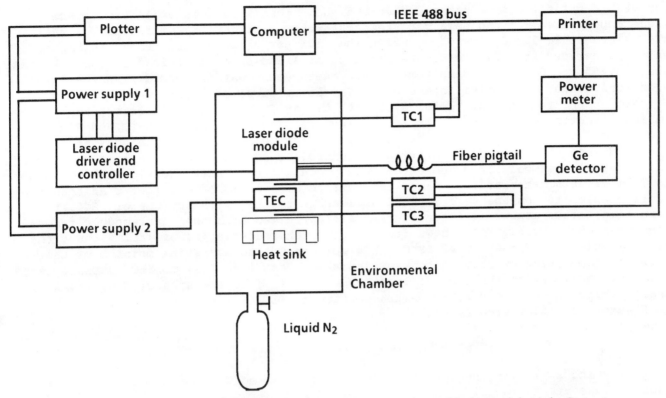

Figure 1. Computer Controlled Set-Up for High Temperature Laser Diode Module Light Output Stabilization Experiment

3. RESULTS FOR LASER MODULE A

A commercial laser diode module (from here on, labelled as laser module A) which is a standard 14 pin DIP package, with a bult-in thermoelectric cooler, back detector, temperature sensor and multimode fiber pigtail, was placed inside the chamber. The laser diode inside module A is an InGaAsP/InP Double Channel Planner Buried Heterostructure (DCPBH) laser with 1.3 µm emission wavelength. The dimensions of this laser module are 0.75"X0.5"X0.25". The CW current vs. voltage (I-V) and light output power vs. current (L-I) characteristics of the laser diode inside the module was tested with the driver and controller turned off before the experiment started. Next, the computer turned on the laser diode driver and controller and started the automatic power control (APC) operation of the module with the chamber ambient temperature (monitored by TC1) varied from -45° C to 70° C. The results of the fiber pigtail output power vs. ambient temperature is shown in Figure 2. The output power of the laser module was stablized at 2 mW which was set at the starting (room) temperature. But over 70° C, output power started to drop. To extend the stable operating temperature of the laser module, an external thermoelectric cooler (from here on, labelled as TEC1) with universal performance graph shown in Figure 3 [1] was used to cool the module. With 4 A of constant current applied to TEC1 the temperature range for stable power output was extended to 110° C as shown in Figure 4. But above 110° C output power started to roll off. At 110° C, the laser diode module case temperature was 70° C as measured by TC2. TC3 measured the temperature at the hot side of TEC1 during the experiment. The results of Figure 2 and 4 indicate that as the ambient temperature increases, the heat load of module A on TEC1 increases. It is also necessary to maintain the module case temperature below 70° C for stable optical output power. Figure 5 shows the difference (ΔT) between the hot side temperature (T_h) and cold side temperature (T_c) of TEC1 at different T_h, where $\Delta T = T_h - T_c$. At $T_h = 50°$ C, $\Delta T = 50°$ C, using the TEC1 performance curve shown in Figure 6 which is derived from Figure 3, operating point A indicates heat load (Q_A) on TEC1 is about 8.255 W. Next, the same temperature measurement was performed with the laser diode driver and controller turned off. The lower curve of Figure 7 shows the ΔT vs. T_h measurement results, at $T_h = 50°$ C, $\Delta T \approx 50°$ C. At $T_h = 140°$ C which corresponds to ambient temperature of $110°C$, the lower curve of Figure 7 shows $\Delta T = 64°C$ and Figure 5 shows $\Delta T = 47°$ C, this indicates that heat load from module A is much higher at $T_h = 140°C$ when the laser diode driver and controller is turned on. This is because the internal thermoelectric cooler of laser module A generates additional heat load to TEC1 at this temperature. Since the surface area of TEC1 is larger than than the laser module, to compensate for the heat leakage to the extra surface of TEC1, the same temperature measurement procedures were performed with the laser module removed. The upper curve of Figure 7 shows its ΔT vs. T_h characteristics of TEC1 without the laser module. At $T_h = 50°$ C, $\Delta T = 58°C$, this corresponds to operating point B of the lower TEC1 performance curve shown in Figure 6. Heat load (Q_B) to TEC1 surface is 3.175 W. Normalizing the area of laser module A (A_{MA}) to the area of TEC1 (A_{TEC1}), heat leakage ($Q_{L,M1A}$) due to the extra surface of TEC1 during the measurement shown in Figure 5 is calculated as follow

$$Q_{L,M1A} = Q_B * (1 - A_{MA}/A_{TEC1}) = 2.738 \text{ W}$$

where A_{MA} and A_{TEC1} are the surface area of the laser module A and TEC1 respectively. Their values are as follow

$$A_{MA} = 0.5" \times 0.75" = 0.375 \text{ in}^2$$
$$A_{TEC1} = 1.65" \times 1.65" = 2.7225 \text{ in}^2.$$

Therefore, the actual heat load (Q_{MA}) of laser module A on TEC1 is obtained as

$$Q_{MA} = Q_A - Q_{L,M1A} = (8.255 - 2.738) \text{ W} = 5.517 \text{ W} \qquad (1)$$

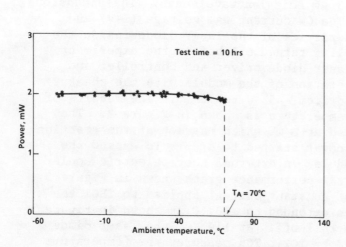

Figure 2. Fiber Output Power Versus Ambient Temperature of Laser Module A With Automatic Power Control (APC)

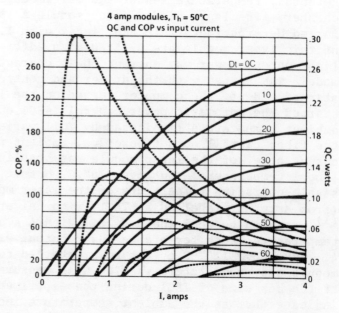

Figure 3. Universal Performance Graph of TEC1

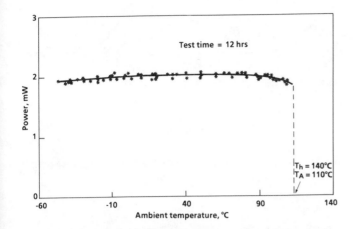

Figure 4. Fiber Output Power Versus Ambient Temperature of Laser Module A With APC and External Cooling of TEC1

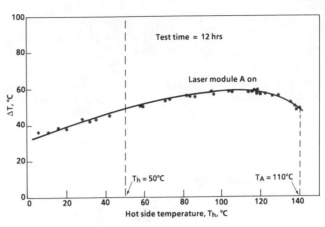

Figure 5. ΔT Versus T_h of TEC1 With Laser Module A Turned On

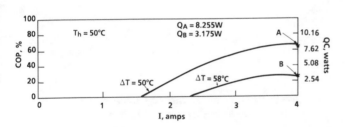

Figure 6. Upper Curve: TEC1 Performance Curve With Laser Module A on TEC1
Lower Curve: TEC1 Performance Curve With Laser Module A Removed

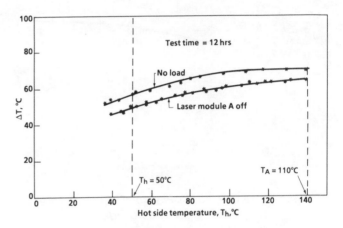

Figure 7. Lower Curve: ΔT Versus T_h Plot for TEC1 With Laser Module A on its Cold Side
Upper Curve: ΔT Versus T_h Plot for TEC1 With Laser Module A Removed

4. RESULTS FOR MODULE B

In a separate experiment, a miniature size laser module (from here on labelled as module B), with dimension about 3/16"X7/8"X1/8" was used for the same temperature measurement procedures using TEC1 again. This miniature laser module has a back detector, temperature sensor and single mode fiber pigtail but no built-in thermoelectric cooler. The laser diode inside module B is an InGaAsP/InP Buried Heterostructure (BH) laser with 1.3 μm emission wavelength. Figure 8 is the ΔT vs. T_h plot for laser module B. At $T_h=50°$ C, $\Delta T=57°$ C, This corresponds to operating point C on the TEC1 performance curve shown in Figure 9 which is also derived from Figure 3. Point C indicates heat load $Q_C=3.81$ W. By the same analysis, heat leakage ($Q_{L,M1B}$) to the extra surface area of TEC1 during the measurement shown in Figure 8 is calculated as

$$Q_{L,M1B} = Q_B(1 - A_{MB}/A_{TEC1})$$
$$= 3.175 * (1 - (7/8"X3/16")/(1.65"X1.65")) \text{ W}$$
$$= 2.984 \text{ W}$$

where A_{MB} is the surface area of miniature laser module B. The actual heat load (Q_{MB}) of module B on TEC1 is calculated as

$$Q_{MB} = Q_C - Q_{L,M1B} = (3.81 - 2.984) \text{ W} = 0.826 \text{ W} \qquad (2)$$

The heat load ratio (H_R) of the two laser module is calculated from results obtained in (1) and (2) as

$$H_R = Q_{MA}/Q_{MB} = 5.517/0.826 = 6.68$$

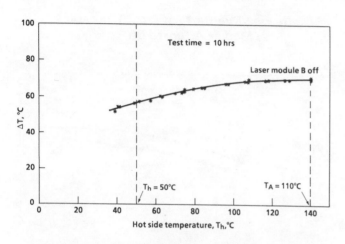

Figure 8. ΔT Versus T_h Plot for TEC1 With Laser Module B on its Cold Side

Figure 9. TEC1 Performance Curve With Laser Module B on its Cold Side

H_R indicates that heat load of module A is almost 7 times higher than module B. Also from Figure 8, at $T_h=140°$ C which corresponds to ambient temperature of $110°$ C, $\Delta T=70°$ C, and laser module B case temperature is about $70°$ C. To extend the ambient operating temperature higher than $110°$ C, a thermoelectric cooler which generates larger ΔT at $125°C$ ambient temperature is needed. Therefore, we replaced TEC1 by a 2 stage cascaded thermoelectric cooler, TEC2, with performance graph shown in Figure 10.[2] Constant current of 7 A was applied to this module, Figure 11 shows the ΔT vs. T_h measurement of laser module B attached to TEC2. At $T_h=143°C$, $\Delta T=83°C$, the ambient temperature is $125°C$, and the laser module B package temperature is $60°C$ which is within the normal operating temperature range of the module. After testing the CW I-V and L-I characteristics of laser diode inside module B, we performed the light output stablization measurement with the laser module B and TEC2 combination. Since laser module B does not have a built-in thermoelectric cooler, back detector monitoring technique was used to adjust the laser diode driving current. Figure 12 is the light output vs. ambient temperature of the laser diode module B. The highest ambient operating temperature is $125°C$. The fiber output power was stablized at 140 μW which was set at room temperature at the beginning of the experiment.

5. POWER EFFICIENCY AT MAXIMUM OPERATING TEMPERATURE

The power efficiency of operating laser module A and module B at the maximum operating temperature are calculated. From Figure 5, the maximun operating

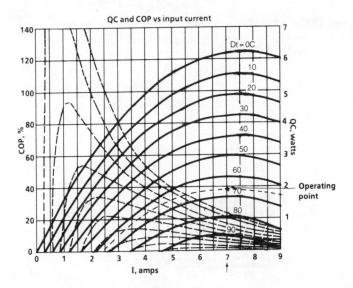

Figure 10. Performance Graph of Cascaded Thermoelectric Cooler TEC2

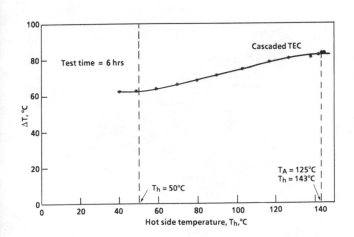

Figure 11. ΔT Versus T_h Plot for TEC2 With Laser Module B on its Cold Side

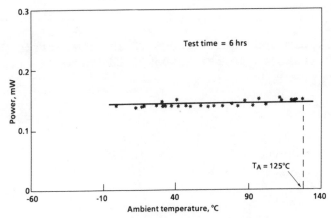

Figure 12. Fiber Output Power Versus Ambient Temperature for Laser Module B on the Cold Side of TEC2

temperature of module A is at 110°C ambient temperature. The power consumption of TEC1 at this temperature is

$$P_{TEC1} = I_{TEC1} * V_{TEC1} = (4\ Amp)*(16.79\ V) = 67.16\ W$$

where I_{TEC1}, V_{TEC1} are the current and voltage applied to TEC1 at $T_h = 140°C$. From Figure 12, at ambient operating temperature of 125°C, laser diode module B is at $T_h = 143°C$. The power consumption is

$$P_{TEC2} = I_{TEC2} * V_{TEC2} = (7\ Amp)*(5.9\ V) = 41.3\ W$$

where I_{TEC2} and V_{TEC2} are current and voltage applied to TEC2 at $T_h = 143°C$. The ratio of power consumption between the two thermoelectric cooler is calculated as

$$P_{TEC2}/P_{TEC1} = 41.3/67.16 = 0.615$$

This indicates that the TEC2 and laser module B combination achieved stable 125°C operation with 38% reduction in power consumption.

6. CONCLUSIONS

An experimental technique to evaluate the heat load of 2 laser diode modules with different size and construction was performed. The results are fully consistent with the geometry and operating conditions of the laser diode modules. Further more, our experimental results also indicate that miniaturization of the laser diode module size allows higher temperature operation and better thermoelectric cooling efficiency. Stable CW power output operation of a miniature size laser diode module with single mode fiber pigtail was demonstrated. The information obtained from the present study will assist our specification of a custom designed thermoelectric cooler which can further minimize the power consumption at high temperature.

7. ACKNOWLEDGEMENT

The authors would like to thank L. Figueroa, C. S. Hong, G. Roome and D. K. Smith for their support of this work.

8. REFERENCES

1. Cambion Series 1500S-CE Thermoelectric Cooler, Part #801-1010.
2. Cambion series 1500MLTI-CU Thermoelectric Cooler, Part #801-1005.

Laser diode cooling for high average power applications

D. Mundinger, R. Beach, W. Benett, R. Solarz, V. Sperry

Lawrence Livermore National Laboratory
P. O. Box 5508, L-487, Livermore, California 94550

ABSTRACT

Many applications for semiconductor lasers that require high average power are limited by the inability to remove the waste heat generated by the diode lasers. In order to reduce the cost and complexity of these applications a heat sink package has been developed which is based on water cooled silicon microstructures. Thermal resistivities of less than 0.025 °C/(W/cm^2) have been measured which should be adequate for up to CW operation of diode laser arrays. This concept can easily be scaled to large areas and is ideal for high average power solid state laser pumping. Several packages which illustrate the essential features of this design have been fabricated and tested. The theory of operation will be briefly covered, and several conceptual designs will be described. Also the fabrication and assembly procedures and measured levels of performance will be discussed.

1. INTRODUCTION

Diode lasers are an attractive alternative to flashlamp pumps for high average power solid state lasers for many reasons including the greatly reduced thermal load placed on the laser host, and the increased pumping efficiency. However, presently the cost of the pump arrays necessary to drive a 100 watt solid state laser is too high to be practical. This high cost is due in part to the large mismatch between the thermal loads generated by the diode lasers and the thermal impedance of the packages currently being used. Essentially, if dollars per average watt is the appropriate figure of merit, as it is in many applications, then conceivably, an order of magnitude reduction in cost could be achieved simply by using a more aggressive heat sink. In addition, schemes for coherently or incoherently combining the outputs of many diodes could benefit in terms of reduced cost and complexity by having heat sinks better matched to the demands of the diodes. Silicon microchannel structures are well suited for this and can be designed to handle the high intensity heat loads. They are also amenable to low cost mass production techniques.

2. CONCEPT/PERFORMANCE GOALS

Microchannel coolers were originally invented to cool wafer scale integrated circuits which generate heat loads on the order of <200 W/cm^2. The concept is schematically illustrated in Fig. 1. Water, or some other coolant, is introduced into the channels through a header and laminar flow is established in the narrow channels. Heat flows flows throughout the solid structure and across the coolant boundary layer into the flowing coolant. The strategy for achieving the very low thermal resistance necessary to handle the kW/cm² type of heat loads generated by diode lasers is to make the channels narrow, say less than 25 μm, to keep the boundary layer thin, and keep the flow path short to maintain sufficient flow to meet the temperature uniformity requirements. This leads to a slightly more complicated header structure which is illustrated in Fig. 1b.

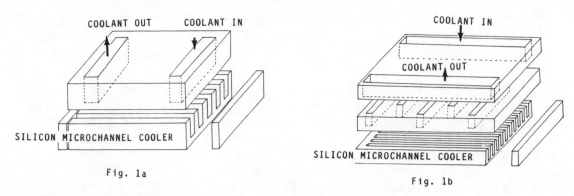

Fig. 1a

Fig. 1b

There are a variety of materials that could be used for these packages. We have chosen silicon. Silicon is a reasonably good thermal conductor ($\kappa = 1.4$ W/°C-cm), it can meet the performance requirements of laser diodes, and perhaps most important it can be inexpensively mass produced using well established techniques. Copper might also be a good candidate.

The two key performance figures of merit are thermal resistance and temperature uniformity. Thermal resistance is defined as the temperature rise at the laser junction relative to the coolant inlet temperature, per watt/cm² of heat load. The temperature uniformity is a measure of the maximum temperature variation across the surface where the heat is applied. This could be due to coolant heating or due to variations in heat load or variations in thermal resistance.

Performance goals were established based on heat loads generated by close packed arrays, that is, the individual laser structures are assumed to be spaced as closely as allowed by considerations other than thermal. Based on devices that are designed for quasi-cw operation, a generic 1 cm long bar with a 500 μm cavity length operating at 50% efficiency puts out about 50 watts of optical power. That translates into a heat flux of 1 kW/cm². For reliable long lived operation our experience has shown that the operating temperature should be limited to less than 40 to 50°C. Based on these considerations a design goal of 0.025 °C/(W/cm²) was set for the thermal resistance.

The temperature uniformity requirement depends somewhat on the application but typically the wavelength shifts about 3 Å/°C and the emission feature is typically 2-3 nm wide so a reasonable goal for temperature uniformity is 5 °C under a 1 kW/cm² heat load. This implies a coolant flow rate of about 50 (cc/sec)/cm².

The theory of microchannel coolers has been worked out in detail in Ref. 1 and to summarize that work very briefly it says that given a material with a certain conductivity, and given a coolant with a certain heat capacity and thermal conductivity and viscosity, then the thermal impedance can be broken into two components: 1) the thermal impedance of the coolant boundary layer which scales linearly with the channel width,

$$\Theta_{bl} \propto W$$

and 2) the coolant heating per unit area heat load which is inversely proportional to the coolant flow rate per unit area, and scales as:

$$\Theta_{cal} \propto 1/\text{flow} \propto W^3/L^2,$$

where L is the length of the channels.

For the specific case of silicon microchannel structures, with water as the coolant, assuming "optimized" geometries (see Ref. 1 pg. 25), Fig. 2 shows the total thermal resistance as a function of channel width. For our design goal of 0.025 °C/(W/cm²) this implies a channel width of about 25 μm.

Figure 3 shows the projected temperature variation due to coolant heating as a function of channel length for several different channel widths. The pressure referred to in this plot is the pressure drop in the microchannels themselves and does not include the header losses. In fact, a pressure drop of 10 to 15 psi is observed in the headers and taking that into account we project that for 25 μm wide channels the channel length, i.e. the distance between inlet and outlet header (see Fig. 1b), should be less than 1 mm.

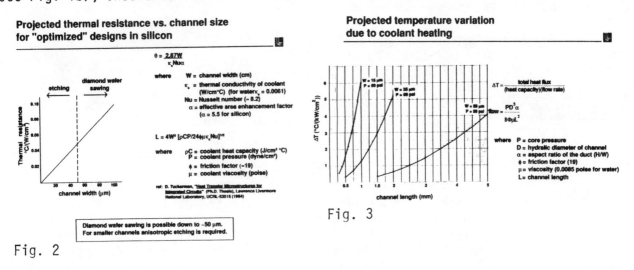

Fig. 2

Fig. 3

3. DESIGNS

A variety of conceptual designs have been considered for different applications. Figure 4 shows a design based on the rack and stack architecture which uses good thermal conductors to carry the heat down to the back plane where it is then carried away in the coolant. Materials that could be used for the racks could be BeO, Cu/W composites, pure copper, or something more thermally conductive such as cubic boron nitride or synthetic diamond. This choice would depend on what kind of duty factor is required. The rack should be as short as possible, slightly longer than the cavity length, to minimize thermal resistance.

Silicon microchannel structures are also well suited to the monolithic surface emitting architecture which is illustrated in Fig. 5. This shows a distributed bragg reflector type of device, but they could be other types of architectures as well. Additionally, a heat spreader such as cubic boron nitride could be used to improve temperature uniformity.

Another alternative that could prove attractive depending on how the fabrication yields improve is illustrated in Fig. 6. Here the microchannel structure is fabricated as the chip carrier itself. So, for example, a single diode bar could be mounted on each silicon structure. These could all be tested and burned in individually before assembling into an array. This modular type structure could also be maintained in the sense that as units failed they could be replaced without having to discard a large expensive component. They could also be kept thin, $\leq$ 1mm to allow a high packing density.

In the illustration a one cm long diode bar is shown on the cooler, but it could in fact be longer than 1 cm, or shorter to optimize yield or lifetime. Another option might be to place a thin expansion matched Cu/W plate between the diode and silicon to reduce mechanical stresses if that proves to be an issue.

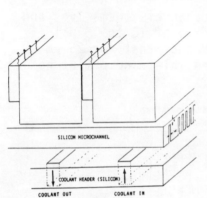
Fig. 4 Rack and Stack Design

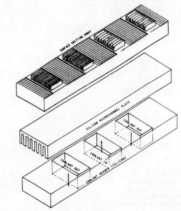
Fig. 5 Surface Emitting Architecture

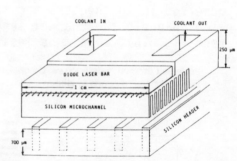
Fig. 6 Single Bar Modular Element

4. FABRICATION

The fabrication techniques we have used are all standard in the microelectronics industry. First a photo process is used to lay down a resist pattern of silicon nitride on a 3 inch undoped silicon wafer that has been sliced perpendicular to the 110 plane. The wafer is then etched in 44% KOH at a temperature of 35°C [2]. The etch rate along the 110 direction is about 5 µm per hour and is 600 times faster than the etch rate along the 111 direction. This allows very precise depth control and very high quality features. The wafers can be etched with different patterns on each side with a registration accuracy of about 5 µm. This two sided etching simplifies the header and plenum structures by reducing the number of layers required.

The etched silicon wafers are then laminated using a field-assisted bonding process that was developed originally for silicon dielectric isolation[3] and consist of first growing an oxide on one surface and then applying a moderate voltage between the wafers at a temperature of 1100-1200°C. This technique generates large fields in the gaps that give rise to strong attractive forces which gives a high strength, void free, permanent bond.

Alternatively, borosilicate glass can be used rather than silicon for the manifold and plenum component. The glass can be machined using an ultrasonic cavitation mill which can produce features of 1 mm or so which is adequate for testing and evaluating assemblies. Also the anodic bond between the glass and the silicon can be done more conveniently at low temperatures. All the diode assemblies that have been tested so far were made with the glass manifold. However, for the more advanced devices etched headers as preferable. The advantages in going to silicon are that finer features can be achieved and it will be cheaper to produce than the glass.

Figure 7 shows a photograph of some 17 μm channels that were etched in silicon. Also shown is a silicon header that illustrates a 2 sided etch and a borosilicate glass header.

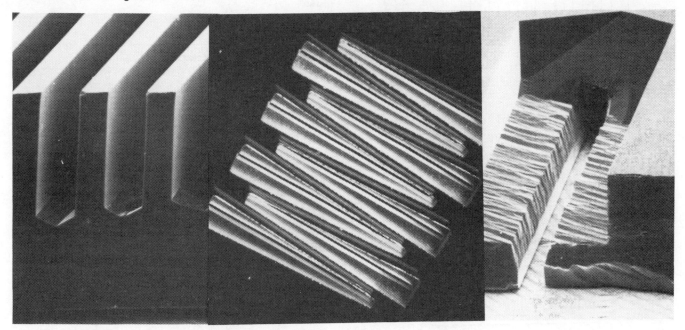

Fig. 7

5. EXPERIMENTS

Several assemblies have been fabricated and the thermal resistivity has been measured using dummy heat loads as well as laser diodes.[4] The diagnostics employed were thermo-couples, a high resolution IR imaging camera, and a gated spectrometer to observe the frequency shift in the output of the diode laser vs. time. Coolant flow rates have also been measured under varying pressure conditions and for different channel dimensions.

Figure 8a shows the geometry of an experiment to measure the thermal response under a purely resistive heat load. This device had 16 μm wide channels, 90 μm deep. The channel length was 1mm and the bulk silicon thickness was 300 μm. The flow rate was measured to be about 20 (cc/sec)/(cm²) under no load conditions

at 15°C, and 50 PSI. Based on our model, this flow rate and these channel
dimensions imply a thermal impedance of 0.04 °C/(W/cm²).

The measured temperature rise is shown in Fig. 8b as a function of applied heat
load. Up to 3 kW/cm² was applied with a corresponding temperature rise of 100 °C,
which corresponds to a thermal resistance of 0.033 °C/(W/cm²), in good
agreement with modeling.

Geometry of experiment

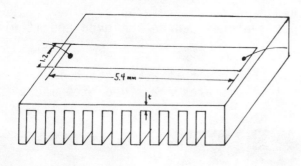

**Temperature vs. Power
measured at the center of the resistor**

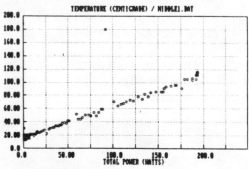

Fig. 8a

Fig. 8b

Integrated assemblies using 3 mm diode bars mounted on synthetic diamond
submounts have also been fabricated. The architecture is illustrated schematically
in Fig. 9a and a functioning device is shown in Fig. 9b.

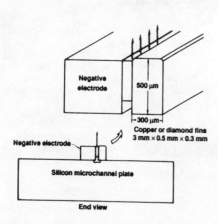

Fig. 9a

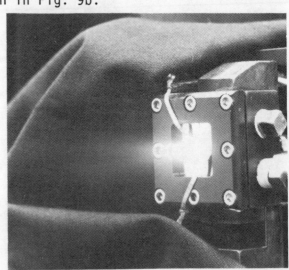

Fig. 9b

Approximately 15 of these devices have been tested to date. Figure 10 shows
the best device which had a slope efficiency of about 1 watt/amp and was emitting
at 770 nm. Under quasi-cw conditions with 100 μsec pulses at 10 Hz a peak output
of 20 watts was measured from the 3 mm aperture. The duty factor was then
increased up to 50% where the peak output dropped to about 12 watts for an average
power output of 5.1 watts.

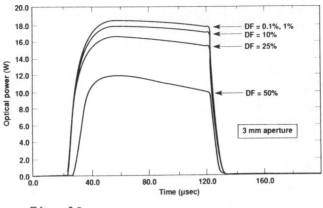

Fig. 10

The thermal resistance was also measured directly on a similar device which had no emission and so was essentially a purely resistive heat load (see Fig. 11). This measurement showed a thermal resistance of 0.013 °C/(W/cm²) which is actually lower that one would expect and is most likely due to some thermal spreading in the silicon which effectively increases the effective footprint of the heat load at the coolant boundary layer.

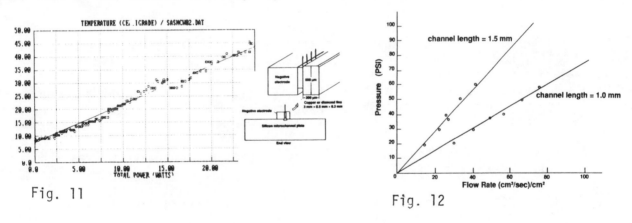

Fig. 11

Fig. 12

Finally, the coolant flow rate has been measured as a function of inlet pressure and channel length. This data is summarized in Fig. 12. The width of the microchannels in this test series was 21 µm and the channel lengths were 1 mm and 1.5 mm. The pressure was varied up to 60 psi which was limited by the pump capacity. These structures should be capable of much higher pressure, although sufficient flow rates can be achieved at 50 psi. These flow rates are consistent with a header loss of 10 to 15 psi which could be reduced, but is adequate to meet the requirements. At 60 psi a flow rate of about 76 (cc/sec)/cm² was measured which corresponds to a caloric heating of only 4 deg/(kW/cm²).

6. CONCLUSIONS

In summary a variety of silicon microchannel structures have been assembled and tested. A thermal resistivity of less than 0.025 °C/(W/cm²) and a coolant flow rate of 76 (cc/sec)/cm² have been demonstrated. This should be adequate for up to 1 kW/cm² of heat flux.

An average output of 5.1 watts from a 3 mm diode bar mounted on a microchannel cooler has been obtained. If these assemblies were close packed that would translate into an average optical power density of over 400 watts/cm^2.

Based on these measurements and our experience in fabrication, we conclude that water cooled microchannel structures are capable of handling the intense thermal loads generated by laser diodes. In applications where dollars per watt of average power is the relevant figure of merit this technology can effectively reduce costs by increasing the duty factor.

In addition fabrication techniques have been developed that should lead to a robust, inexpensive package and could form the basis for a modular architecture that would be convenient for a broad range of applications.

7. ACKNOWLEDGMENTS

This work was done under the auspices of the U.S. Department of Energy by the Lawrence Livermore National Laboratory.

8. REFERENCES

[1] D. Tuckerman, "Heat-Transfer Microstructures for Integrated Circuits", (Ph.D. Thesis), Lawrence Livermore National Laboratory, UCRL-53515 (1984).

[2] R. C. Frye, J. E. Griffith, Y. H. Yang, "A Field-Assisted Bonding Process for Silicon Dielectric Isolation", J. Electrochem. Soc.: Solid State Science and Technology, vol. 133, pp. 1673-1677 (1986)

[3] D. E. Kendall, Ann. Rev. Mat. Sci. vol. 9, Huggens, Bube, Vermilyea, Editors, pp 373 (1979)

[4] D. Mundinger, R. Beach, W. Benett, R. Solarz, W. Krupke, R. Staver, D. Tuckerman, "Demonstration of High Performance Silicon Microchannel Heat Sinks for Laser Diode Array Cooling", Appl. Phys. Lett. 53, pp. 1030 (1988).

Wafer thin coolers for continuous wave (CW) aluminum gallium arsenide/gallium arsenide (AlGaAs/GaAs) monolithic linear diode laser arrays

S.M. Stazak Kastigar, R.E. Hendron, J.R. Lapinski, Jr., and G.R. Hertzler

McDonnell Douglas
P.O. Box 516, St. Louis, MO 63166

Export authority: 22 CFR 125.4(b)(13)

ABSTRACT

The attractive prospect of CW AlGaAs/GaAs monolithic linear diode laser arrays (aka bar arrays) arises from the continuing improvement of the attributes of pulsed diode lasers, such as external quantum efficiency, lifetime, and coherence capabilities. Unfortunately, for close packed arrays, CW operation of an array at ambient temperature is limited to a few watts of optical power. Wafer thin coolers (on the order of 1mm thick) that have been designed to remove heat fluxes of over 100W/cm^2 from laser array packages (a diode bar soldered directly to the coolers via a 'sandwich' package) which operate more effectively in a CW mode. Tests were conducted to compare the thermal and optical performance of five types of such wafer thin coolers; a double pass microchannel cooler, two types of single pass microchannel coolers, and two versions of a compact high intensity cooler (CHIC). Thermal tests were conducted on the coolers alone at heat fluxes from 5 to 125W/cm^2. CW power vs. current (P-I), uniformity of emission, and wavelength vs. current measurements were made for each cooler/bar package. The optical experiments were conducted at 5 and 15kg/hr flow rates, and at 15° and 25°C inlet temperatures, using water as the cooling fluid. Results of the optical tests performed on 0.9cm linear arrays mounted on the wafer thin coolers showed impressive performance, such as 19.4W CW at 30 amps input current, and a very small wavelength spread across a bar. Such performance levels warrant these cooler/bar packages as a standard in CW bar operation.

1. INTRODUCTION

Wafer thin coolers allow linear diode laser arrays to operate more effectively in CW mode. These coolers have been designed to remove the high localized heat fluxes that are generated by GaAs/AlGaAs diode bar packages. This cooling improvement, along with the continuing improvement of laser bar attributes; such as external quantum efficiency, lifetime, and coherence capabilities; make CW operation of GaAs/AlGaAs diode bars an attractive prospect for optical systems.

Five types of wafer thin coolers; a copper double pass microchannel cooler, a copper single pass microchannel cooler, a beryllia single pass microchannel cooler, and two versions of Sundstrand's CHIC; were tested to compare their thermal performance and the optical performance of mounted laser arrays.

The thermal performance tests were conducted on each cooler at heat fluxes from 5 to 125W/cm^2, using the front square centimeter as the heat active zone and providing a uniform heat input on that area[1]. The thermal tests provided cooler heat removal and surface temperature data, which characterize each cooler. These thermal test results provide a guide as to how each different cooler will compare when a diode bar is mounted to its surface.

The optical performance tests were conducted by mounting a diode bar on each cooler and measuring the electro-optical characteristics of the array of importance for pump source application.

The optical performance tests were conducted with the diode bar / cooler package operating in the CW mode at fluid inlet temperatures from 15 to 25°C, and mass flow rates of 5 to 15 kg/hr. Uniformity of emission, wavelength, and power vs. current (P-I) measurements were made. In this test configuration, the waste heat generated by the CW operation of the diode bars exceeds the thermal test condition of 125W/cm^2. CW test results show performance of the bars is far superior to those mounted on a passive large copper heatsink.

This paper will first present thermal considerations and subsequent mechanical design of the coolers; second, a summary of the thermal testing; and finally, resulting optical performance of diode bar/cooler packages operating in the CW mode.

2. THERMAL AND MECHANICAL DESIGN

This study shows the development of thermal control devices for GaAs/AlGaAs diode laser elements used in our Laser Communications programs. The semiconductor lasers are used to pump solid state lasers (Nd:YAG, Nd:YLF, etc.) or as direct sources. The overall optical conversion efficiency of these diode bars in a pumping application is related to the operating wavelength of each stripe on the bar. The operating wavelength is, in turn, related to junction temperature. For maximum efficiency, all diodes must be nearly the same temperature (within 1°C) and must operate below or near 25°C. To prevent condensation on the lasers in a laboratory environment, it is desirable to keep the temperature at least 15°C at all times.

The heat removal levels of an average bar, which are in excess of 25W/cm^2, require special cooler designs for active thermal control. The wafer thin cooler designs were based on an average heat flux over a 1 cm^2 wafer of 25W/cm^2. The design goal of these coolers is to maintain the cooler-to-diode interface temperature variations less than 1°C. In addition, the coolers be very thin (about 1mm) to allow the cooler/diode pairs to be packaged into a compact 2-dimension array configuration.

To address these problems, three types of microchannel coolers and two versions of the CHIC cooler were built, fabricated and tested. The microchannel (MC) coolers were a double pass and a single pass unit made of copper, and a single pass unit made of beryllium oxide (BeO) and Kovar. The BeO/Kovar unit was built because BeO is a close match to the thermal expansion coefficient of GaAs and minimizes the internal stresses within the diodes due to temperature. The two copper CHIC coolers were thinned versions of Sundstrand's original CHIC design. All units were designed for a 1 cm by 1 cm heat input area and a thickness goal of 1mm. The CHIC coolers met the thickness goal of 1 mm, while both single pass MC coolers were 1.3 mm thick and the double pass MC cooler was 1.8 mm thick. The microchannel coolers could be made thinner with post-fabrication machining. All units were designed to operate with water cooling, although other fluids could be used. The designs of the various coolers are described below.

2.1 Microchannel coolers

The microchannel cooler concept has been applied to heat removal of Very Large Scale Integration (VLSI) using compact silicon coolers. Removal of heat fluxes up to 790W/cm^2 have been tested and it is projected that the coolers have heat removal capabilities[2] up to 1000W/cm^2. By flowing water through very narrow channels and maintaining the flow within the laminar regime, high heat transfer coefficients are obtained. The heat transfer coefficient increases with either an increase in the channel aspect ratio or a decrease in the hydraulic diameter of the flow channels.

The double pass MC design, shown in Figure 1, uses the microchannel concept in the top flow path (heat input side) along with the lower regenerative flow path (coolant inlet side) to reduce the surface temperature gradients at the heat input surface. The regenerative path contains the inlet header, which is designed to have a low pressure loss and to provide uniform flow distribution. At the end of the regenerative channels; the flow mixes, turns upward, and enters the narrow flow passages of the microchannel path adjacent to the heat input surface. Note that the water flows through these narrow upper channels in the opposite direction as the lower passage, thus allowing heat transfer between the two channels. In fact, the regenerative lower flow path absorbs the majority of the heat, thus reducing the temperature change in the water adjacent to the heat input surface and the temperature gradients at the interface plane.

The single pass MC cooler design is shown in Figure 2 and is essentially the same for the copper version and the BeO/Kovar version, except for material selection and bonding techniques. The design is similar to the basic plate/fin coldplate, where the inlet and outlet headers are in the same plane as the primary flow path. Since the water flows across the cooler through the microchannels from one header to the other, the surface temperatures are expected to duplicate the rise in fluid temperature across the flow path.

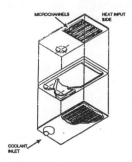 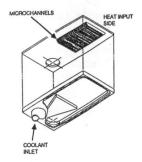

Figure 1. Double pass microchannel cooler design   Figure 2. Single pass microchannel cooler design

Both copper microchannel coolers are constructed from machined parts that are diffusion bonded together, and then the inlet and outlet tubes are soldered on. The BeO/Kovar MC cooler is constructed of two machined parts. The BeO top plate, which includes the microchannel fins, is brazed to the lower frame made of Kovar.

2.2 Compact high intensity coolers (CHIC)

The CHIC concept was developed for heat removal of high power density electronics and high energy laser mirrors, while maintaining high surface temperature uniformity. Removal of heat fluxes up to $50 W/cm^2$ has been tested for the basic design and it has been projected that the CHIC coolers have heat removal capabilities[3] up to $1000 W/cm^2$. By flowing the water through very small orifices, creating a jet flow, and forcing the jet flow to impinge on the following orifice plate, high heat transfer coefficients are obtained. Since the fluid flow is perpendicular to the heated surface, the fluid, striking each orifice plate and finally the heated surface, is approximately at a constant temperature near the surface, as reflected by the small surface temperature gradients.

For our application, a 1mm thick version of the basic CHIC was developed. Shown in Figure 3 is the basic CHIC concept. The first version proved the feasibility of fabricating the scaled down version of the basic CHIC. Based on test results from the first unit, a second version was built to increase the thermal performance and reduce the pressure losses. The jet impingement concept was not used for the second version. Instead, it used a multipass microchannel concept in which the flow is divided into 36 separate paths and winds its way up to the heat input surface. The first version had 42 small circular orifices in each of six flow paths. Both CHIC designs were constructed from seven plates, which were fabricated by photolithography and chemical milling, and assembled by diffusion bonding.

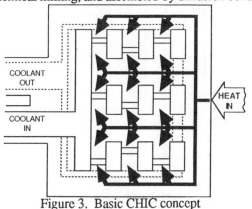

Figure 3. Basic CHIC concept

3. THERMAL TEST RESULTS

The five coolers were tested at heat fluxes ranging from 5 to $125 W/cm^2$ over a range of flow rates, using identical test procedures. A summary of performance results is shown in Figure 4 for a flow rate of 10kg/hr, a heat flux of $25 W/cm^2$, and a fluid inlet temperature of 15°C. The lowest surface temperatures and surface temperature variations are found in the double pass microchannel and CHIC 2 coolers. The double pass microchannel cooler has a large pressure drop, but a redesign of the inlet and outlet manifolding should reduce it considerably. The double pass and CHIC 1 have the same manifolding technique and CHIC 2 has a redesign of that manifold, which yeild approximately 60% reduction in pressure drop.

A projection of how each of the coolers will perform with a diode bar mounted based on the thermal performance results is shown in Figure 4. The projection is based on a flow rate of 10 kg/hr, a heat flux of 125W/cm^2, and a fluid inlet temperature of 15°C. The double pass microchannel and the CHIC 2 are expected to be the best performers. Only edge effects, which may have been smoothed out during thermal testing, are the most probable problems in this mounting configuration.

The projection is based on a centimeter long diode bar of 60 micron stripes on 250 micron centers operating at 9 amps with an overall efficiency of 20%. Using a 300 micron cleave length and a 2 volt drop, which translates to a heating rate of almost 500W/cm^2 directly under the diode bar. However, the cooler material is thermally very conductive and will allow a considerable amount of heat spreading. If a heat spreading angle of 45° and the thickness of the cooler top is 0.01 inches, the heat flux is approximately reduced by one fourth. This then approximately corresponds to the maximum heat rate tested of 125W/cm^2.

The predictions in Figure 4 are based on the expected wavelength shift of 1 nm/4°C and assume that at a surface temperature of 30 °C, the diode bar wavelength is 804 nm. The expected wavelength across the diode bar due to temperature effects, as shown, is less than 2 nm in all cases; however, this needs to be added to the wavelength variation due to manufacturing techniques, which is typically 2 nm.

THERMAL TEST RESULTS --- Q/A=25W/CM2, M=10KG/HR, T_{INLET}=15°C

COOLER TYPE	HA (W/°C)	ΔP (PSI)	$\Delta T_{SURFACE}$ (°C)	$T_{SURFACE}$ (°C)
DOUBLE PASS	5.3	29.5	0.26	20.8
Cu SINGLE PASS	4.9	12.0	1.36	21.2
BeO SINGLE PASS	3.0	6.1	0.94	24.5
CHIC #1	3.1	30.7	0.81	24.1
CHIC #2	4.4	11.5	0.54	21.8

OPTICAL PREDICTIONS --- Q/A=125W/CM2, M=10KG/HR, T_{INLET}=15°C

COOLER TYPE	HA (W/°C)	ΔT_{BAR} (°C)	T_{BAR} (°C)	$\Delta \lambda_{BAR}$	λ_{BAR}
DOUBLE PASS	6.5	0.7	34.2	0.2	805
Cu SINGLE PASS	5.5	7.6	37.7	1.9	806
BeO SINGLE PASS	3.9	6.1	47.1	1.5	808
CHIC #1	3.4	3.6	51.8	0.9	810
CHIC #2	5.1	3.4	39.5	0.9	807

Figure 4. Summary of thermal performance results

4. OPTICAL TESTING

Metallo-organic chemical vapor deposition (MOCVD)-grown GaAs/AlGaAs graded-index, separate confinement heterostructure (GRIN-SCH), single quantum well (SQW) diode laser arrays, 0.9 cm long, with 60μm stripes on 250μm centers, 300μm cavity length with HR/passivation coatings on the facets, were mounted in the standard MDAC-MDE 'sandwich package', where the bar is soldered down and sandwiched between two thin sheets of copper. The bars were then pre-tested, burned in for 46 hours at 9 amps, 150μs pulsewidth and 10Hz repetition rates, and post-tested in the Bar Burn-In and Test Station. "Good" bars, exhibiting post-test characteristics of similar values for lasing wavelength (804nm), bar uniformity of emission, slope efficiency and threshold current (about 4A pulsed) were chosen, and indium-soldered to the gold-plated coolers. Plumbing to a Neslab HX-75 chiller bath filled with deionized water was attached, and a thermocouple was placed near the inlet of the cooler under test. Inlet temperatures to the coolers were set and stabilized at 15°C and 25°C, in turn. Mass flow rates of 5 and 15 kg/hr were run. Based on the thermal results, this range exhibited little to no change in the maximum temperature difference, even for high heat fluxes. Each bar/cooler configuration was optically tested at each of these 4 conditions (15°C and 5 kg/hr, 15°C and 15kg/hr, etc.) utilizing our CW-capable bar test station. A measurement system was set up to characterize the electro-optic parameters of diode laser bar devices. The parameters measured include optical power output vs. current, current vs. voltage, and wavelength of emission.

4.1 Optical output power vs. current

The test system for this measurement is illustrated in Figure 5. The optical output of the lasing device is directed into a calibrated integrating sphere/optical detector combination. The voltage output of the optical detector is directly sampled by the digital oscilloscope. The current to the device is increased slowly, while the digital oscilloscope simultaneously captures power and current data points. The data points are held by the oscilloscope, or transferred back to the computer by IEEE 488 bus. The computer can print the power vs. current plot, and calculate a least squares fit to derive current threshold and slope efficiency.

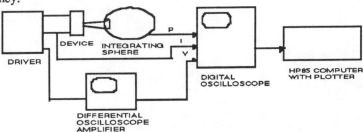

Figure 5. Optical output power vs. current test setup

4.2 Current vs. voltage

The optical output of the device is sampled the same as for the power vs. current data. The voltage across the device is measured by a differential oscilloscope amplifier. The output of the oscilloscope channel is fed into the input of the digital oscilloscope. Again, the data points are captured simultaneously while the current is slowly increased. The data may be displayed in x-y format on the oscilloscope, or transferred back to the computer. The computer can print the current vs. voltage plot, and calculate a least squares fit to derive voltage threshold and slope resistance.

4.3 Wavelength of emission

The test system for this measurement is illustrated in Figure 6. The emission of the device is focussed onto the variable inlet slit of a spectrometer, with spectral resolution of 2nm. The long dimension of the slit lines up with the long dimension of the extended emission source. The output slit of the spectrometer has been removed and the dispersed output strikes a television camera tube. The TV image displayed is a two dimension picture of emission wavelength vs. position on the device. This data representation is capable of detecting substandard thermal interfaces, by looking for the shift in emission wavelength at higher temperatures.

Tests were run on each of the bar/cooler packages using this described setup. Each cooler was run at 5kg/hr and 15kg/hr mass flow rates, and at inlet temperatures of 15°C and 25°C, making for 4 tests. CW P-I curves were taken, the wavelength across the bar was recorded at currents of 5, 7 and 9 amps, and uniformity scans were also made.

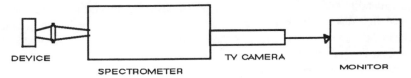

Figure 6. Wavelength of emission test setup

5. OPTICAL TEST RESULTS

In order to best compare the effectiveness of the coolers, the results are displayed for maximum and minimum stress conditions, i.e., 5kg/hr mass flow rate at 25°C inlet temperature worst-case, and 15kg/hr mass flow rate at 15°C inlet temperature best-case.

To display the heating effects of the diode bar, the peak wavelength vs. input current was observed at each of the aforementioned test conditions and is shown in Figure 7. Assuming that the characteristics of the diode bars are similar, being that they're from the same wafer, an observed lower operating wavelength indicates a lower diode junction temperature. The double pass cooler, corrected for improper fluid inlet temperature, provided the lowest wavelengths as projected from the thermal test data. The lower wavelength is either due to a more efficient cooling technique or a lower heat generating (more efficient) diode bar. The wavelength or temperature trends, shown in this figure, follow the results of the thermal testing except for the CHIC 1, which is performing better than expected, especially at the higher flow rate of 15 kg/hr.

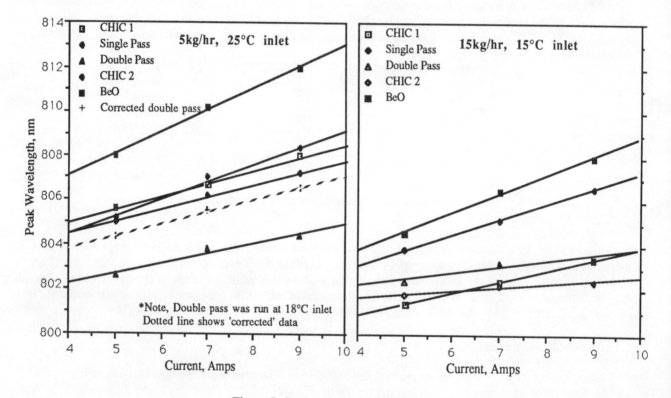

Figure 7. Peak wavelength vs. current*

In Figure 7, the slope of the peak wavelength curve indicates the measurement of the cooling capacity. Again assuming that the diode bar material is constant for each cooler, the more efficient cooler (high HA, a measure of total heat transfer coefficient in W/°C, from thermal testing) will have a slower change in wavelength as current is increased. At the 5 kg/hr flow rate, the BeO single pass and CHIC 1 have a considerably higher slope (lower HA) than the other three coolers and this agrees with the optical predictions of Figure 4. The copper single pass cooler has a similar slope to the BeO and CHIC 1 at the higher flow rate which differs from the thermal test results.

The coolers' capability to cool the bar uniformly is demonstrated by plotting the change in lasing wavelength across the bar. A typical diode bar would show approximately 2nm variation in wavelength due manufacturing techniques or nonuniformities in the diode material. Figure 8 shows the wavelength variation across the diode bars for the five coolers at the two extreme testing conditions. Once again, the double pass cooler was the best performer and agrees closely with the predictions made from the thermal test results. At the low flow rate, the wavelength variations followed the predictions, except for CHIC 2. However at the high flow rate, the CHIC 2 results were more favorable but still a little worse than expected.

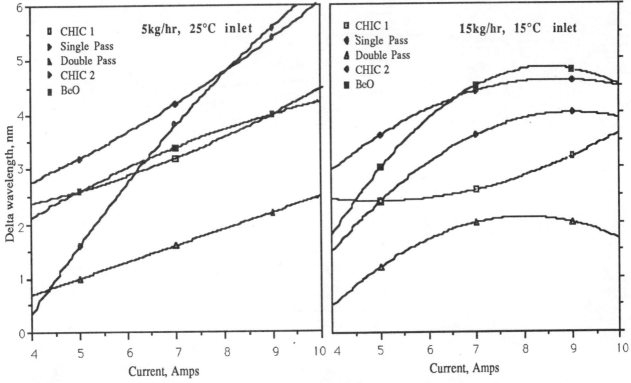

Figure 8. Wavelength variation vs. current

To better show this spread in wavelength, Figure 9 exhibits the scans made for each of the diode bars at 15kg/hr mass flow rate and 15°C inlet temperature, at 9 amps CW input. As can be seen, the double pass cooler shows superior performance in that the wavelength variation across the bar is minimal.

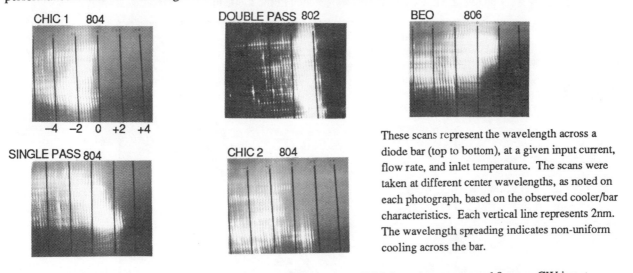

These scans represent the wavelength across a diode bar (top to bottom), at a given input current, flow rate, and inlet temperature. The scans were taken at different center wavelengths, as noted on each photograph, based on the observed cooler/bar characteristics. Each vertical line represents 2nm. The wavelength spreading indicates non-uniform cooling across the bar.

Figure 9. Wavelength scans at 15kg/hr mass flow rate, 15°C inlet temperature, and 9 amps CW input

In an effort to understand the differences between the thermal test results and optical test results, a measurement of the amount of waste heat is required. The heating is a function of the overall electrical to optical conversion efficiency of the diode bars and is shown in Figure 10 for coolers. The BeO and copper single pass coolers had the most efficient diode bar, however, they did not perform the best in terms of wavelength variation and junction temperatures. The double pass cooler had an efficiency which was relatively low yet it outperformed all coolers, both in wavelength and junction temperatures.

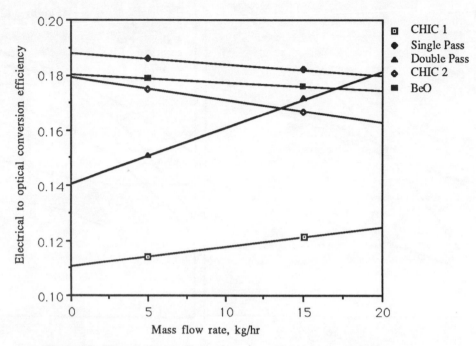

Figure 10. Electrical to optical conversion efficiency vs. mass flow rate

Another measurement of the amount of waste heat per cooler is the optical output and is shown in Figure 11 versus input current. Since the voltage drop of each diode bar is approximately the same, the cooler with the highest optical output (most efficient diode bar) has to remove the lowest amount of waste heat for a given current. The 9 amp data in this figure directly corresponds to 15kg/hr data in Figure 10, thus confirming the expected heated trends. However, Figure 11 provides more information about the quality and consistancy of the diode bar material used.

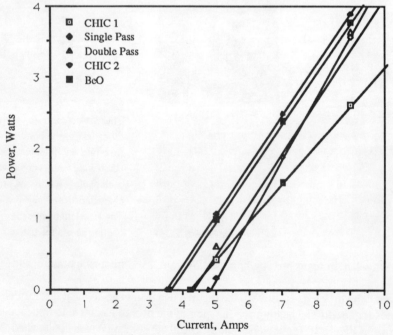

Figure 11. Optical power vs. current

The diode slope efficiency (the actual slope of these lines) is shown in this plot and is very consistant for all coolers, except for CHIC 1. Therefore, the major difference in the diode bar material is the threshold current, the current required at zero watts optical output or x-intercept. The threshold currents, except for CHIC 1, are directly proportional with the heating rates; for example, lowest for the cooler with lowest heating rates and highest for the cooler with the highest heating rates.

6. CONCLUSIONS AND FUTURE WORK

The diode bar material characteristics, as shown in Figures 10 and 11, show that the wavelength results were affected more by the cooler characteristics. Since the wavelength results, as shown in Figures 7 and 8, did not merely reflect the diode bar characteristics, the double pass cooler clearly outperformed the other four coolers, despite the fact that the diode bar material on the double pass was the second worst of the diode bar material tested. Note that the worst material was on CHIC 1, and it had approximately the same heating (same electrical to optical conversion efficiency at 15kg/hr) as the double pass, but lacked in wavelength performance.

Overall, the cooler exhibiting the most consistent characteristics is the double pass cooler. It has the least amount of wavelength drift across the bar, and thus would be a good candidate for cooling of a pump source, which depends on single wavelength input. This cooler/bar package has a low peak wavelength, so that one can depend on pulsed test results to determine lasing wavelength cw for this cooler. The value of electrical to optical conversion efficiency on this cooler is also quite good, being around 15%. The most power observed before catastrophic damage occurred was 19.4W at 30 amps input current on the double pass cooler. Recalling the diode sandwich is soldered on a 'dead zone' of the coolers, we were most encouraged by these results.

More diagnostic tests are planned for these coolers. We would like to optimize the coolant; only DI water has been used to date. The use of other fluids, Freons or coolants, will further separate the coolers when comparing wavelength spread across the bars, since thermally water is an excellent coolant. We would also like to model the diode bar/cooler configuration for heat removal levels. We plan to use longer diode bars (1mm cavity length), so we may better utilize the cooler's surface. We are happy with the results to date, and see such coolers as integral parts in CW diode bar operation.

7. ACKNOWLEDGEMENTS

The work described herein was performed under McDonnell Douglas Corporation Independent Research and Development Project 2-300 and 2-225. The single pass and double pass microchannel coolers were designed and their components fabricated by McDonnell Douglas. These units were assembled by the Sundstrand Energy Systems Division of the Sundstrand Corporation. The BeO/Kovar microchannel cooler was fabricated by Accuratus Corp. of Washington, N.J. The CHIC coolers were designed and fabricated by Sundstrand.

We would first like to thank Dave Begley, now at Ball Aerospace Systems Division, for his inspiration and help on getting the optical study funded, and for his subsequent consultation. We would like to thank Chip Chandler of Sundstrand for his work in fabricating the CHIC coolers, for the diffusion bonding of the copper microchannel coolers, and for the soldering of the inlet and outlet tubes to those coolers, and to Bruce C. Cunningham of Accuratus Corp. for developing the BeO fabrication techniques. We would like to thank Doug Leapley and Bill Vivian for their assistance in testing and data collection, and Larry Long for a test set description.

8. REFERENCES

1. M.G. Grote, R.E. Hendron, H.W. Kipp, and J.R. Lapinski, "Test Results of Wafer Thin Coolers at Heat Fluxes from 5 to 125 W/cm^2", SAE Paper #880997, 18th Intersociety Conference on Environmental Systems (1988).

2. D.B. Tuckerman, and R.F.W. Pease, "High Performance Heat Sinking for VLSI", IEEE Electron Device Letters, Vol. EDL-2 #5 (1981).

3. T.J. Bland, R.E. Niggemann, and M.B. Parekh, "A Compact High Intensity Cooler (CHIC)", SAE Paper #831127, 13th Intersociety Conference on Environmental Systems (1988).

SCREENING TEST PROCEDURE FOR LONG LIFE
SINGLE MODE STEP INDEX SEPARATE CONFINEMENT HETEROSTRUCTURE
SINGLE QUANTUM WELL (SINSCH-SQW) LASER DIODES

WILLIAM FRITZ

MCDONNELL DOUGLAS ASTRONAUTICS COMPANY
P. O. BOX 516
ST. LOUIS, MO 63166

ABSTRACT

An experiment was conducted to establish an effective burn-in and screening procedure for long life SINSCH-SQW laser diodes. The laser diodes were grown by MOCVD and processed with 20μm wide oxide defined stripes. The devices had a high reflective back facet coating with a small etalon bonded to a passivated front facet to ensure single mode operation. The laser diodes were bonded p-side up to copper heat sinks using indium solder.

A total of 48 devices were selected prior to burn-in and were operated at 200mA constant current for 2000 hours at an average heat sink temperature of 55°C. The average initial output power was 45mW per device. At the end of the test, the output powers ranged from 1mW to 85mW. Most of the devices with the low final power failed catastrophically within 24 hours from the start of the test. Many laser diodes showed very little change in output power while others degraded gradually by varying amounts. Failure analysis showed that failures were facet, bulk, or heat sink related. The temporal output power degradations (i.e., gradual degradation, etc.) can be explained by the identified failure mechanisms.

From the test results and failure analysis, a screening strategy based on inspection and burn-in can be devised to reject devices that may fail early. Also, improvements in processing can provide potential yield improvements. After accounting for degradation related to processing, a very long material lifetime is predicted for these SINSCH-SQW laser diodes.

1. INTRODUCTION

Semiconductor lasers are being used for various applications such as in communication systems, optical recording, consumer electronics and as a solid state laser pump source. Some applications of these devices, for example for use in space communications, require high output power in addition to long-term, reliable operation. SINSCH-SQW and graded index separate confinement heterostructure single quantum well (GRINSCH-SQW) laser diodes (LDs) can provide the high output power required by these systems. They offer an improvement over more conventional LD structures such as double heterostructure (DH) since they are more efficient and less sensitive to temperature. In addition, initial reliability studies regarding quantum well structures have been extremely promising.[1]

To obtain reliable, long life semiconductor lasers correct design, growth, processing and testing procedures must be followed.[2,3] Also, burn-in and screening procedures must be utilized to select long-life devices.[2,4] These procedures have been established for many laser structures such as DH lasers.[2] The general procedure for obtaining reliable, long life semiconductor devices consists of utilizing results from step stress tests, burn-in definition tests, life tests and field tests to develop screening criteria to select long life devices. The results from a burn-in definition test which were used in the process for obtaining long life SINSCH-SQW and GRINSCH-SQW laser diodes are presented in this paper. The following first describes the details and results of the test. Next, analysis of the devices from the test is presented. Based on the test results and failure analysis, a screening strategy is suggested to yield long life devices. Finally, a rough lifetime estimate for these devices is determined.

2. TEST CONDITIONS

The laser material used in this experiment was separate confinement heterostructure material with a 100-Å-thick single quantum well (SQW) active layer sandwiched between two step refractive index barrier layers. The SINSCH-SQW material was grown in a conventional metalorganic chemical vapor deposition (MOCVD) vertical reactor. The specifics of the seven layer wafer, grown at a susceptor temperature of 750°C on an n-type GaAs substrate (Si@2×10^{18}/cc), are as follows: a 1.0μm GaAs buffer layer (Se@1×10^{18}/cc), a 2μm $Al_{0.4}Ga_{0.6}As$ confining layer (Se@1×10^{18}/cc), a 0.22μm $Al_{0.2}Ga_{0.8}As$ barrier layer(Se@5×10^{17}/cc), a 100 Å GaAs active layer (undoped), a 0.22μm $Al_{0.2}Ga_{0.8}As$ barrier layer (Zn@1×10^{17}/cc), a 2μm $Al_{0.4}Ga_{0.6}As$ confining layer (Zn@1×10^{18}/cc), and a 0.15μm GaAs zinc-doped cap layer.

The devices made from this material had 20μm wide oxide defined stripes. The devices had a high reflective back facet coating and a small etalon attached with epoxy to a passivated front facet to ensure single mode operation. The laser diodes were bonded p-side up to a copper block (heat sink) with indium solder. The copper blocks were then mounted on an alumina substrate. A total of ten LDs were mounted to each substrate. The devices were electrically connected in series and each ten LD string was driven by a separate power supply.

A total of 48 LDs with no prior operation were tested at an average heat sink temperature of 55°C and at a constant current of 200mA for 2000 hours in a laboratory environment. The output power and spectral content for each laser diode were monitored at regular intervals during the test. The heat sink temperature varied by no more than 10°C throughout the test. A failure was defined as a device with an output power less than 50% of the initial output power.

3. TEST RESULTS AND FAILURE ANALYSIS

Analysis of the output power versus time curves showed that each of the 48 tested devices could be placed into one of four categories describing the type of power decrease with time. A complete description of each type of temporal power degradation, a discussion of failure analysis performed on devices from each category and a correlation between failure mechanisms and temporal power degradation category follows.

3.1 Catastrophic Failure Type I

A catastrophic failure was defined as a device that degrades at a rate greater than .25% of initial output power per hour. A Type I catastrophic failure was categorized as a device that failed within 168 hours from the start of the test. There were 5 devices (10% of the test population) that failed catastrophically before 168 hours. Of these devices, 3 (6%) failed within the first 24 hours of test. Figure 1 shows the output power versus time for a typical device from this group. The LD had an initial output power of 43mW and had a decrease in power to 19mW (failed catastrophically) in the first 24 hours of the test. After 48 hours the power was down to 3mW, and at the end of test (2000 hours) the power was less than 1mW.

An examination of the post test output power versus current (P-I) curve (in both the pulsed and CW mode) for the device documented in Figure 1 showed the LD had a very low pulsed slope efficiency and very high pulsed threshold current. Based on analysis of devices from previous tests, it was identified that typically, tested laser diodes that had low pulsed slope efficiencies and high pulsed threshold currents had failed due to bulk degradation. One of the more common types of bulk degradation that can cause early catastrophic failure is the dark line defect (DLD). To confirm the failure mechanism for this device, the LD was examined with electron beam induced current (EBIC). Figure 2 shows the results of the EBIC analysis. There were numerous <100> DLDs through the stripe located at the center of the device. The EBIC analysis confirmed the failure mechanism to be dark line defects.

An examination of the overall die, die bond, p-side surface, p-side metals and GaAs surface with chemical etches and optical examinations disclosed no anomalies or source of excessive mechanical stress. Since the device failed early and there were no obvious anomalies, it is suspected the cause of failure was inherent bulk material defects probably formed during growth. Analyses to date of other devices from this category has produced similar results.

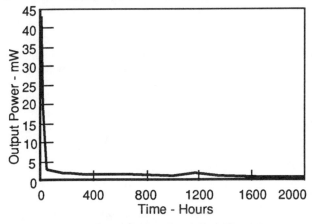

Figure 1. Output power versus time for device from Catastrophic Failure Type I Category.

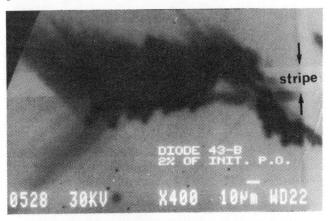

Figure 2. EBIC image shows DLDs in stripe for device from Catastrophic Failure Type I category.

3.2 Catastrophic Failure Type II

A Type II catastrophic failure was categorized as a device that failed after 168 hours from the start of the test. There were 4 devices (8% of the test population) that failed catastrophically after 168 hours. Figure 3 show the output power versus time curve for a typical device from this group. The LD had an initial output power of 62mW. There was an initial, rapid decrease in power to 45mW during the first 400 hours of the test. This was followed by a gradual decrease in power to 40mW for the next 800 hours. The device then failed catastrophically after the 1200 hour test point.

An examination of the post test P-I curve for the device documented in Figure 3 showed the LD had a low pulsed slope efficiency and high pulsed threshold current. As mentioned previously, this is indicative of bulk degradation.

To confirm bulk degradation, the LD was examined with EBIC. Figure 4 shows the results of the EBIC analysis. There are numerous <100> DLDs through the stripe. The DLDs are located from the front facet to about 100 microns into the device. Due to their location at the facet and since the device operated for over 1000 hours before failing catastrophically, it is suspected surface anomalies at the facet caused the failure. The absorption of light and concomitant heating that can be caused by a surface defect could account for the <100> DLDs forming at the facet late in the test. Examination of the facet with a scanning electron microscope (SEM) did identify anomalous particles, but it is not conclusive these caused the problem since the particles could be debris left on the facet after removal of the etalon.

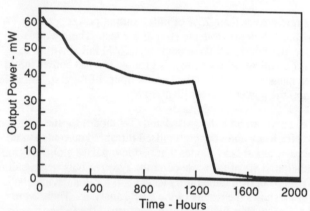

Figure 3. Output power versus time for device from Catastrophic Failure Type II Category.

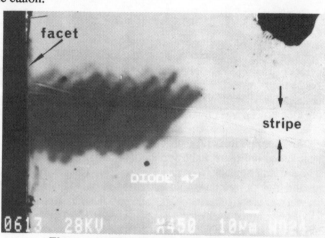

Figure 4. EBIC Image shows DLDs behind facet for device from Catastrophic Failure Type II Category.

Not all devices from this category failed due to DLDs behind the facet. One device failed due to gross bulk degradation as indicated by a completely darkened stripe with EBIC. The cause of failure for this device has not been determined to date.

3.3 Gradual Degradation Type I

Devices placed in this category had an overall gradual decrease in output power. However, during the test they would have abrupt, and sometimes large, increases or decreases in power at a particular time. For most devices these abrupt changes occurred more than once. To be placed in this category the power change had to be greater than 5mW between measurements. Fluctuations in power greater than 5mW was chosen for this category because it indicates real degradation in power. Fluctuations in power less than 5mW could be due to changes in heat sink temperature. The final output powers for these devices ranged from 99% of the initial power to 1% of the initial power. There were 29 devices (61% of the total test population) in this category. Of the 29 devices, 7 devices (15%) were failed devices (i.e., output power less than 50% of the initial output power). Figure 5 shows the output power versus time for one device from this category. This device had slightly greater abrupt changes in power than the typical device. However, this device illustrates the effect more clearly. There was an initial rapid drop in power during the first 50 hours of the test for the device shown in Figure 5. There was relatively little change for the next 100 hours of test. After 200 hours of test, there was a sudden drop in power of nearly 10mW. However, after 300 hours of test, there was an increase of nearly 20mW. This was followed by a drop in power greater than 20mW. After a slight increase in power after 600 hours of test, the device had a jump in power of over 30mW to return it to the start of test output power of 58mW after 1000 hours of test. From this point on there were alternate increases and decreases in power until an end of test output power of approximately 5mW.

An examination of the post test P-I curve for the device documented in Figure 5 showed the LD had a moderate pulsed slope efficiency value and a high pulsed threshold current value. Since evaluation of the electro-optical data did not clearly indicate the failure mechanism, the device underwent extensive failure analysis.

Examination of the device with EBIC showed no dark areas in the stripe. This indicated the device did not degrade due to gross bulk degradation. It is possible some minor, gradual, uniform bulk degradation could have occurred but this would not be revealed by a cursory EBIC examination. A SEM examination of the facets disclosed a blistered (contaminant) area on the front facet in the stripe area of the active region as shown in Figure 6 (arrow).

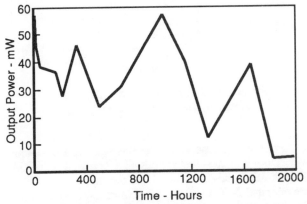

Figure 5. Output power versus time for device from Gradual Degradation Type I Category.

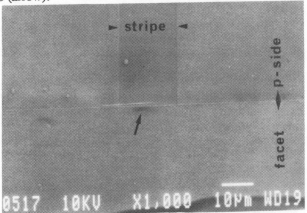

Figure 6. SEM micrograph shows blistered area in stripe area of active region.

A contaminant material on the facet can cause a decrease in output power by lowering the reflectivity and absorbing the emitted light. The abrupt swings in power can be accounted for by a contaminant film on the facet growing with time. Figure 7 shows how the output power theoretically changes with film thickness for an oxide growth. Regardless of the type of contamination, as a film grows on the facet, the output power will cycle through a minimum and maximum. If the film also absorbs light, there will be an overall decrease in power as the film thickness increases. The output power versus time curve shown in Figure 5 exhibits the characteristics of an absorbing contaminant film growing with time.

To determine the composition of the contaminant, the device was examined with Auger electron spectroscopy (AES). The AES analysis determined the contaminant to consist primarily of silicon (Si), iron (Fe) and possibly carbon (C) as shown in Figure 8. The aluminum (Al) and oxygen (O) are from the passivation layer. The carbon could be from normal exposure to the ambient. The epoxy used to bond the etalon consists of Si so the contaminant could be the result of a photochemical reaction with the epoxy at the emitting region. However, the exact cause and source of the Si/Fe blistered area has not been clearly established. Nonetheless, as will be shown in the following, it clearly caused a decrease in output power.

To show that the contaminant caused at least part of the power decrease, the facet was argon (Ar) plasma etched. The solid line in Figure 9 shows the P-I curve before etching. The output power at 300mA is 28mW. After 40 minutes of etching the device was remeasured. The dashed line in Figure 9 shows the P-I curve after etching. The output power at 300mA is 47mW which is nearly a 20mW increase from before etching. The fact that the device did not completely recover to its initial power could be because the Ar plasma etch did not completely remove all the contaminant. So, these results show the contaminant did cause some, if not all of the power decrease for this device.

Another cause for the fluctuations in power was also identified. Numerous devices showed a rollover in the CW mode at moderate currents as identified in the P-I curves measured at 30°C. The P-I curve for a typical device is shown in Figure 10. Usually, differences between pulsed and CW operation are a result of junction heating due to a heat sink degradation. For the device in Figure 10 though, after an initial rollover in the CW curve, there is a large jump in power (approximately 40mW) at 320mA. The reason for the jump in power is that the device begins lasing at the n=2 transition in addition to the n=1 transition. The transition change was verified by wavelength measurements. It has been suggested that by increasing cavity losses (such as by raising device temperature) the n=2 transition can be achieved[5]. Consequently, the fact that the n=2 transition sometimes occurs in these devices when there is rollover in the CW mode is consistent with a heat sink degradation causing a heating of the junction. The large, abrupt increases or decreases in power for some devices during the test can be explained by the device suddenly shifting to the n=2 transition during operation. For example, for the device shown in Figure 10, operation near 320mA would produce an output power of 112mW. However, if the junction temperature were to change slightly so there was

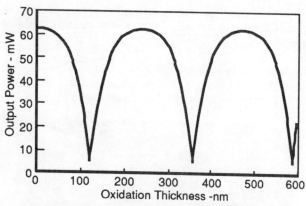

Figure 7. Plot of output power versus film thickness (where in this example an oxide film is examined).

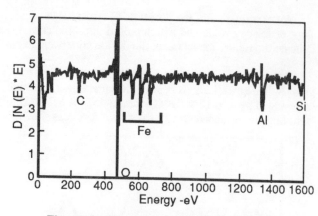

Figure 8. Survey of elements found in contaminant on the facet by AES.

no lasing at the n=2 transition, the device would produce an output power of 64mW. Operation near this point with excursions in temperature could cause erratic swings in the measured output power. During the test the devices were operated at 200mA which would place the device in Figure 10 well below the transition. However, those devices with the transition near 200mA would show large fluctuations in output power. Also, the devices were operated 20°C to 30°C higher in temperature than the temperature at which the P-I measurements were made. Consequently, this higher operating temperature could have caused the transition to occur at a different operating current than that determined by the P-I measurements. In fact, operation at different heat sink temperatures during post test measurement of devices shifted the current at which the transition occurred. Although, in some cases, the transition was shifted towards higher current for higher temperatures.

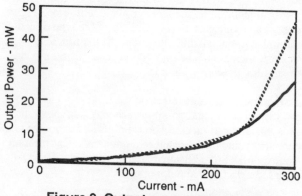

Figure 9. Output power versus current before plasma etching (solid line) and after (dashed line).

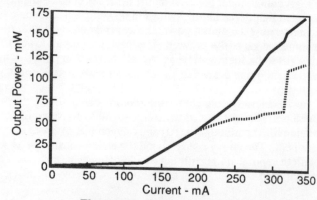

Figure 10. Output power versus current in both the pulsed (solid line) and CW(dashed line) modes.

3.4 Gradual Degradation Type II

Devices placed in this category had an overall gradual decrease in output power. The final output powers for these devices ranged from 48% to 95% of the initial power. There were 10 devices (21% of the total population) in this category. There was only one failed device in this group. Figure 11 shows the output power versus time for a typical LD from this category. There is an initial rapid decrease in power from 56mW to 47mW during the first 200 hours of test. Although there were some flucuations in the output power (<5mW), the device degraded gradually (from 200 hours to the end of test) to a final output power of 44mW. The fluctuations in power were probably due to variations in heat sink temperature and measurement instabilities.

An EBIC examination of the device documented in Figure 11 showed no dark areas. An examination of the facet disclosed no obvious contamination. However, since an initial rapid decrease in power can indicate facet degradation, and EBIC showed no gross bulk degradation, it is suspected the cause for the small decrease in power was due in part to minor facet

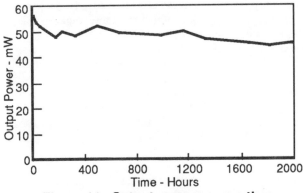

Figure 11. Output power versus time for device from Gradual Degradation Type II Category.

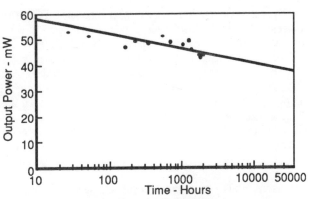

Figure 12. Plot of logarithmic curve fit to data with logarithmic curve fit extended in time.

degradation. It is possible that minor, gradual, uniform bulk degradation could be occurring. Also, analysis of post test P-I curves (pulsed and CW) indicated minor heat sink degrdation to be occurring. Analyses to date of other devices from this category has produced similar results.

4. DISCUSSION

The previous section identified the various degradation mechanisms that had occurred in the tested devices. It was found that the devices could be placed into one of four categories based on the manner the device's output power decreased with time. Ten percent of the devices failed catastrophically in the first 168 hours of test (Catastrophic Failure Type I). The primary failure mechanism was <100> DLDs in the stripe probably caused by bulk defects formed during material growth. Eight percent of the devices failed catastrophically after 168 hours (Catastrophic Failure Type II). The primary failure mechanism was <100> DLDs behind the facet probably caused by particulate matter on the facet. Sixty-one percent of the devices degraded gradually overall but showed erratic changes in power (Gradual Degradation Type I). The primary degradation mechanisms were facet degradation caused by a contamination on the facet and heat sink degradation. Twenty-one percent of the devices degraded gradually (Gradual Degradation Type II). The cause of the degradation is suspected to be minor facet degradation due to contamination on the facet and minor heat sink degradation. Gradual, uniform bulk degradation could be occurring in both gradual degradation categories. In the following, the results from the test and failure analysis are used to develop a burn-in and screening procedure. Next, process changes to improve yield are discussed. Finally, a projected lifetime is determined based on devices from the Gradual Degradation Type II category.

4.1 Burn-in strategy and screening procedure

The goal of a burn-in is to operate devices under stress conditions such that the failure mechanisms in weaker devices are accelerated while aging mechanism-free devices as little as possible. Consequently, for an effective burn-in, one must identify conditions to accelerate those mechanisms. Some of these conditions can be defined a priori when there is a good understanding of the physical basis of the failure mechanisms that are likely to occur. As an example, DLDs are known to grow as a function of nonradiative electron-hole recombination density and mechanical stress.[6] Consequently, conditions can be set to accelerate this mechanism such as operating at a high current density. Analyses of burn-in failures are then conducted to confirm the anticipated mechanism is occurring in the weaker devices and also that the burn-in conditions are not removing sizeable portions of the good devices' lifetime. However, previously unidentified or new failure mechanisms can exist with new structures. Consequently, it is necessary to select burn-in conditions to identify possible new failure mechanisms in addition to accelerating established failure mechanisms. From this point, further tests can be conducted to refine the burn-in conditions if necessary (i.e., to sufficiently accelerate new failure mechanisms). The test discussed in this paper falls into the new structure burn-in category. In this test and subsequent analyses, several, but not all burn-in conditions were defined.

All catastrophic failures must be removed from the device population designated for use or life test. Analysis of devices from the Catastrophic Failure Type I category indicated the primary failure mechanism to be DLDs probably due to material defects. Analysis of devices from the other failure categories indicated non-material defects to be the cause. Consequently, this test shows the effectiveness of a 168 hour burn-in at moderate output power and current levels in eliminating virtually all devices prone to catastrophic failure due to material defects.

Heat sink degradation was another mechanism identified from this test (primarily from the Gradual Degradation Type I devices). A gradual decrease in power (and change in wavelength) due to the increased junction temperature might be tolerated in a system that can compensate for the shift. However, the fluctuations in power found in these devices due in part to the heat sink degradation probably would not be acceptable. Examination of the P-I curves in Figure 10 for a typical device showed some, but not a large amount of heat sink degradation. Consequently, the n=2 transition, which is a function of junction temperature and which caused the erratic changes in power for some devices, could still occur well above the operating point as for the device in Figure 10. Nonetheless, if there is continued heat sink degradation, the transition could be brought near the operating point with the subsequent instability in output power and wavelength. So, the test results, while not establishing the specific conditions, indicate there is a need to develop a burn-in condition to eliminate devices prone to heat sink degradation. One possible cause of heat sink degradation is intermetallic formation at the die bond. One way to accelerate this formation is to operate the devices at high temperature and high current.

As previously mentioned, erratic changes in power were also due to facet degradation in addition to heat sink degradation. As a consequence of the facet degradation, the power was found to decrease precipitously at one test measurement time and then recover to near its initial power at the next measurement time for several devices. This result indicates that during a burn-in the power of the devices must be continuously monitored. The continuous monitoring is necessary because periodic measurements might occur at the times when the device's power has undergone an erratic increase. Consequently, it would appear the device had undergone little degradation, when in fact considerable degradation could have occurred.

Finally, the cause of failure for most of the devices from the Catastrophic Failure Type II category is suspected to be surface anomalies (such as particulate matter) on the facet causing DLDs to form behind the facet. Consequently, a high magnification visual examination of the facets before the burn-in would provide a screen to remove these devices. Also, a high output power burn-in could be designed to eliminate devices that had facet anomalies but slipped through the visual examination. The absorption of a high output would cause significant heating and the quick formation of <110> or <100> DLDs behind the facet.

4.2 Yield improvement

From tests, data analysis, and design specifications parametric criteria is established to determine if a device is good or bad. Also, from tests, etc. acceptable changes in parameters during burn-in are developed to determine whether to pass or reject a device. For the devices from this test, if a change in output power of less than 20% of the initial power is the criteria for a passed device, then there would be 17 of the 48 (35%) LDs in this category. However, if the acceptance criteria included no erratic changes in power, then only 8 of the 48 devices or 17% (all from Gradual Degradation Type II) would pass.

This 17% yield can be improved by eliminating fabrication/processing problems. The two main causes of degradation for devices from the gradual degradation categories were facet and heat sink degradation. The components of the contamination suspected to be causing the facet degradation were identified as iron and silicon. Removal of the source of this contamination should eliminate the facet degradation. Some of the typical causes of heat sink degradation are flux trapping, intermetallic formation and delamination. With the elimination of the facet and heat sink degradation, most of the devices from the gradual degradation categories would pass. This would increase the yield to 39 of 48 devices (81%), which is a considerable improvement over 17% yield. Furthermore, the devices from the Catastrophic Failure Type II category are suspected to have failed primarily due to facet anomalies. Some causes of facet anomalies are poor cleaving or solder splattering during bonding. With the elimination of the facet anomalies, the yield for this group of devices would be 43 of 48 (89%).

So, elimination of the identified problems with processing, testing, and design would result in a yield of 89%. The remaining decrease in yield is due to the growth process. The devices making up this group are primarily the Type I Catastrophic Failures. With all other problems eliminated, the yield will fluctuate depending on the quality of the laser material. Designing the simplest device required for the application, choice of the best growth process, etc. will result in ease of growth, improved material and consequently a very high yield.

4.3 Lifetime estimate

One method to estimate lifetime is to operate the devices at an accelerated stress condition (e.g., temperature) and use an established relation (e.g., Arrhenius) to extrapolate the lifetime at use conditions.[4] Because the devices in this test were not operated at several accelerated stress conditions, this method could not be used. Another approach is to empirically fit the data to a curve and extrapolate the curve in time to project a lifetime. However, the assumption made when using this technique is that the device will continue to degrade in the manner exhibited during operation. One consequence of this assumption is that the device will not fail catastrophically at some point after the actual test time. For the devices discussed in this paper, the number tested and length of test time are not enough to provide overwhelming support to the assumptions. However, continued testing will add support to the lifetime determined from this work or redefine the method of extrapolation to determine lifetime for the LDs from this test. So, to provide an initial estimate for the lifetime of these devices, LDs from the Gradual Degradation Type II category were examined.

Figure 12 shows the output power versus time for a typical device (the device documented in Figure 11) from the Gradual Degradation Type II category fit to a logarithmic curve. The curve is plotted as output power versus log time. A visual examination indicates a reasonably good fit. However, the curve fit resulted in a low (.7) r^2 value. This is due to the slight fluctuations in power for this device. If the device were to follow the logarithmic degradation trend, then the extrapolated lifetime shown in Figure 12 for this device would be in excess of 50,000 hours.

5. CONCLUSIONS

The results from a test in which 48 SINSCH-SQW LDs were operated at 200mA for 2000 hours to develop burn-in and screening criteria were presented. The devices could be placed into one of four categories depending on how the output power decreased with time. There were two categories in which the devices failed catastrophically. In one category, devices failed catastrophically in the first 168 hours of test due to DLDs throughout the stripe. Devices in the other category failed catastrophically after 168 hours of test primarily due to DLDs behind the facet. Devices degraded gradually in the remaining two categories. In one category, the devices degraded gradually overall, but showed erratic changes in power. The primary degradation mechanisms were facet and heat sink related. In the final category, devices had a well-behaved, gradual decrease in power.

The test results showed these operating conditions successfully removed devices with material defects within 168 hours of operation. A high magnification visual inspection of the facet probably could remove most of the devices that failed catastrophically after 168 hours of operation. Also, processing improvements could eliminate the facet and heat sink degradation mechanisms. With these mechanisms eliminated, most of the decrease in power for the gradually degraded LDs would be eliminated. This would result in more devices passing burn-in and thus increase burn-in yield in addition to producing devices with long lifetimes.

An initial estimate for the lifetime of the well-behaved devices that degraded gradually was projected to be greater than 50,000 hours. It should be noted no failure mechanism unique to quantum well material was identified in this test. Consequently, the burn-in conditions developed here are similar to those established for more conventional structures such as double heterstructure laser diodes.

6. ACKNOWLEDGEMENT

The author would like to thank A. Chenoweth and T. Ganley for initiating and conducting the test. L. Bauer and J. Yahl for SEM/EBIC analysis, M. Lee and S. Stazak for electro-optical measurements and T. Faltus for comments on the manuscript.

7. REFERENCES

1. G. L. Harnagel, T. L. Paoli, R. L. Thornton, R D. Burnham, D. L. Smith,"Accelerated aging of 100mW CW multiple-stripe GaA1As lasers grown by metalorganic chemical vapor deposition", Appl. Phys. Lett., 46, 118 (1985).

2. D. Dreisewerd, W. Fritz, D. Begley, S Schwedt, G. Elliott, "Reliability of A1GaAs/GaAs Laser Diodes Grown by Metal Organic Chemical Vapor Deposition", Proc. SPIE, 885, 111 (1988).

3. A. R. Goodwin, I. G. Davies, R. M. Gibb, R. H. Murphy, "The Design of a High Reliability Semiconductor Laser for Single-Mode Fiber-Optical Communication Links", IEEE J. Lightwave Tech., Vol. 6, No. 9, September, 1988, p.1424.

4. B. G. King, R. L. Hartman, Eds., "Assuring High Reliability of Lasers and Photodetectors for Submarine Lightwave Cable Systems", AT&T Technical Journal, vol. 64, No. 3, March, 1985.

5. P. S. Zory, A. R. Reisinger, R. G. Waters, L. J. Mawst, C. A. Zmudzinski, M. A. Emanuel, M. E. Givens, J. J. Coleman, "Anomalaus temperature dependence of threshold for thin quantum well A1GaAs diode lasers", App. Phys. Lett., 49,16 (1986).

6. G. B. H. Thompson, "Physics of Semiconductor Laser Devices", New York, 1980, John Wiley and Sons, p. 26.

LASER DIODE TECHNOLOGY AND APPLICATIONS

Volume 1043

ADDENDUM

The following papers, which were scheduled to be presented at this conference and published in this proceedings, were cancelled.

[1043-36]   **Multi-mode, star coupled fiber optic data bus with 1300 nm laser sources**
C. E. Polczynski, Lockheed Aeronautical Systems Co.

[1043-41]   **Laser diode system for geostationary satellite ranging and communication**
R. Seshamani, Y. K. Jain, T. K. Alex, ISRO Satellite Ctr. (India)

The following papers were presented at this conference, but the manuscripts supporting the oral presentations are not available.

[1043-01]   **Semiconductor quantum wells for optoelectronics**
A. Yariv, California Institute of Technology

[1043-22]   **Coherence properties of diode laser arrays**
N. W. Carlson, R. Amantea, J. K. Butler, G. A. Evans, J. M. Hammer, M. Lurie, S. L. Palfrey, David Sarnoff Research Ctr.

[1043-30]   **Low-threshold lasers for optoelectronic integration**
P. D. Dapkus, K. M. Dzurko, E. Menu, J. S. Osinski, S. P. Denbaars, C. A. Beyler, Univ. of Southern California

LASER DIODE TECHNOLOGY AND APPLICATIONS

Volume 1043

AUTHOR INDEX

Alex, T. K., Laser diode system for geostationary satellite ranging and communication (Cancelled), Addendum

Amantea, R., Coherence properties of diode laser arrays (Oral only), Addendum

Anderson, E. R., Monolithic two-dimensional arrays of diode lasers (Invited Paper), 69

Aoyagi, T., Transverse-mode-controlled wide-single-stripe lasers with loading modal filters, 81

Appelbaum, A., High frequency characteristics of 1.3-μm lasers (Invited Paper), 300

Ash, R. M., Laser-based optoelectronic integrated circuits for communications (Invited Paper), 214

Bailey, R. J., Two-dimensional surface-emitting arrays of GaAs/AlGaAs diode lasers (Invited Paper), 92

Baillargeon, J. N., Influence of In on the performance of (Al)GaAs single quantum well lasers (Invited Paper), 310

Ballantyne, J. M., Influence of In on the performance of (Al)GaAs single quantum well lasers (Invited Paper), 310

Beach, R. J., Laser diode cooling for high average power applications, 351

Beausoleil, R. G., Diode laser radar system analysis and design for high precision ranging, 228

———, Semiconductor laser stabilization by external optical feedback, 167

Begley, D. L., Applications and requirements of laser diodes for free-space laser communications (Invited Paper), 274

Benedict, M. K., Reliability of single-element diode lasers for high performance optical data storage applications, 318

Benett, W., Laser diode cooling for high average power applications, 351

Beyler, C. A., Low-threshold lasers for optoelectronic integration (Oral only), Addendum

Bossert, D. J., Focused-ion-beam micromachined diode laser mirrors (Invited Paper), 25

Brueck, S. R. J., Optical cavity design for wavelength-resonant surface-emitting semiconductor lasers (Invited Paper), 111

Buckley, D., Quantum well ridge waveguide lasers optimized for high power single spatial mode applications, 61

Bull, J. G., Diode laser radar system analysis and design for high precision ranging, 228

Burrus, C. A., Compound-cavity lasers for medium-range lidar applications, 238

Butler, J. K., Analysis of double-heterostructure and quantum well lasers using effective index techniques (Invited Paper), 148

———, Coherence properties of diode laser arrays (Oral only), Addendum

Cabrita Freitas, J. C., Radiation pattern of a laser diode collimator as a function of driving current and frequency, 291

Cadete, L., Radiation pattern of a laser diode collimator as a function of driving current and frequency, 291

Carlson, N. W., Coherence properties of diode laser arrays (Oral only), Addendum

Carter, A. C., Laser-based optoelectronic integrated circuits for communications (Invited Paper), 214

Carvalho Rodrigues, F., Radiation pattern of a laser diode collimator as a function of driving current and frequency, 291

Cassarly, W. J., Phase control of coherent diode laser arrays using liquid crystals, 130

Chan, E. Y., High performance 1.3-μm buried crescent lasers and LEDs for fiber optic links, 221

———, Self-consistent heat load evaluation of laser diode modules for high temperature operation, 344

Chen, C. C., Self-consistent heat load evaluation of laser diode modules for high temperature operation, 344

Cheng, W. H., High frequency characteristics of 1.3-μm lasers (Invited Paper), 300

Chinn, S. R., Computer modeling of GRIN-SCH-SQW diode lasers, 157

Chuang, Z. M., Compound-cavity lasers for medium-range lidar applications, 238

Chung, H. F., Laser-patterned desorption of GaAs in an inverted MOCVD reactor (Invited Paper), 36

Chung, K.-H., Measurement of semiconductor laser linewidth enhancement factor using coherent optical feedback, 175

Cohen, D. A., Compound-cavity lasers for medium-range lidar applications, 238

Coldren, L. A., Compound-cavity lasers for medium-range lidar applications, 238

Coleman, J. J., Influence of In on the performance of (Al)GaAs single quantum well lasers (Invited Paper), 310

Crow, G. A., Focused-ion-beam micromachined diode laser mirrors (Invited Paper), 25

D'Amato, F. X., Mode control of an array of AlGaAs lasers using a spatial filter in a Talbot cavity, 100

Dahlhauser, K. J., Optical cavity design for wavelength-resonant surface-emitting semiconductor lasers (Invited Paper), 111

Daniel, D. R., Quantum well ridge waveguide lasers optimized for high power single spatial mode applications, 61

Dapkus, P. D., Low-threshold lasers for optoelectronic integration (Oral only), Addendum

da Silva, M., Radiation pattern of a laser diode collimator as a function of driving current and frequency, 291

DeFreez, R. K., Focused-ion-beam micromachined diode laser mirrors (Invited Paper), 25

DeJule, M., Phase control of coherent diode laser arrays using liquid crystals, 130

de La Chapelle, M., Diode laser radar system analysis and design for high precision ranging, 228

Denbaars, S. P., Low-threshold lasers for optoelectronic integration (Oral only), Addendum

Donnelly, J. P., Two-dimensional surface-emitting arrays of GaAs/AlGaAs diode lasers (Invited Paper), 92

Dzurko, K. M., Low-threshold lasers for optoelectronic integration (Oral only), Addendum

LASER DIODE TECHNOLOGY AND APPLICATIONS

Volume 1043

Eaton, L. R., Monolithic two-dimensional arrays of diode lasers (Invited Paper), 69

Elliott, R. T., Packaging considerations for semiconductor laser diodes, 330

Elliott, R. A., Focused-ion-beam micromachined diode laser mirrors (Invited Paper), 25

Enochs, S., Optomechanical packaging for extended temperature performance, 338

Epler, J. E., Laser-patterned desorption of GaAs in an inverted MOCVD reactor (Invited Paper), 36

Evans, G. A., Analysis of double-heterostructure and quantum well lasers using effective index techniques (Invited Paper), 148

———, Coherence properties of diode laser arrays (Oral only), Addendum

Fekete, D., Influence of In on the performance of (Al)GaAs single quantum well lasers (Invited Paper), 310

Fenner, W. R., Coupling of index-guided lateral modes in three-stripe gain-guided laser diode arrays, 138

Figueroa, L., Leaky-guided channeled substrate planar laser with reduced substrate radiation and heating, 197

Finlan, J. M., Phase control of coherent diode laser arrays using liquid crystals, 130

———, Scanning single-slit and double-slit phase measurements of grating surface emitter diode laser arrays, 123

Fischer, S. E., Influence of In on the performance of (Al)GaAs single quantum well lasers (Invited Paper), 310

Fried, D. W., Reliability of single-element diode lasers for high performance optical data storage applications, 318

Fritz, W. J., Screening test procedure for long-life single-mode step index separate confinement heterostructure single quantum well laser diodes, 368

Fu, R. J., High performance 1.3-μm buried crescent lasers and LEDs for fiber optic links, 221

Garrett, B., Quantum well ridge waveguide lasers optimized for high power single spatial mode applications, 61

Giewont, K. J., Reliability of single-element diode lasers for high performance optical data storage applications, 318

Gleckler, A. D., Reliability of single-element diode lasers for high performance optical data storage applications, 318

Goodfellow, R. C., Laser-based optoelectronic integrated circuits for communications (Invited Paper), 214

Goodhue, W. D., Two-dimensional surface-emitting arrays of GaAs/AlGaAs diode lasers (Invited Paper), 92

Goodwin, F. E., Utilizing GaAlAs laser diodes as a source for frequency-modulated cw coherent laser radars, 245

Grattan, K. T. V., All fiber laser low cost "rangefinder" for small vibration measurements, 284

Hagman, R. L., Semiconductor laser stabilization by external optical feedback, 167

Hamada, H., Monolithic four-beam semiconductor laser array with built-in monitoring photodiodes, 17

Hamilton, S. M., Scanning single-slit and double-slit phase measurements of grating surface emitter diode laser arrays, 123

Hammer, J. M., Coherence properties of diode laser arrays (Oral only), Addendum

Harding, C. M., Influence of In on the performance of (Al)GaAs single quantum well lasers (Invited Paper), 310

Harnagel, G. H., Recent advances in high power semiconductor lasers, 2

Heflinger, D. G., Coupling of index-guided lateral modes in three-stripe gain-guided laser diode arrays, 138

Heflinger, L. O., Monolithic two-dimensional arrays of diode lasers (Invited Paper), 69

Hendron, R. E., Wafer thin coolers for cw AlGaAs/GaAs monolithic linear diode laser arrays, 359

Hertzler, G. R., Wafer thin coolers for cw AlGaAs/GaAs monolithic linear diode laser arrays, 359

Hess, K. L., High frequency characteristics of 1.3-μm lasers (Invited Paper), 300

Hinata, S., Transverse-mode-controlled wide-single-stripe lasers with loading modal filters, 81

Hjelme, D. R., Semiconductor laser stabilization by external optical feedback, 167

Hong, C. S., High performance 1.3-μm buried crescent lasers and LEDs for fiber optic links, 221

Huang, J., Monolithic two-dimensional arrays of diode lasers (Invited Paper), 69

Ikeda, K., Extremely low threshold InGaAsP DFB laser diode by the MOCVD/LPE (Invited Paper), 10

———, Transverse-mode-controlled wide-single-stripe lasers with loading modal filters, 81

Inoue, Y., Monolithic four-beam semiconductor laser array with built-in monitoring photodiodes, 17

Iyotani, R., High power AlGaAs broad-area laser diodes for a light-triggered thyristor valve system, 107

Jain, Y. K., Laser diode system for geostationary satellite ranging and communication (Cancelled), Addendum

Jansen, M., Design of multiple quantum well lasers for surface-emitting arrays, 192

———, Monolithic two-dimensional arrays of diode lasers (Invited Paper), 69

Kakimoto, S., Extremely low threshold InGaAsP DFB laser diode by the MOCVD/LPE (Invited Paper), 10

Kaneno, N., Transverse-mode-controlled wide-single-stripe lasers with loading modal filters, 81

Katz, J., Monolithically integrated two-dimensional arrays of optoelectronic threshold devices for neural network applications, 44

Kim, J. H., Monolithically integrated two-dimensional arrays of optoelectronic threshold devices for neural network applications, 44

Komeda, K., Monolithic four-beam semiconductor laser array with built-in monitoring photodiodes, 17

Lapinski, J. R., Jr., Wafer thin coolers for cw AlGaAs/GaAs monolithic linear diode laser arrays, 359

Lau, K. Y., Short-pulse and high frequency signal generation in semiconductor lasers (Invited Paper), 206

Lee, S. J., Leaky-guided channeled substrate planar laser with reduced substrate radiation and heating, 197

Lehman, J. G., Jr., Scanning single-slit and double-slit phase measurements of grating surface emitter diode laser arrays, 123

Lin, C., Semiconductor laser-based multichannel analog video transmission using FDM and WDM over single-mode fiber, 260

Lin, S. H., Monolithically integrated two-dimensional arrays of optoelectronic threshold devices for neural network applications, 44

Liou, K.-Y., Compound-cavity lasers for medium-range lidar applications, 238

———, Novel device functions and applications of two-electrode distributed feedback lasers (Invited Paper), 252

Lundgren, C. W., Semiconductor laser-based multichannel analog video transmission using FDM and WDM over single-mode fiber, 260

Lurie, M., Coherence properties of diode laser arrays (Oral only), Addendum

Lutes, G. F., High stability frequency and timing distribution using semiconductor lasers and fiber optic links, 263

Mahbobzadeh, M., Optical cavity design for wavelength-resonant surface-emitting semiconductor lasers (Invited Paper), 111

McClure, J. D., Diode laser radar system analysis and design for high precision ranging, 228

McGarvey, J. A., Diode laser radar system analysis and design for high precision ranging, 228

———, Semiconductor laser stabilization by external optical feedback, 167

McInerney, J. G., Measurement of semiconductor laser linewidth enhancement factor using coherent optical feedback, 175

———, Optical cavity design for wavelength-resonant surface-emitting semiconductor lasers (Invited Paper), 111

Meggitt, B. T., All fiber laser low cost "rangefinder" for small vibration measurements, 284

Menu, E., Low-threshold lasers for optoelectronic integration (Oral only), Addendum

Mickelson, A. R., Semiconductor laser stabilization by external optical feedback, 167

Mihashi, Y., Transverse-mode-controlled wide-single-stripe lasers with loading modal filters, 81

Minakuchi, K., Monolithic four-beam semiconductor laser array with built-in monitoring photodiodes, 17

Morrison, C. B., Reliability of single-element diode lasers for high performance optical data storage applications, 318

Mundinger, D. C., Laser diode cooling for high average power applications, 351

Nagai, Y., Transverse-mode-controlled wide-single-stripe lasers with loading modal filters, 81

Nakatsuka, S., Fundamental lateral-mode operation in broad-area lasers having built-in lens-like refractive index distributions, 87

———, High power AlGaAs broad-area laser diodes for a light-triggered thyristor valve system, 107

Namizaki, H., Extremely low threshold InGaAsP DFB laser diode by the MOCVD/LPE (Invited Paper), 10

Natarajan, P. S., Semiconductor laser-based multichannel analog video transmission using FDM and WDM over single-mode fiber, 260

Niina, T., Monolithic four-beam semiconductor laser array with built-in monitoring photodiodes, 17

Ning, Y. N., All fiber laser low cost "rangefinder" for small vibration measurements, 284

Orloff, J. H., Focused-ion-beam micromachined diode laser mirrors (Invited Paper), 25

Osinski, J. S., Low-threshold lasers for optoelectronic integration (Oral only), Addendum

Osiński, M., Measurement of semiconductor laser linewidth enhancement factor using coherent optical feedback, 175

———, Optical cavity design for wavelength-resonant surface-emitting semiconductor lasers (Invited Paper), 111

Ou, S. S., Design of multiple quantum well lasers for surface-emitting arrays, 192

———, Monolithic two-dimensional arrays of diode lasers (Invited Paper), 69

Palfrey, S. L., Coherence properties of diode laser arrays (Oral only), Addendum

Palmer, A. W., All fiber laser low cost "rangefinder" for small vibration measurements, 284

Paoli, T. L., Laser-patterned desorption of GaAs in an inverted MOCVD reactor (Invited Paper), 36

Perryman, A. J., Packaging considerations for semiconductor laser diodes, 330

Peterson, G. P., Design of multiple quantum well lasers for surface-emitting arrays, 192

Polczynski, C. E., Multi-mode, star coupled fiber optic data bus with 1300 nm laser sources (Cancelled), Addendum

Pooladdej, J., High frequency characteristics of 1.3-μm lasers (Invited Paper), 300

Prina, R. D., Radiation pattern of a laser diode collimator as a function of driving current and frequency, 291

Psaltis, D., Monolithically integrated two-dimensional arrays of optoelectronic threshold devices for neural network applications, 44

Puretz, J., Focused-ion-beam micromachined diode laser mirrors (Invited Paper), 25

Raja, M. Y. A., Optical cavity design for wavelength-resonant surface-emitting semiconductor lasers (Invited Paper), 111

Ramaswamy, R. V., Leaky-guided channeled substrate planar laser with reduced substrate radiation and heating, 197

Rauschenbach, K., Two-dimensional surface-emitting arrays of GaAs/AlGaAs diode lasers (Invited Paper), 92

Regan, J. D., Packaging considerations for semiconductor laser diodes, 330

Reinhold, S. L., Scanning single-slit and double-slit phase measurements of grating surface emitter diode laser arrays, 123

Reisinger, A. R., Computer modeling of GRIN-SCH-SQW diode lasers, 157

Renner, D. S., High frequency characteristics of 1.3-μm lasers (Invited Paper), 300

Roychoudhuri, C., Mode control of an array of AlGaAs lasers using a spatial filter in a Talbot cavity, 100

Sakamoto, M., Recent advances in high power semiconductor lasers, 2

LASER DIODE TECHNOLOGY AND APPLICATIONS

Volume 1043

Schaus, C. F., Optical cavity design for wavelength-resonant surface-emitting semiconductor lasers (Invited Paper), 111

Scifres, D. R., High power single-mode laser diodes (Invited Paper), 54

———, Recent advances in high power semiconductor lasers, 2

Seiwa, Y., Transverse-mode-controlled wide-single-stripe lasers with loading modal filters, 81

Sergant, M., Monolithic two-dimensional arrays of diode lasers (Invited Paper), 69

Seshamani, R., Laser diode system for geostationary satellite ranging and communication (Cancelled), Addendum

Shibayama, K., Extremely low threshold InGaAsP DFB laser diode by the MOCVD/LPE (Invited Paper), 10

Shigihara, K., Transverse-mode-controlled wide-single-stripe lasers with loading modal filters, 81

Shimizu, H., Long-life GaAlAs high power lasers with nonabsorbing mirrors (Invited Paper), 75

Siebert, E. T., Mode control of an array of AlGaAs lasers using a spatial filter in a Talbot cavity, 100

Silvestre, V. M., Radiation pattern of a laser diode collimator as a function of driving current and frequency, 291

Simmons, W. W., Design of multiple quantum well lasers for surface-emitting arrays, 192

———, Monolithic two-dimensional arrays of diode lasers (Invited Paper), 69

Simonson, D. L., Utilizing GaAlAs laser diodes as a source for frequency-modulated cw coherent laser radars, 245

Slotwinski, A. R., Utilizing GaAlAs laser diodes as a source for frequency-modulated cw coherent laser radars, 245

Solarz, R. W., Laser diode cooling for high average power applications, 351

Soltz, B. A., Influence of In on the performance of (Al)GaAs single quantum well lasers (Invited Paper), 310

Sperry, V., Laser diode cooling for high average power applications, 351

Stazak Kastigar, S. M., Wafer thin coolers for cw AlGaAs/GaAs monolithic linear diode laser arrays, 359

Stein, C., Phase control of coherent diode laser arrays using liquid crystals, 130

Streifer, W., High power single-mode laser diodes (Invited Paper), 54

———, Recent advances in high power semiconductor lasers, 2

Strzelecki, E. M., Compound-cavity lasers for medium-range lidar applications, 238

Susaki, W., Extremely low threshold InGaAsP DFB laser diode by the MOCVD/LPE (Invited Paper), 10

———, Transverse-mode-controlled wide-single-stripe lasers with loading modal filters, 81

Tabuchi, N., Monolithic four-beam semiconductor laser array with built-in monitoring photodiodes, 17

Tanaka, C., High power AlGaAs broad-area laser diodes for a light-triggered thyristor valve system, 107

Tatsuno, K., Fundamental lateral-mode operation in broad-area lasers having builtin lens-like refractive index distributions, 87

Treat, D. W., Laser-patterned desorption of GaAs in an inverted MOCVD reactor (Invited Paper), 36

Tzou, A. J., Reliability of single-element diode lasers for high performance optical data storage applications, 318

Vahala, K. J., Effects of fabricational variations on quantum wire laser gain spectra and performance, 184

Venkatesan, P. S., Semiconductor laser-based multichannel analog video transmission using FDM and WDM over single-mode fiber, 260

Vertatschitsch, E. J., Diode laser radar system analysis and design for high precision ranging, 228

Wang, C. A., Two-dimensional surface-emitting arrays of GaAs/AlGaAs diode lasers (Invited Paper), 92

Waters, R. G., Influence of In on the performance of (Al)GaAs single quantum well lasers (Invited Paper), 310

Welch, D. F., High power single-mode laser diodes (Invited Paper), 54

———, Recent advances in high power semiconductor lasers, 2

Wilcox, J. Z., Design of multiple quantum well lasers for surface-emitting arrays, 192

———, Monolithic two-dimensional arrays of diode lasers (Invited Paper), 69

Wilson, G. A., Focused-ion-beam micromachined diode laser mirrors (Invited Paper), 25

Ximen, H., Focused-ion-beam micromachined diode laser mirrors (Invited Paper), 25

Yamaguchi, T., Monolithic four-beam semiconductor laser array with built-in monitoring photodiodes, 17

Yang, J. J., Design of multiple quantum well lasers for surface-emitting arrays, 192

———, Monolithic two-dimensional arrays of diode lasers (Invited Paper), 69

Yariv, A., Effects of fabricational variations on quantum wire laser gain spectra and performance, 184

———, Semiconductor quantum wells for optoelectronics (Oral only), Addendum

Yodoshi, K., Monolithic four-beam semiconductor laser array with built-in monitoring photodiodes, 17

York, P. K., Influence of In on the performance of (Al)GaAs single quantum well lasers (Invited Paper), 310

Zarem, H., Effects of fabricational variations on quantum wire laser gain spectra and performance, 184

Zehr, S. W., High frequency characteristics of 1.3-μm lasers (Invited Paper), 300

Zory, P. S., Computer modeling of GRIN-SCH-SQW diode lasers, 157